The
Longevity
Code

The Longevity Code

Your Personal Prescription for a Longer, Sweeter Life

ZORBA PASTER, M.D.

with Susan Meltsner

THREE RIVERS PRESS • NEW YORK

Author's Note: Many of the names used in this book are pseudonyms or composites. In addition, identifying characteristics of people and places may have been changed.

For updates about information in this book, visit www.longevitycode.com

Published by Three Rivers Press, New York, New York.
Member of the Crown Publishing Group.

Random House, Inc. New York, Toronto, London, Sydney, Auckland
www.randomhouse.com

THREE RIVERS PRESS and the Tugboat design are registered trademarks of Random House, Inc.

Originally published in hardcover by Clarkson Potter/Publishers in 2001.

Grateful acknowledgment is made to the following for permission to reprint previously published material: "Birth Is a Beginning" from Gates of Repentance, Central Conference of American Rabbis, copyright © 1978 by Rabbi Alvin I. Fine is used by permission.

Printed in the United States of America

Design by Maggie Hinders

Library of Congress Cataloging-in-Publication Data
Paster, Zorba.
    The longevity code : your personal prescription for a longer, sweeter life /
by Zorba Paster, with Susan Meltsner—1st ed.
    1. Longevity. 2. Health. 3. Medicine, Preventive. I. Meltsner, Susan. II. Title.
RA776.75.P377 2000
612.6'8—dc21   00-027864

ISBN 0-609-80814-1

10 9 8 7 6 5 4 3

First Paperback Edition

To Penelope, Zak, DeeDee, Eli, and Vanessa

Whose laughter and insight skillfully
weave the five spheres together

Contents

Acknowledgments

I WOULD LIKE TO THANK MY LISTENERS, viewers, and patients for their provocative questions and their continual support.

Many thanks to my medical and scientific colleagues and friends, whose invaluable acumen was both diversified and honest. They include Drs. Bob Mendelsohn, Bob Auerbach, Dan Barry, Dave Okada, Adam Balin, Marshall Fields, Ken Robbins, Dave Hahn, and the medical librarians at St. Mary's Hospital Medical Center. Thanks to Pat Remington for our early morning chats. Thanks to Dan Levy for his thoughtful Preface and his many astute suggestions. Special thanks to Karen Prager, whose creative and timely contributions were invaluable.

Thanks to my media friends from radio and television who have contributed so much to my professional and personal life. Monika Petkus, my producer at Wisconsin Public Radio, and Tom Clark, my cohost, clearly were pivotal in my becoming comfortable sharing my thoughts on the radio. Our weekly public radio show is a joy to produce because of their wit, humor, and tenacity. Tom Bier and the crew at WISC-TV3, our CBS affiliate, were always encouraging and insightful for the decade I have given my medical commentary. They have taught me so much.

Lifelong thanks to my good friends Ben Sidran, Rita Mendelsohn, Nancy Ross Ryan, Amy Kogut, Rhea Rubin, Lois Wackner Solomon, Jacques Lemelin, Howard Gelman, and Hannah Rosenthal Phelps, who motivated me to see medicine as both an art and a science.

A giant thank-you to Susan Meltsner, my cowriter, whose attention to detail is unparalleled, and whose ability to turn disparate concepts into coherency always amazed me. And thank you, Pam Krauss, my first editor, for transforming this book into the readable work that it is. You are masterful. And thanks to Chris Pavone, my second editor, whose insight and skill with the editing pencil were exemplary.

Heartfelt thanks to my agent and friend, Carl DeSantis, for believing in my vision of wellness and longevity, but more important, for your example of living the five spheres. Your tireless efforts on my behalf have gone beyond the boundaries of this book.

Most humble thanks to His Holiness the Dalai Lama of Tibet, Tenzin Gyatso, whose compassion, humor, warmth, and wisdom were always present when I wrote. Thank you so much for writing the Foreword.

And many thanks to my large, passionate, multigenerational family, who have always served as my model. To my wife, Penelope, whose influence can be seen throughout this book in heart, thought, and action, and to our four fabulous, intuitive, loving children. Your vitality is the future. May you all live beyond one hundred.

Foreword by The Dalai Lama

IN *THE LONGEVITY CODE,* Dr. Paster refers to the five spheres of influence in our lives and the importance of finding a balance among them. While it is becoming increasingly obvious that material success alone does not provide genuine happiness, it is also true that without mental peace, mere physical good health is insufficient. The importance of generating a warm heart and behaving with kindness and compassion toward others is that those qualities bring us inner peace. According to Dr. Paster's findings, they increase longevity as well. This makes sense to me, since I believe that inner peace is definitely of benefit to good health.

All of our actions have consequences. Dr. Paster has found that our positive and negative actions, whether they are physical, mental, social, material, or spiritual, have a direct consequence on both the quality and duration of our lives. He suggests that you are not a completely healthy person if you pay attention only to your physical well-being.

This is not so surprising, for in my experience, when, for example, we develop the ability to patiently forbear with frustrating situations, we find that we develop a proportionate reserve of calmness and tranquility. We tend to be less antagonistic and more pleasant to associate with. This, in turn, creates a positive atmosphere around us so that it is easy for others to relate to us. And being better grounded emotionally through the practice of patience, we find that not only do we become much stronger mentally and spiritually, but we also tend to be healthier physically. Certainly I attribute the good health I enjoy to a generally calm and peaceful mind.

On the other hand, not only do negative thoughts and emotions destroy our experience of peace, they also undermine our health. In the Tibetan medical system, anger is a primary source of many illnesses, including those associated with high blood pressure, sleeplessness, and degenerative disorders—a view that seems increasingly accepted in allopathic medicine.

I am sure that readers of this book will find much to encourage the development of what I think of as our basic human qualities of kindness, compassion, and a warm heart. If we put these into practice, not only will we find a greater sense of calm and happiness in our day-to-day lives, but also the hope that we can live longer too, as Dr. Paster offers.

Preface

CONTEMPORARY LITERATURE IS REPLETE with recipes for the prevention of disease and the prolongation of life. For example, for heart disease and stroke—the first and third leading causes of death in the United States—we have learned a great deal about causal factors and approaches to prevention. The resultant lessons of the past several decades have contributed to a 50 percent decline in death rates from heart disease, and a 60 percent decline in deaths from stroke.

While we have a great deal of information to help us live longer lives and live them more free of disability, there has been precious little authoritative literature to guide us in living *fuller* lives. In *The Longevity Code,* Dr. Zorba Paster provides numerous pearls of wisdom made possible by twenty years of clinical experience and a keen interest in keeping up with the latest medical discoveries. Not only does Dr. Paster embrace the treatment of such severe conditions as high blood pressure and elevated cholesterol levels, but he also has integrated an evidence-based strategy into a broad lifestyle scheme to prepare us to better enjoy the longer lives we are likely to face.

Unlike the quick fixes recommended by some, Dr. Paster's approach is one of reasoned moderation. Wisely, he does not promote extreme diets or radical means by which one can prolong life or fight disease. Instead, the steps he advocates are simple, and he provides concise summaries of the evidence (or lack thereof) supporting each one.

In *The Longevity Code* we are reminded, "Wellness is not defined entirely by those factors your doctor can measure at your annual checkup." Indeed, our wellness is a complex interplay of factors, some of which can be examined by a doctor or determined in a laboratory, and others that are not amenable to measurement. For instance: among his prescriptions for wellness, Dr. Paster emphasizes the importance of establishing social-support networks and pursuing lifelong learning. These are secrets of wellness that doctors are not taught in medical school, nor can they be prescribed.

Through improvements in hygiene in the early part of the twentieth century, the introduction of antibiotics in the middle of the century, and the development of prevention strategies for heart disease and stroke in the latter part of the century, life expectancy in the United States has increased dramatically and to a greater degree than in any period in the history of mankind. The commonsense steps spelled out in *The Longevity Code* are designed to allow us to better enjoy our longer lives and infuse them with greater meaning.

—Daniel Levy, M.D.
Director, Framingham Heart Study
National Heart, Lung, and Blood Institute

Introduction

WHEN THE CLOCK STRUCK MIDNIGHT on December 31, 1999, ushering in a new millennium, it was a wake-up call for many of us. "How much of the new century will I see?" we asked ourselves. "Will I be like the sage centenarians profiled in the media as we looked back on the past century—vital, sharp-minded, and eager to experience more of what life has to offer? How can I achieve that kind of longevity? Is it too late to make significant changes that will alter the course of my life?"

Longevity has become the medical buzzword of the moment as we all, young and old, contemplate how we would most like to live out our lives. We all want to know the tricks for prolonging our life spans, and physicians, researchers, and scientists have devoted thousands of pages to the topic. For the most part they address the benefits of attending to the body by physical means: slash your cholesterol, reduce your weight, don't forget about exercise, stop smoking, and have your blood pressure checked every year.

While these measures are important contributors to longevity—and they are *very* important—there's much more. To make an analogy: When you bring your child to the family doctor or pediatrician for a checkup, the doctor's findings give you only part of the picture. Your child might need some immunizations, and perhaps you might discuss eating habits. But as the parent, you know how your child does in school, what sort of friends she or he has, whether she or he is happy or sad, and what kind of self-image your child has. All these things are truly important, too. They are what make our children whole.

The same is true of you. Diet, exercise, smoking, and cholesterol are important, but they are not the total you. Just as critical are how much you like your job, whether you have a good or rotten relationship with your parents and children, what sort of friendships you have, whether you're depressed or happy, angry or delighted, abusive or kindhearted.

We would all agree that these factors count indisputably in quality of life. The fact is that they count in longevity, too—perhaps even as much as the physical factors your doctor can treat. Happy, satisfied people with strong social relationships live longer *regardless of their cholesterol, eating habits, weight, or exercise pattern.* It's a scientific fact.

The truth is that being well does not simply mean getting a clean bill of health from your physician. Overall good health is composed of five unique and interrelated spheres of wellness: the physical, the mental, the family and social, the spiritual, and the material. Picture the Olympic symbol of five interlocking rings in your mind, with each ring overlapping and interacting with the others, and you'll have a good sense of how the five spheres relate to one another. In order to achieve your longevity plan and a happy, satisfied, fulfilling, vivacious life, you must find balance and good health in all five spheres. Identifying which areas need the most improvement and which are already robust is the key to unlocking your personal longevity code and will ultimately guide you in devising the most effective plan for enhancing your life span.

Longevity is a two-sided coin, with quantity on one side and quality on the other. Just as no one wants a great life that's cut short prematurely, no one wants a life that's simply long and not satisfying on many levels. We want to have it both ways: long *and* great. And in fact we can.

No matter where you are in your life, you can improve your lot. Studies have shown that smokers get years from quitting, whether they do it at twenty-five or sixty-five; that mammograms can add years to the life of a seventy-year-old, just as they can for a forty-year-old; that having a spiritual path, be it time with Mother Nature, personal meditation, or going to church, can add a perspective that you don't get from reading the *Wall Street Journal* or the *New York Times.*

The questions, then, are these: How do you find your path? What are your first steps? Which will make the most profound differences in your life—and in your longevity?

When you make a longevity plan, you need one that is as specific and unique as you are. One size does not fit all, any more than one restaurant or one occupation is right for all of us. There are some general rules that should probably be a part of each person's plan—reducing the amount of red meat you eat, consuming more fruits and veggies, wearing seat belts all the time, getting screened for cancer, and so on. But having an occupation that you love reaps you quality benefits and boosts your longevity, too. Practicing kindness and compassion not only brings you more mental peace than anger and hatred but reduces your risk of premature heart disease and stroke. Only you know if these are changes you need to implement in your life—right now.

Every aspect of the life you live—from the genetic factors that predispose you to certain diseases to the personal choices you make each day—can be seen as either a longevity *buster* or a longevity *booster*. The goal of this book is to help you identify and eliminate as many of the former while adopting as many of the latter that apply to you as possible. To this end I've devised an easy-to-follow system for identifying which longevity boosters are most vital to your continued good health. And what you find may surprise you, because you'll see that there is more to your longevity plan than the typical doctor's visit has to offer. It's broader, deeper, and much more fulfilling than that.

In this book I will give you a method for finding all of the missing pieces in your search for a longer, sweeter life. I won't discount the significance of diet and exercise or smoking and cholesterol. But I will put them into perspective with the other factors that we know contribute equally to your longevity plan: happiness, friends, controlling anger, managing debt, looking at toxins, and dealing with family stress. A plan that balances quantity *and* quality.

I promise you a life that is not just long but filled with optimism and hope. Longevity is satisfying, vibrant, and challenging when you balance the five spheres of wellness.

PART I

Cracking the Code

Identifying the Factors That Contribute to—or Threaten—Your Longevity

1

How We Age Today

Can We All Live to One Hundred?

ONE-HUNDRED-YEAR-OLD ALEX HARDY grows fresh herbs and glorious perennials in the window boxes of the cottage he shares with his "child bride," Eleanor, a mere youngster at eighty-three. I often see the two of them out for a stroll on warm summer evenings, and I miss them when they head south to Arizona each November. By March I find myself wondering if Alex made it through another winter. But then I drive past his home, spot new seedlings beginning to sprout in his window boxes, and smile. My friend is alive—and still well enough to continue doing what he loves most.

Alex is one of a dozen or so centenarians I've had the good fortune to know. Another is Betty Ellis. At 102 she is by far the oldest of my patients, and a true original. A farmer's daughter who became a farmer's wife, Betty raised five children before she and her husband, Ed, sold their farm and opened a restaurant, which she ran right along with him until 1951. That's when Ed, who was twenty years her senior, died. Betty kept the restaurant going and did most of the cooking for another thirty-plus years. At seventy-five, she sold the place to her nephew but hardly retired. She cooked for and took care of "old folks" (many of them a decade or more younger than she) for the next seventeen years.

With her hundredth birthday approaching, Betty briefly considered moving into an assisted-living facility, but not because her ability to handle the tasks of daily living was slipping away. No, Betty was simply tired of cooking. She wanted her meals prepared for her for a change. "Only their food was terrible," Betty grumbled. "And the time went too slowly." So she took a room in the home of a local minister and was soon supervising food preparation for his church's soup kitchen. As of this writing, she's still at it and showing few signs of slowing down.

While Alex and Betty are casual acquaintances, I've known Emma Axelrod my entire life. Hers is the name that conjures the most fondness when I think of people who have lived a long, long time.

Emma was eight when her family came to this country from Russia. They landed on Ellis Island, then traveled by train to Chicago, where they lived with relatives until they found a place of their own. It was a fairly typical immigrant story, one that played itself out again and again as each new wave of Emma's family arrived in the region.

Despite being a bright girl who did well in school, Emma dropped out at thirteen to help support a household nearly bursting at the seams with hopeful relatives. She went to work in a spice factory putting peppercorns in little boxes for fancy shops to sell to wealthy women. Although she sometimes peered into those shops, feeling a mixture of awe and envy, she would not have traded her life for anybody else's. "A little hard work never hurt anyone" are words that Emma lives by. As far as she was concerned, the key to happiness was to "keep busy."

A real beauty, young Emma modeled for magazine advertisements until 1917, when she married Harry Axelrod—and continued to keep busy. Emma "helped out" with her husband's carpet business and devoted herself to raising her son and daughter, "100 percent American." All three predeceased her, and each death was a tremendous blow. But Emma coped by involving herself in other people's lives. She filled her days by "doing this and that" for her synagogue, visiting shut-ins, chatting with neighbors, organizing card parties at the senior center, and calling in to radio talk shows.

At eighty she was as sharp and spry as any sixty-year-old, and at ninety-five she was still living on her own in a meticulously maintained apartment. But at ninety-eight she broke her hip, was hospitalized, then was transferred to a rehabilitation facility, where the staff determined that she was no longer able to function safely in an apartment.

Reluctantly she moved to a nursing home, a very nice place where residents are treated with grace and dignity, but still a regimented institution with fixed schedules, preset menus, and minimal freedom of choice. The very idea made Emma profoundly unhappy. But after a brief adjustment period, she has found that she likes the place.

In the nursing home she has a roommate to talk to. The nurses are pleasant, and the afternoons spent conversing with fellow residents or reminiscing with visitors are a joy. Indeed, being back in a social milieu has been a real longevity booster for Emma, who celebrated her hundredth birthday in 1997. Surrounded by friends and family and looking as if she would be around for at least another decade, she joined the exclusive club consisting of the world's longest-living men and women.

What's the secret to Alex's, Betty's, and Emma's longevity? Why have they lived for more than a century while more than 99 percent of their peers died at sixty or seventy or eighty-four? Did they have a genetic advantage, a better upbringing, healthier lifestyles, an exceptional outlook? Was it just a matter of chance? Or all of the above?

Longer and Better—The Story of Our Lives Today

For centuries we humans have been fascinated with the idea of immortality and driven by the desire to stay young indefinitely. Countless quests have been fueled by the hope of finding the mythical fountain of youth whose waters were purported to make the old young again.

Over the years we've also tried to locate a "cure" for aging in various foods, drinks, minerals, lotions, potions, injections, and incantations. Thus far no magical elixir has been discovered, although biologists, sociologists, and other scientists have accumulated an impressive—and still expanding—body of knowledge. We now know a lot about how people age, what kills us prematurely, and how to prevent or avoid those killers, which substances and behaviors undermine health and which promote it. While this may not be enough know-how to put a lifetime of one hundred within everyone's grasp, I believe it gives most of us a chance to reach our nineties.

We're already living longer than any generation that came before us. Since the start of the twentieth century, average life expectancy in this country has climbed from forty-nine to seventy-six. The number of people surviving to one hundred or older (one out of every ten thousand Americans) has increased fivefold during that same period and is expected to triple again by the year 2020. Naturally, the ranks of men and women in their eighties and nineties have swollen, too, and those octogenarians and nonagenarians tend to be healthier and to do more for longer than they've ever done before. Active life expectancy—the number of years people remain in a vital, independent state—is on the rise.

Today, athletes run marathons well into their seventies. Grandmothers graduate from college. Downsized employees in their forties, fifties, and sixties start their own businesses. Senator and former astronaut John Glenn returned to space as a septuagenarian. The late comedian George Burns continued to perform long past his ninetieth birthday.

And in Arles, France, Jeanne Calumet was still living in her own apartment at 110. She rode a bicycle and handled all daily living activities independently until her 115th year and might have gone on longer if she had not injured herself in a fall. When she died in August 1997 at the age of 122, she had lived longer than any person on record.

Some of these folks are exceptional individuals, having been trendsetters and fearless adventurers since childhood or recipients of remarkable genetic heritages. But most are everyday folks, more like us than not. They simply do not treat getting older as if it were a one-way express-train ticket to illness, infirmity, and inactivity. They go right on skiing, swimming, running companies, running for Congress, fathering children, painting masterpieces, tending to abandoned babies in hospital nurseries, and more. Their achievements are evidence that there is no statute of limitations on travel or learning or continuing any life-enhancing activity—no designated birthday when we must stop listening to rock and roll, start "acting like senior citizens," give up superhot chili peppers, or take up needlepoint. Of course, you're free to do any of those things if that's what you desire. But you don't have to.

The John Glenns, George Burnses, and Jeanne Calumets of the world give us hope. They become our role models. And so do regular people such as Alex Hardy, Betty Ellis, and Emma Axelrod. "If they can still do what they love at their ages, why can't we?" we wonder. Many of us can. What's more, you can add to your lifestyle—a form of physical exercise such as resistance training or a mental challenge such as learning a foreign language. If you think your muscles or mind won't be up to the task when you're sixty, seventy, or eighty-five, think again.

In Maryland or Minnesota, Sweden or Japan or elsewhere, researchers have been keeping their eyes trained on average citizens who represent a cross section of races, religions, occupations, and socioeconomic statuses. They are participants in decades-long studies to identify and measure how humans age. They have allowed themselves to be poked, prodded, observed, evaluated, and questioned on a wide range of topics, some of them extremely personal.

These studies—conducted separately and sometimes for different reasons—all seem to support the same general conclusion: *Although biological aging may be one of nature's givens and, at present, an unavoidable phenomenon, disease, disability, and decline are not.*

In a cluster of research projects initiated by the MacArthur Foundation, a multidisciplinary team of scholars confirmed that the world is full of people whose risk for disease and disease-related disabilities is low, whose physical and mental functioning are high, and who remain actively engaged in life. Medicare, which has tracked the characteristics of folks over sixty-five for nearly two decades, reports that the percentage of older people who are significantly disabled has dropped by nearly 1 percent per year since 1983. That means that seniors today are 15 percent less likely to be disabled than seniors during Ronald Reagan's presidency. They're healthier, more energetic, and doing more for themselves than their parents or grandparents did.

The Baltimore Longitudinal Study of Aging (BLSA), a forty-year federally funded project involving nearly twenty-five hundred participants, has observed that many losses of function once thought to be age-related, including decreased joint mobility and memory lapses, can be slowed or stopped. Strength, stamina, and muscle mass do decrease with time—you need only swing a tennis racket or hike with your son's college classmates to be convinced of that. But if you've stayed even moderately active, more than enough physical prowess remains to meet the demands of daily living. And even couch potatoes can regain some of what they lost. After ten weeks of weight lifting, a group of one hundred nursing home patients whose mean age was eighty-seven significantly increased the muscle strength in their legs. Clearly, any limits nature might set for us are not as fixed as we once believed.

Behind Every Centenarian: Technology, Medicine, and Personal Choice

If longer, healthier lives are the rule these days, medical science and public health measures can take a good deal of the credit. With the advent of industrialization came the wealth, science, and technology to separate drinking water from sewage, resolve housing shortages, and see that people got adequate nutrition. These changes alone marked the beginning of the end for certain diseases: tuberculosis was virtually obliterated when nutritional and overcrowding problems were eliminated; diseases such as cholera, dysentery, and typhoid fever, all spread by contaminated water, as well as airborne diseases including whooping cough, measles, diphtheria, and scarlet fever have all but disappeared in the developed world.

The introduction of vaccinations and antibiotics further reduced the damage done by infectious diseases, dramatically decreasing the number of deaths from polio, influenza, meningitis, and hepatitis. An international effort spearheaded by the World Health Organization literally eradicated smallpox worldwide.

While early gains went to infants and children, whose mortality rates had been many times higher than they are today, more recent developments have improved our odds of surviving conditions that strike the middle-aged. New equipment, medications, and procedures, including angioplasty and coronary bypass surgery, contributed to a drop in premature deaths from heart disease of almost 50 percent since the Beatles first appeared on the *Ed Sullivan Show* in 1966. Stroke deaths have decreased by nearly 60 percent as well. And we're more successful at managing chronic conditions, from diabetes and high blood pressure to atherosclerosis and asthma.

We've even made strides toward remedying the problem of injured or worn-out joints. The ability to replace knees and hips (more than a hundred thousand of them last year alone) has returned pleasure and mobility to many people's lives. I have patients who are now dancing, fishing, walking in the woods, or eating out for the first time in years.

New measures for extending or enhancing lives seem to arrive daily. Synthetic estrogens are being developed so that women can ward off osteoporosis and heart disease after menopause without increasing their risk for breast or uterine cancers. Faster computers and other advances are enhancing the effectiveness of mammograms, CAT scans, and MRIs. These are vital for the early detection of diseases that would be fatal if diagnosed at later stages. And the medical establishment is finally seeing the value of vitamin E, vitamin C, and folic acid supplements, touted for years by natural healers.

By doing their part to curb premature death and disabling conditions, all of the advances I've mentioned lengthen life span and improve life quality. But they're not the whole show. Technology doesn't operate in a vacuum. Indeed, it is rendered valueless if we don't elect to use it.

Take the screening test for cervical cancer, which you know as a Pap smear: a simple, inexpensive diagnostic test that successfully detects very early signs of a disease that once struck down young women by the tens of thousands, killing them in their twenties and thirties. Early detection makes it possible to treat the condition at a stage where it can be readily cured. However, the test, which saves thousands of lives every year, would do no good whatsoever if women didn't go to their doctors to get Pap smears. Because so many do go and the test does work, cervical cancer deaths have decreased by 90 percent since 1950. They could be wiped out almost completely if more women were tested every one to three years.

Likewise, the people who heeded the surgeon general's warnings about cigarettes when they were first made public more than thirty years ago are in much better shape today than those who didn't. Back then, nearly half of all adult Americans smoked. A decade later, only one-third did. And currently, among the college-educated, the number of smokers has dropped to less than 15 percent. This single change made as much impact on health as modern sanitation did.

Check Your Lifestyle

There is no alchemist's key to longevity, no foolproof formula or one-size-fits-all strategy for living longer and loving it. But that doesn't mean life is a crapshoot, with its length and quality determined by nothing more than a toss of the dice. There are proven ways to extend life expectancy (although not to eternity) and highly effective measures we can take to stay healthy, active, alert, and happy (if not forever young).

Although genetics, early childhood experiences, random acts of violence, and other circumstances beyond our control all contribute to health and longevity, the length and quality of our lives are in large measure shaped by the actions we take and the choices we make as adults. We can be sun worshipers and increase our odds of developing skin cancer. Or we can practice safe sex and reduce our risk of contracting AIDS and other sexually transmitted diseases. We can smoke or not, take advantage of mammograms and other early detection measures or not, buckle up or not, allow drivers to enrage us or not. Our daily choices influence how long we live and how well.

In a landmark long-term study conducted for the Human Population Lab in the San Francisco Bay area, Dr. Lester Breslow and Dr. Lisa F. Berkman looked at mortality among men and women between thirty and sixty-nine, homing in on seven high-risk practices: (1) smoking, (2) excessive alcohol consumption, (3) physical inactivity, (4) obesity or unusually low body weight, (5) sleeping fewer than seven or more than eight hours per night, (6) skipping breakfast, and (7) snacking. To varying degrees, all seven had an adverse impact on longevity. Subjects who engaged in these risky practices had death rates from 25 to 115 percent higher than those who did not.

Healthy practices (essentially reversals of the unhealthy factors) had the opposite effect. And the more healthy behaviors someone adopted, the better. A forty-five-year-old man who observed six healthy practices could expect to live eleven or more years longer than someone who observed only one or two.

Personal actions with the potential to prolong life and promote health are not limited to these seven. There are scores more. And they clearly wield considerable clout. Indeed, if we could eliminate all the lifestyle factors known to cause us harm and replace them with conditions and behaviors linked to health and longevity, we would prevent two-thirds of the premature deaths and disabling conditions that occur in this country. Half of all heart problems, 65 percent of all cancers, 75 percent of liver failure, and up to 90 percent of lung diseases such as emphysema and bronchitis would be eliminated. Twenty or more years could be added to our average life expectancy.

Achieving such lofty objectives would require draconian measures. Everyone would have to live perfectly. We could take no chances, make no move without weighing its long-range effect on our life expectancy, and do little if anything just for the fun of it. That's not going to happen. It's not what we want to happen. And it doesn't have to.

Just look at the centenarians I introduced earlier. They didn't lead perfect lives. Emma has never, ever done twenty consecutive minutes of vigorous, aerobic exercise. Betty has started off nearly every morning of her adult life with a breakfast of bacon, eggs, and fried potatoes. And Alex, who worked for decades as a telephone lineman, risked injury and death each time he scaled a pole or came across a downed electrical wire. He tempted fate even further by purchasing a sports car at age fifty and driving as if he were trying to qualify for the Indy 500 whenever he got behind the wheel. Clearly they had enough going for them and did enough of what they individually needed to do for themselves to outlive the majority of their peers. But they didn't have vice-free, totally safe lifestyles—or cookie-cutter ones identical to the others'.

We Each Have Our Own Code

We each bring a unique life résumé to the task of improving our well-being and extending our stay on the planet. It contains our medical histories, habits, likes, dislikes, disabilities, and family histories. Age, socioeconomic status, the medications we take, the environments we live or work in, and the skills we use to cope with stress are all found on these personal vitae. Clearly no two are the same. And because they aren't, every measure aimed at extending and enhancing life simply cannot be applied across the board.

Even a measure that has been scientifically tested and proven effective in the general population may not be right for you. There's plenty of evidence that drinking in moderation (roughly one glass of wine or its equivalent per day, and no more than two) can help prevent heart attacks, for example. Yet someone in recovery from alcoholism would be foolish to adopt the practice.

Likewise, there are benefits to be derived from taking estrogen, or more commonly estrogen/progesterone combinations, after menopause. Hormone replacement therapy (HRT) has been shown to reduce one adverse effect of menopause: osteoporosis. For many years, we thought that it significantly reduced the risk from heart disease, but new research has called that into question. And HRT has also been linked to increased risk for breast and uterine cancer and therefore may pose a threat to women, especially those with a personal or family history that predisposes them to those diseases. As a result, any woman considering HRT must factor in her own background information. And so should all of us when we're trying to decide which longevity-boosting lifestyle changes to make.

The key to both prolonging and enhancing your life is to first determine which longevity-boosting actions and attitudes best address your goals, needs, and circumstances—and then to adopt them at a reasonable pace. To accomplish this you'll need to crack your longevity code—to figure out what you have going for or working against you today, not only physically but mentally, socially, spiritually, and materially. You'll want to take credit for what you've already accomplished and zero in on the aspects of your life that may need adjustments.

In fact, you may want to visualize your longevity code as a page from a bookkeeper's ledger. On one side of the page are debits, or what I call longevity busters. They are the conditions, circumstances, and activities that tend to decrease life expectancy and diminish life quality. On the other side are credits, or longevity boosters, which tend to extend and enhance our lives. Once you decipher the code, you can use that information to initiate not just any lifestyle changes but the specific changes that will do you the most good.

Cracking your code is what the first part of this book is all about. In Chapter 2 you'll take a closer look at the five spheres of wellness and the boosters and busters in each. Some of these will fall under the heading of "life's givens"—the subject of Chapter 3. They include inherited predispositions, events that influenced our early development, the impact of race, gender, or socioeconomic status, and the residual effects of past ill-advised behavior. Although these factors can't be altered appreciably, you can certainly overcome or compensate for their adverse effects (as well as build on their positive features).

If diabetes runs in your family, for example, and you've been putting on weight (a controllable factor for adult-onset diabetes), then one of your top priorities is to keep an eye on your blood sugar levels and lose ten or twelve pounds. Neither of those would be necessary for someone with a different background and body fat level.

The influence of life's givens also means that our personal longevity profiles reflect our individual differences even when the same longevity boosters and busters turn up. Take the generally good idea of limiting exposure to direct sunlight by wearing a hat and sunscreen when you're outdoors. Because this precaution can reduce anyone's risk of developing skin cancer, I recommend it for everyone. But for folks who have the shadow of a previous malignancy hanging over them, there's more urgency. If you have had malignant melanoma, the skin cancer that can kill you, wearing a hat and using a good sunscreen is something you absolutely must do immediately, continue doing indefinitely, and try to do every single time you go out in the sun.

But remember, at least half and possibly as many as three-quarters of all longevity boosters and busters are not dealt to us by history or heredity. They are the by-products of lifestyle choices, choices that can be corrected or reversed if they're harming us and repeated or reinforced if they're enhancing our lives. Some of those choices predispose us to (or protect us from) conditions such as cancer and heart disease and events such as motor vehicle accidents that tend to bring about our early demise. These are profiled in Chapter 4.

Any action in any sphere that maximizes a longevity booster or neutralizes a longevity buster will prove beneficial in the long run. But some of the biggest gains may come from targeting known risk factors for major killers. These lethal events and diseases don't just shave a year or two off your life. They cut it down by decades. And they don't do it nicely. Stroke, emphysema, cirrhosis of the liver, AIDS, and other lingering illnesses rob you of life quality as well as life expectancy. If you avoid them (by reducing or eliminating the things that make you more vulnerable to them), you'll dramatically increase your chances of living a longer, sweeter life.

Finally, our personal longevity codes contain several crucial attitudes that anyone can't do without. Along with your mental picture of how you'd like your life to be at various points down the road, these must-have elements motivate, inspire, and focus our efforts to extend and enhance our lives.

It's Never Too Late

As a family physician, I'm constantly pointing my patients in the direction of longevity. Whether I'm seeing them about a specific health problem or conducting a periodic, preventive tune-up, I find a way to touch on the topic. Our casual conversation about the high school soccer team often switches to a low-key discussion about the benefits of taking a daily aspirin or the adverse effects of limiting our vegetable intake to french fries and ketchup. I ask about my patients' jobs, families, stress levels, or exercise programs and not just their medical histories. Then I mention a new study or cite a statistic or make a suggestion. You never know when a bit of new data, a word of advice, or a show of concern will start the ball rolling for someone.

Just ask Harry Winston. When I met him, he was forty-eight, working for a shipping company, and from all outward signs speeding toward an early grave. He came to me with a nagging backache, but it quickly became apparent that he suffered from a multitude of other, not strictly medical maladies. His boss, who believed Harry's pain was all in his head, was pressuring him to "get up to speed" or resign. His wife, who had been sleeping in the guest room for months, was threatening divorce. And his two grown children were always in some kind of trouble. It wasn't difficult to understand why Harry, whose worries woke him up at night, described himself as depressed. He showed up for appointments listless and lethargic, his eyes glazed over and heavy-lidded from the codeine-based pain medication he was overusing, his breath reeking of brandy.

Although Harry vehemently denied it, his growing dependence on alcohol and pain pills was deepening his depression, impairing his judgment, and bringing him closer and closer to death's door. He had gotten into several motor vehicle accidents, and late one afternoon at work he had nearly plummeted down a flight of concrete steps.

I tried and tried to convince Harry to tackle this obstacle first, but he wasn't budging. There was no way he could bear his back pain without medication, he insisted, and nothing else could help: physical therapy hadn't "done a darn thing"; biofeedback was "a bunch of hokum." Then, during an office visit, I handed him a flyer advertising yoga classes and gave him some background on the instructor, a registered nurse who was once nearly incapacitated by back pain herself. Hesitantly he agreed to "give it a try."

Much to Harry's amazement, yoga's gentle stretching and fluid movement did indeed work wonders for his back. As some of his pain subsided his disposition softened. "I didn't realize how tense and grouchy I had been," he says. After the first round of classes ended, he signed up for another. And another. Before long he felt good enough to start weaning himself from his pain pills. Then he checked into an alcohol rehab program, "joined the ranks of the clean and sober," went to couples counseling, and marveled at the results.

"Life just keeps getting better," Harry reported the last time I saw him—in a hospital lobby awaiting the birth of his second grandchild. Four years had passed since I handed him the yoga flyer, and not a trace of his drugged expression or downtrodden demeanor remained. He looked years younger—and delighted to be alive.

Harry may never set any longevity records. Yet he has clearly increased his life expectancy, because he took a series of action steps, some planned, others incidental, but all suited to his unique personal makeup. He now has a real shot at reaching a ripe old age and savoring life's sweetness all along the way.

Can You Really Add Years (and Quality) to Your Life Span?

Time and time again, people like Harry have appeared to remind me that even when our words and actions seem to indicate the opposite, most of us really do want to "live long and prosper," as Star Trek's Mr. Spock used to say. We just need to find our way there.

Our aim is not merely to accumulate extra years but rather to live in a sound, satisfying, and self-sufficient state for as long as possible. Mountains of research and years of practical medical experience have convinced me that this outcome is definitely within our grasp. There is no magic to longevity, no foolproof formula. But there are proven ways to extend life expectancy and highly effective measures we can take to stay healthy, active, alert, and happy. All of us may not be at the same point in our lives now or have the same obstacles to conquer. But each of us can increase our longevity in some way.

For Harry, yoga, new friendships, and recovery from alcoholism were the keys. For you, an exercise regimen, meditation, or a new job could open the door. There are plenty of ways to boost longevity.

The most extensively studied and widely publicized routes involve

SEVEN SIMPLE STEPS FOR PEOPLE WHO HOPE TO LIVE A CENTURY (OR LONGER)

1. Drink Juice Daily

Maintaining a varied, nutritionally balanced diet is still one of the best ways to promote health and prevent life-shortening conditions that have been linked to dietary deficiencies or excesses. Drinking a six-ounce glass of juice contributes to that balance. Whether you choose orange, apple, grape, guava, carrot, cranberry, tomato, or others, juice is great for getting fruit and vegetables into your system. We need at least five servings from that food group daily. In addition, certain juices offer specific health benefits, from combating constipation to reducing the risk of urinary tract infections. And most are excellent sources of antioxidants such as vitamin C, vitamin E, and beta-carotene, which have been shown to slow the aging process.

2. Add Physical Activity at Every Opportunity

Take the stairs instead of the elevator. Park farther away from the office, mall, or train station and walk. Do ten minutes on your stationary bike while you're waiting for the pasta to cook. Rake leaves. Vacuum carpets. Mow the lawn. Play Marco Polo in the neighborhood pool with a bunch of eight-year-olds. Exercise, whether vigorous and intentionally scheduled or moderate and incidental, is a measure with multiple benefits: promoting heart health, facilitating weight loss, reducing stress, relieving depression, improving your sex life, and more. Of particular interest to those of us who may never willingly enter a health club are two recent studies showing that moderate activity (such as walking or gardening) in short sessions throughout the day is as beneficial as thirty minutes of sustained, intense exercise three to five times weekly.

3. Learn Something

Read up on a subject. Attend lectures. Take a class. Join a book club. Do crossword puzzles. It is more and more apparent that our brains need to be exercised as much as our muscles do. Those of us who put our minds through their paces regularly, challenging them with new ideas, are far more likely to retain our faculties. What's more, numerous studies show a clear correlation between education and life expectancy. The more we know, the longer we're likely to live.

4. Floss

And see your dentist regularly. Include at least one annual cleaning session with a hygienist. You'll improve the odds of keeping your own teeth into old,

old age. But more than that, by keeping your gums healthy you could be preventing a coronary. Periodontal disease is a risk factor for heart problems.

5. Grow Something

Herbs in a window box. Tomatoes in the backyard. Silver bells, cockleshells, and an occasional petunia. Gardening is a wonderful, often relaxing pastime that is also good exercise and emotionally soothing and spiritually replenishing. It takes our minds off our worldly worries and puts us in touch with nature. Even if serenity can't be proven to extend life, it most certainly enhances it.

6. Roll Coins

Turn spare change into a nest egg, a fund for emergencies, or a savings account. Simply empty your pockets or purse into a coin jar every evening. Then periodically fill wrappers. You'll be amazed by the amount you can accumulate, especially if you make a point not to use coins smaller than a quarter for routine purchases. You can use this "found money" to fill in the gaps in your monthly budget, assuaging some of your financial worries and the stress levels they create. You can pay for massages, aerobics classes, or other health-promoting extras that you might not otherwise indulge in. You can invest. Or derive social, emotional, and spiritual benefits by donating to a charity or supporting a cause.

7. Look Ahead Hopefully

Compile a list of things you want to learn, accomplish, or experience before you die—either totally new endeavors or current activities. Former pastimes are fair game, too. Add to your list periodically. Keep track of the goals and accomplishments. The prospect of actually learning to speak Italian or traveling by train across Canada or raising money for cancer research fuels our will to live as long—and stay as well—as possible. Whether they're fun and frivolous or serious and formidable, having goals to pursue gives us a reason to greet each new day with a sense of purpose and optimism. Both longevity researchers and exceptionally long-lived individuals mention that kind of outlook as a powerful force.

physical changes. Giving up tobacco, improving our eating habits, and getting more exercise lead the pack. But other things—self-confidence, goals to pursue, lifelong learning, hope for the future, a social support system—are important, too.

The state of our psyches, marriages, work lives, social ties, spiritual beliefs, and finances all add to or subtract from our life expectancy, multiplying the number of action steps available to us. And that's a mixed blessing when it comes to deciding which steps to take: You can't do everything, and things are not of equal value. So what do you choose? How do you judge? How far must you go?

Most of us are willing to do something for the chance to someday blow out a hundred birthday candles. But following a superstrict, ultra-low-fat, vegetarian diet for the next fifty years may be too much. Never eating another steak or slice of cheesecake, never savoring another cigar or snifter of brandy, not stopping to enjoy a spectacular sunset because our evening run must be done at a certain pace to maintain an optimal heart rate . . . this may be more than we care to give up.

Most of us also have busy lives, many of them already overflowing with demands and obligations and things we do for pleasure. Developing a new habit will shake things up. It will require adjustments. So the million-dollar question is this: Will the outcome of whatever you do to boost your longevity justify the time, money, or effort you invest in it? And because of your personal background or lifestyle, will some measures be a better investment than others? How can you tell? These are precisely the kinds of questions this book was designed to answer.

You Are the Secret Ingredient

Cooking is one of my passions, and I'm constantly fine-tuning recipes. One week you'll find me pursuing the ultimate pasta primavera with my daughter DeeDee, the next a near-perfect puff pastry. I once tinkered with a cheesecake recipe for a month, trying a new twist every few days. I added chocolate chips, tried a low-fat version, and experimented with different crusts until I finally had a version with just the right flavor and texture for my palate. It was *my* definitive cheesecake. Yet I didn't expect everyone to love it.

Our personal longevity codes are a lot like definitive recipes or ideal home decors or individualized investment plans. There are some basic ingredients that work for just about everyone. But other features are a much better fit for one person than another. Indeed, the same piece of advice can be anything from an answered prayer to a living nightmare.

Take my friend Arlene. She has a number of food sensitivities. Certain kinds of fish make her break out in a rash. Products with wheat or refined sugar in them bring on headaches and mood swings. So she has scrupulously avoided these items for years. As a concession to her hips and her heart, she has followed the USDA's guidelines and cut down her consumption of meat and other high-fat foods.

"Now I read that I shouldn't eat potatoes, rice, carrots, and most dairy products because they could cause breast cancer," she declares incredulously. "For Pete's sake, what's left?" The answer, in Arlene's case, is to take a step back and see what is truly scientifically based. If she continued to follow every food guru's advice, she could wind up undermining her well-being rather than improving it.

Similarly, many of us would benefit from aerobic exercise at 60 to 80 percent of our maximum heart rate for at least twenty minutes three days per week—if we could get ourselves to do it. But what if *you* can't? What if you hate the handful of activities that get your heart rate up that high? What if you don't have a twenty-minute block of time available? What if you have family commitments and can't just say, "I'm going out to jog now. You take care of the kids"? Well, then, this particular longevity-boosting measure may not be for you.

And what if you actually have twenty minutes to spare but want to use it to meditate or tend your rosebushes or cut out paper snowflakes with your five-year-old daughter? Then do those things. If they calm and relax you, bring you pleasure or make you laugh, they might ultimately have a more positive impact than forcing yourself to complete a vigorous workout. Maybe getting your exercise in brief (five- to ten-minute) bursts of activity is a better option.

Then there's the preoccupation with cholesterol. I can't tell you how many of my patients and radio listeners drive themselves crazy trying to cut cholesterol. Many of them come to me requesting cholesterol-lowering drugs when their cholesterol levels are normal. Cholesterol counts, but it's only one star in the constellation we call heart disease.

When we sign on to seek longevity, we don't sign away our rights to self-determination, peace of mind, pleasure, and spontaneity. And we should not place so much pressure on ourselves to live longer and feel better that we wind up elevating our killer stress levels. We want to take in the scenery, enjoy the company of friends and family, learn, love, or

leave our mark in some way. What may appear at first glance to be frivolous side trips sometimes influence life expectancy even more than
the precise amount of cholesterol in our bloodstream or our hours of
aerobic exercise.

Overall, some behaviors have more impact on life expectancy than
others. Likewise, some measures are more important to us because
they're linked to conditions such as breast cancer or kidney failure,
which we find particularly frightening. We are willing to go to great
lengths to avoid them. However, much of what we could conceivably
do to live fully for longer is neither clearly right for us nor obviously of
no use. Where should you start? What should your priorities be?

I believe you are the only one who can answer that question.
Not you alone, of course. You will need information and assistance
and encouragement from books such as this one or from knowledgeable organizations such as the American Cancer Society or the
American Heart Association. You may benefit from medical supervi-
sion or the support of a self-help group. But ultimately, which steps
you're willing and able to take, in what order, and at what pace will
be your call.

There was a time when we depended on doctors to have all the
information about health and longevity. We often took their advice
without asking questions. Now we look to doctors and medical experts
for information that we can use to help us make health decisions for
ourselves. Gone are the days when doctors rendered their opinion and
we obeyed. Today, as consumers of health care, we want to be, deserve
to be, and have the personal insight to be part of that process.

Studies have shown that regardless of their level of education,
socioeconomic status, race, or gender, people have a fairly accurate
sense of how they are doing healthwise. They have a sense of their own
weak points and a pretty good idea of what they need to do to correct
them. I'm sure you are no exception.

And whether your doctor recommends a course of action or your
spouse insists upon it, you are the one who has to carry it out. If you
don't see its value or consider it important or feel up to the challenge,
you aren't going to do it.

You could try to process all the medical and scientific information
on longevity that's available right now. But the sheer volume is mind-

boggling. The task of evaluating it generally and then applying it to your life specifically would paralyze you with indecision. I've seen this happen all too often. Helping people avoid that fate is what I had in mind when I set out to write this book.

I approached the task by doing what you would expect your doctor to do. I studied the presenting problem—lives that weren't as long or as sweet as they could be. I looked at the history of those problems, their causes and remedies, and the things that seemed to help. I pored over medical journals, talked to hundreds of fellow professionals, compared and critiqued until I was able to distill the information into a compendium of what I consider to be the best longevity-boosting measures around.

If you read and consider all of this book's information and suggestions, you will end up with a detailed prescription for getting from where you are today to wherever you want to be in the future. Like a customized Trip-Tik from AAA, it will guide you along the route to longevity that suits you best.

But you don't have to use this book that way. You can use it as a reference to look up physical, mental, social, spiritual, or material conditions that threaten longevity and learn how to avoid them. You can use it as an idea book to help you locate solutions to actual problems or find new and different ways to lengthen and enrich your life. Or you can use it simply for inspiration.

2

The Five Spheres of Wellness
Aiming for Total Health

WHEN ALL IS SAID AND DONE, the quest for personal longevity boils down to a simple formula: Start eliminating the longevity busters you've accumulated and build up your supply of longevity boosters. But it's important to remember that wellness is not defined entirely by those factors your doctor can measure. Our sense of well-being derives as much from factors that lie outside the physical realm as it does from those things we most commonly associate with good health: absence of disease, physical fitness, appropriate weight, and the like. Though your doctor can't write you a prescription for a less stressful job, a closer relationship with your parents, or confinement to a national park for a day spent enjoying the beauty of nature, each of these has an appreciable and profound effect on your overall wellness.

The Big Picture

Ralph Peters, an advertising executive who recently turned fifty, was one of the first people I met when my wife, Penny, and I moved to the small Wisconsin town where we still live. He is also a patient, although his wife practically has to drag

BUSINESS REPLY MAIL

FIRST-CLASS MAIL   PERMIT NO. 1099   SKOKIE IL

POSTAGE WILL BE PAID BY ADDRESSEE

ARCHITECTURE

PO BOX 2099
SKOKIE IL 60076-9355

NO POSTAGE
NECESSARY
IF MAILED
IN THE
UNITED STATES

him into my office when he's due for a checkup. Medical exams take time, and until recently Ralph never had any to spare.

Once a classic workaholic who routinely put in eighty-hour work-weeks, Ralph was known to have business on his mind from breakfast through bedtime. He owned a pleasure boat and a lakeside vacation home but rarely used either, and was the father of four sons he rarely saw. He was also a type A personality—ambitious, impatient, and usually juggling a half-dozen tasks at once. Quick to anger, he had fits of temper that were legendary—and frequent enough for his colleagues to avoid meeting with him if they got wind that he was in "one of his moods."

To his credit, Ralph had given up cigarettes. And he stopped at the Y most mornings to swim laps. But then he was off to another day of deadlines, demands, and doughnuts. His lopsided lifestyle was taking its toll. Ralph was plagued by tension headaches, chronic heartburn, and bouts of insomnia. Both his blood pressure and blood sugar levels were approaching their respective danger zones. And for what?

Ralph wasn't strapped for money. His expenses were covered, and his retirement, savings, and investment accounts had substantial balances. He didn't experience the thrill of starting a new project or the satisfaction of finishing one anymore. Indeed, for the past year all that had kept him going were daydreams about taking a leave of absence and motorcycling to Alaska, "just me, my camping gear, and my Harley."

"Then do it," I advised him. "Take that trip." I telephoned occasionally to see if he'd set his plan in motion. I sent him full-color travel brochures. And I was thrilled when he finally took off for two and a half months this past summer.

For Ralph, who thought he would miss "always having people around to talk to," the solitude of his ride was surprisingly enjoyable. "Sometimes I would pull off the road, find a log or a tree stump to use as a seat, and just sit there quietly until something moved me to move on. It was almost religious," he added. On Sundays he found himself drawn to small-town churches. "Even though I hadn't been in one in years. I'd stop and attend a service wherever I happened to be."

At various points in his journey, when he was near a city or a town big enough to support an airfield and hotel-like accommodations, Ralph would fly family members up for visits: first his wife alone; then his wife with their two kids; and finally his adult sons, offspring from his first tumultuous marriage, with whom he had not spent an extended period of time since they were infants. "They stayed for a week of day trips and wilderness tours and just hanging out together," Ralph recounts. "I really got to know them. We've never been as close."

"I feel like those ten weeks added ten years to my life," Ralph says now. And they very well may have. He returned twelve pounds lighter and with lower blood pressure, far fewer headaches, and a more balanced approach to daily living. He's working less, becoming more involved with all of his kids, and taking time off just to do things he loves. He's even ready to tackle two more health hazards—his hot temper and the eating habits behind his chronic heartburn and elevated blood sugar level.

Now, that's a remarkable turnaround—achieved to this point without a single medical intervention! Like most gains in longevity and life quality, Ralph's came about through the combined influence of several different, not exclusively physical, factors. The extended vacation from his tension-filled profession, the luxury of sitting quietly with his mind uncluttered, the opportunity to reconnect with his religion, and the chance to get closer to his wife and children all played roles.

An effective personal longevity code covers lots of bases. Yes, longevity busters such as working too much or flying into rages at the slightest provocation may seem inconsequential when compared to obvious dangers such as high blood pressure or living next to a toxic-waste dump. And yes, going to church, hanging out with your kids, or communing with nature in Alaska may seem like far-fetched ways to boost longevity. Yet these kinds of things can be just as important to our well-being as the treatment and prevention of bodily ailments.

There's More to Health Than Not Being Sick

The World Health Organization defines health as "complete physical, mental, and social well-being, not merely the absence of disease." Being healthy, according to this definition, encompasses the obvious—being at your physical best, capable, mobile, adaptable, alert, and involved—as well as many things that might not leap to mind when you hear the words *longevity* or *health*. Marriage is one of them. Several research projects, including the Stanford University–based Terman Life Cycle Study, have shown that happily married people live longer.

Socioeconomic status is another example. In fact, your social class—as evidenced by your income, education, job title, and other status symbols—is as good a predictor of future health and longevity as genetics, diet, or exposure to toxins. Research out of Duke University has also shown that churchgoing men significantly outlive their non-churchgoing counterparts. And in Milwaukee, a study involving elderly nuns linked longer life spans to mental exercise, the kind you get by working on crossword puzzles, word games, and vocabulary-building exercises.

Strong social ties and regular, meaningful contact with other people prolong life. Hermits, who lack both, die younger from heart disease and commit suicide more often than the general population. Among the Human Population Laboratory research subjects, women without close ties to friends, family members, community groups, and such were three times more likely to die from heart disease than women who had those ties.

Life quality is influenced by multiple factors as well. Researchers now know that the people most likely to retain strong mental abilities as they get older are those who (1) are physically active, (2) have a social support system, and (3) believe in their own abilities. And anyone who has ever been on the brink of bankruptcy or forced to borrow money in order to buy their kids new clothes can tell you how financial matters wear you down mentally. Money worries also push things such as routine dental care or potentially life-saving medical screening onto a back burner, sometimes with disastrous results.

It's All Connected

Our minds and our bodies, our social ties and outlook, our jobs, our stress levels, and our susceptibility to heart disease—they're all connected. The physical, mental and emotional, social, spiritual, and material aspects of our lives interact constantly. Take the case of thirty-eight-year-old Grant Lewis, who was diagnosed HIV-positive almost a decade ago and developed full-blown AIDS five years later.

A self-described "party person," Grant is the kind of guy you can count on to liven up a boring bar mitzvah or add a new twist to the typical backyard barbecue by digging a pit and roasting a pig. Everything he does, he does dramatically. And in 1996 he was all set to die.

Wracked by various infections, Grant's body was failing. But thanks to AIDS counseling and support groups, he was in pretty good shape mentally. Socially, his life was resplendent with friends, family, and an uninfected lover. They rallied around him, ministering to his every need. Spiritually, Grant was a blank page. He believed that when his life ended, it ended. "No heaven, no white light, no angels come to carry me home," he would say. And financially? You might say he was unencumbered. Believing that his death was imminent, he had spent every last penny he had (not counting the small cache he had set aside to pay for his funeral and the party to be held afterward).

Luckily, triple-drug therapies came along. This protocol, which combines newer medications, known as protease inhibitors, with existing drugs such as AZT and DDI, does not cure AIDS the way penicillin cures strep infections. But for most patients, continual use seems to keep the virus in check in much the same way that blood pressure medication controls hypertension.

Whether the triple-drug therapies will work indefinitely without the AIDS virus finding a way to resist them is a big question mark. But there was no question about the impact on Grant. In just a few months he had gained twenty pounds and was able to travel, eat out, even hike. He literally had a new lease on life, and you'd think he would have been happy about it. Yet just half a year after being pulled back from the brink of death, Grant attempted suicide.

"Why on earth would he do such a thing?" you may wonder, as I did myself. The explanation lies with the way different facets of existence, or spheres of wellness, as I like to call them, influence one another.

There are five such spheres, one each for our bodies, minds, social ties, spirituality, and material side. If they had mass and volume, they might resemble soap bubbles. When two such bubbles bump into each other, they meld into one double-humped blob. Five bubbles colliding would produce a cluster of five distinct curves, with individual bubbles still discernible, but whole sections of each absorbed by the larger cluster.

If you popped one of the original orbs, the entire cluster would explode. Dye or smoke captured by a single bubble would soon permeate the whole. Spheres of wellness behave in much the same way. *Anything that happens in one sphere directly or indirectly affects at least one other area and often our lives as a whole.*

In Grant's case, the dramatic improvement in his physical health stirred up "survivor guilt." He would lie awake at night wondering why had he stayed around long enough to be "saved" by a medical breakthrough when so many others had not.

Being "saved" physically also forced Grant to face the extremely sorry state of his material sphere, which was a mess. He had government medical assistance but no income, no immediate job prospects, and creditors calling constantly. Every time he thought about this financial fiasco, he felt hopeless and depressed.

In the meantime, his social support system was falling apart. Attending to Grant's needs had drained his friends and family members. Once he no longer needed their constant care, companionship, and sympathy, they had gotten on with their own lives. Even his AIDS support groups told him he should start doing more for himself. But he didn't think he could. And with no sense of purpose (a spiritual issue) to speak of, he didn't see why he should bother.

Although triple-drug therapy's impact on Grant's physical sphere was entirely positive, the changes it instigated in his mental, material, and kinship spheres made the prospect of a prolonged life look decidedly unappealing. "An uphill battle," Grant called it. In comparison, "suicide didn't seem like such a big deal."

The Ripple Effect

Systems theorists will tell you that I've been talking about the "reciprocal interrelationship between elements of a system." They would say that the ripple effect Grant's physical progress caused in nonphysical spheres or the toll Ralph's job pressures and workaholic tendencies took on his blood pressure and sleep patterns were proof that "the disruption of the status quo at any level requires the entire system to adapt." Well, systems theory is one of the underpinnings of the wellness sphere discussion you've been reading. But so are common sense and firsthand experience. Whether in our own lives or other people's, most of us have witnessed the interplay I've been describing.

Perhaps a head cold hampered your concentration or made you forgetful, leaving your coworkers to pick up the slack for you—a fact that took them a week to let you live down. Maybe mental stress triggered a physical rash, which embarrassed you so much you backed out of social plans, which meant you spent Saturday night at home alone eating a half gallon of high-fat ice cream straight from the carton.

Naturally, the interplay among the spheres isn't always negative. Any external event or action on your part that makes a positive impact in a single sphere also reverberates throughout the system. A peaceful walk along the beach that you initiate for spiritual purposes also calms the mind, relaxes tension in your body, affords you the benefits of physical exercise, promotes better sleep, makes you more pleasant to be around, and so on. The seminar you attend for your mind's sake may stimulate a career change or trigger a moneymaking idea for your material sphere, connect you with a social support group, or tip you off to an herbal remedy for a physical ailment. Once we understand the give-and-take among spheres of wellness, we can consciously use it to enhance our lives and extend our life spans.

For Grant, the same interplay that dragged him downhill from successful triple-drug therapy to utter despair would pull him back up to health and happiness—one step at a time. I know this because after Grant's suicide attempt I took on the task of coordinating his care. The first order of business was therapy. To prevent future suicide attempts and to improve Grant's mental state, I arranged for him to see a counselor. Once he was feeling a bit more motivated and optimistic (depression can really sap your strength and blind you to the positive alternatives available to you), he started to tackle his money issues. This included filing for bankruptcy with the help of a credit counselor and obtaining part-time employment designing brochures and advertising for a small marketing company.

As Grant grew stronger emotionally and less dependent, his social life began picking up again. But he found himself hungering for something more, something that would allow him to feel wanted and valued and part of a group effort. I suggested that he become a hospice volunteer, and he was soon giving folks with terminal illness some of the same assistance and compassion that had been given to him. In return, Grant got a spiritual boost from one of his patients, an old, old man who had taken up Zen when he was in his fifties and in his final months seemed to draw strength from "just sitting." Impressed, Grant located a local Zen group and started sitting, too.

With all of his spheres humming the same tune, Grant now breathes in more of life's joy. He still sees a therapist, still takes the pharmaceutical "cocktail" that keeps the HIV in check, and won't be done untangling his finances anytime soon. But he's here and he's content, and he hopes to stay that way for many more years.

Therapy alone would not have accomplished this feat. If Grant had *only* gotten his financial affairs in order or *only* volunteered at the hospice or *only* learned about Zen, he would not have netted the same results. What's more, he could have attended to *all* of those spheres but still failed to noticeably increase his life expectancy if he had not been taking medications to control his physical illness. What worked for Grant, for Ralph, and indeed for everyone whose success stories you'll read in this book was a holistic approach, one that took their entire lives—not just isolated attributes or a single sphere—into account. The more spheres you involve in your personal longevity code, the greater your chances for a longer, sweeter life.

The Spheres of Wellness

All aspects of our existence matter. All five spheres of wellness influence longevity. They are linked together, with each offering us a potential starting point for our efforts to lengthen and enrich our lives. The spheres also serve as a framework for your personal longevity profile. As you'll see, each includes its own set of longevity boosters and longevity busters that can contribute to or detract from a long, sweet life.

SPHERE #1: PHYSICAL

The physical, or body, sphere incorporates anything that directly pertains to your body and how it works—or doesn't. It is made up of four components—physical health, physical fitness, nutrition, and safety strategies—with the best-known being physical health, which commonly means the absence of disease.

Well, *physical health* is certainly a good thing. It's also a pretty good predictor of longevity, since physically healthy people tend to live longer (and enjoy life more) than folks with debilitating medical problems. However, all you learn when you're given a proverbial clean bill of health is that nothing is *taking away* from your active life expectancy.

You still don't know what you could do to add years to it. In other words, if a wellness point was deducted for each illness, ailment, or disabling condition you had, the best score you could get would be zero (no deductions), and zero isn't much of a wellness measure. It's not detrimental. But it's not optimal, either.

There's also *physical fitness*—a combination of strength, stamina, agility, lung capacity, and heart rate. It is a direct reflection of our activity level. The more we use our muscles to lift, push, pull, bend, stretch, and move us from place to place, the more physically fit, full of energy, and long-lived we're likely to be. Physical fitness and the activities that promote it, including moderate amounts of daily exertion (the kind we get from brisk walks and leaf raking) or vigorous exercise (such as running or step aerobics) are definitely physical sphere pluses. But not engaging in them doesn't just keep you from entering 5K races or being picked for a starting position on the company softball team. Sedentary lifestyles limit longevity. They're a definite debit—and one of the top ten contributors to premature death. In the Human Population Lab study, men between the ages of thirty and forty-nine with the lowest level of physical activity had mortality rates three times higher than their more active counterparts.

Nutrition refers to what and how much we consume. The "what" should be based on general USDA and National Institutes of Health guidelines and then shaped by our personal likes, dislikes, and food sensitivities. The "how much" should be enough to obtain the nutrients we need without consuming more calories than our bodies can use. Taking in too many calories can lead to obesity, a medical condition in its own right as well as a significant risk factor for adult-onset diabetes, breast cancer, and other medical conditions. Eating too little also undermines wellness and longevity. It has been linked to malnutrition, impaired immune systems, and osteoporosis.

Some of our deadliest habits (smoking, driving drunk, unsafe sex, etc.) can be remedied by *safety strategies.* But luckily for us, most can be corrected and their ill effects at least partially, and in some instances completely, reversed. These four components contain the steps we take to avoid potential health hazards. From getting regular screening mammograms and not smoking to wearing seat belts and not driving drunk, safety-conscious lifestyle choices address known risk factors for deadly or disabling conditions. By doing so, we improve our odds of living well for a long, long time.

SPHERE #2: MENTAL

Ellie Wilder, a divorced computer programmer, showed up at my office early one afternoon complaining of crushing chest pains. They had started a few minutes earlier, as she was leaving her bank, and she had driven straight over, convinced that she was having a heart attack.

However, Ellie wasn't much of a candidate for a coronary, especially at age forty, which is exceptionally young for a woman without a family history of heart disease. It was only after I admitted her to the hospital for observation and diagnostic testing and got a chance to really talk with her that I learned about the psychological stress that could have been causing her symptoms.

A longtime sufferer of seasonal affective disorder (SAD), Ellie became depressed from late October to early March, when the days were shortest and the skies were often gray. Her illness had contributed to the demise of her marriage but only once interfered with her ability to care for her three children. That was during an exceptionally severe episode at Christmastime two years ago. Believing that she was doing what was best for the youngsters, ages nine, ten, and twelve, Ellie sent them to stay with their father—temporarily, she thought. Only her ex-husband sued for permanent custody and the right to take the kids with him when he and his new wife moved to another state. One expensive, emotionally draining court battle after another had ensued since then.

When the loan officer at her bank informed her that he couldn't approve the refinancing of her home, it was more than her beleaguered system could take. As she thought about the legal fees and other bills she had hoped a second mortgage would pay, Ellie's head began to throb. Her face flushed and her hands turned ice cold. "Then the chest pains started," she recalled, "and I was sure I was going to die."

However, Ellie was in no physical danger, at least not from coronary disease. She was having a panic attack. Her mental state was playing total havoc with her physical being—which is not an uncommon situation. Up to 25 percent of all coronary intensive care unit admissions are the result of panic, not heart problems.

PHYSICAL SPHERE LONGEVITY BUSTERS

❑ Smoking

❑ A diet of fried and processed foods, with few fruits and vegetables

❑ Very little or no physical activity

❑ Unprotected sex with multiple partners or with any partner with an unknown sexual history

❑ Forgoing routine medical care or allowing too much time to elapse between screening for early signs of disease

❑ Ignoring significant changes in your body such as shortness of breath or a sore that doesn't heal

❑ Not using seat belts, life vests, safety goggles, and such

❑ Prolonged, direct exposure to health hazards such as polluted air, toxic materials, radiation, or sunlight

❑ Drinking to excess (more than two drinks containing alcohol daily) or regularly using recreational drugs

❑ Driving a motor vehicle or operating machinery while under the influence of alcohol or drugs

PHYSICAL SPHERE LONGEVITY BOOSTERS

❑ Not smoking (extra credit if you never used tobacco products or stopped using them ten or more years ago)

❑ A diet low in fat and high in fiber with lots of fruits, vegetables, and grains

❑ Maintaining a reasonable weight

❑ At least thirty minutes of moderate activity daily

❑ Exercising vigorously three or more times weekly

❑ Resistance training to build muscle strength

❑ Protecting yourself from the sun with sunscreens, hats, sunglasses

❑ Regular medical and dental checkups, including the screening tests recommended for someone of your age, gender, and background

❑ Safe sex

❑ Doing what's necessary to manage diabetes, high blood pressure, and other chronic conditions, including taking medication as directed

❑ Using safety equipment: seat belts, life vests, safety goggles, helmets

❑ Consuming alcohol in moderation (a daily drink can reduce the risk of heart disease)

❏ If you do take sedatives, tranquilizers, or sleeping pills, using them as sparingly as possible

❏ An aspirin a day to cut the risk of stroke and repeat heart attacks

❏ Vitamins and other dietary supplements, including folic acid, vitamin C, and vitamin E to ward off various maladies and reduce the cell damage that seems to come with the territory of aging

Like the sphere that encompasses the body, the mind sphere includes more than one component. The first, *psychological health,* concerns itself with psychiatric illness or its absence. Among the most dramatic longevity busters in this category is depression, which affects 5 percent of Americans and each year costs billions of dollars for therapy, medications, hospitalization, lost productivity, and more. More than a dozen clinical studies have linked depression to higher mortality rates and lower life quality.

Another psychological state with a negative impact on longevity is *anxiety,* that sense of foreboding and worry that grips us when we anticipate failure, rejection, or some other unwanted outcome. It can cause us to avoid activities that might otherwise add pleasure and richness to our lives. Sometimes anxiety strikes for no discernible reason. Sometimes it is linked to terrifying experiences from earlier in our lives. And when it occurs in sudden, unpredictable bouts complete with heart-attack-like physical symptoms (the hallmarks of a panic disorder), anxiety can be particularly debilitating. People with panic disorders, who live in fear of their next attacks, often limit where they will go and what they'll allow themselves to do.

Other forms of *mental illness,* including schizophrenia, bipolar disorder (manic-depression), and obsessive-compulsive disorder, also take their toll. They affect our ability to sleep or eat properly, get medical problems taken care of, maintain mutually supportive relationships, and more. Smoking, drinking to excess, and other high-risk habits tend to be prevalent among the mentally ill.

Although its influence can be dramatic, psychological health is only a small portion of what the mind sphere covers. There is also *emotional health,* which I define as the ability to appropriately respond to emotional situations. The emotionally healthy people I see in my practice feel a full range of emotions—sadness, betrayal, joy, love, excitement, frustration, elation. They experience each under the circumstances that would be expected to elicit that particular feeling—for instance, sadness over a loss, delight when a child is happy, disappointment when an expectation is not met, or excitement in anticipation of an upcoming event.

Emotionally healthy individuals also react with reasonable intensity. They don't deny or minimize the pain of a painful situation, for example, or magnify minor upsets and "blow their stacks" in response. Becoming furious or extremely agitated over small frustrations every time they occur is truly deadly.

Anger and hostility studies indicate that bouts of anger, especially the face-reddening, fist-clenching, furniture-pounding, tirade-emitting kind, cause adrenaline, cortisol, and other biochemicals to surge through our bloodstreams. Frequent surges wear our bodies down. Worse yet, each surge can put a life-threatening strain on our hearts. Following a fit of anger, the risk of having a heart attack is more than twice as high.

Attitudes are also within the mind sphere's domain. "Never let anyone know how you're feeling," "Once your mind is made up don't let anything change it," "Anything that can go wrong, will"—these are examples of rigid, pessimistic, self-degrading, unduly harsh attitudes that detract from longevity and life quality. They have been linked to heart disease, depression, suicide, interpersonal problems, difficulty holding down a job, resistance to medical advice, and more.

Optimism, characterized as expecting positive outcomes from life circumstances, has the opposite effect. So do flexibility and self-efficacy—the belief that you have what it takes to accomplish what you set out to do. Thinking "I can" or "This will work out" helps you reach your goals. Then success motivates you to reach higher. What's more, when you believe in yourself and like who you are, you want to take care of yourself and are more likely to take actions that positively influence your physical health.

The mind sphere's final component—*cognitive health*—pertains to your brain's capacity to learn, calculate, remember, concentrate, solve problems, evaluate, think, and so on. Debits and credits in this area are determined by what you do or don't do to keep your mind sharp, your memory clear, and your cognitive abilities continually challenged.

Unlike our bodies, which eventually collapse from exhaustion, our minds never stop, not even when we sleep. Mental chatter, worry, and insistence follow us everywhere. Our minds always seem to be under the influence of fluctuating emotions: stress, relief, comfort, fear, joy. But sometimes our minds seem to be speaking to us with special urgency—"Notice me, help me, care for me"—and our perceptions are not always our best friends. Depression, anger, panic attacks, and self-destructive activities can cheat us of a calm mental attitude. Sometimes our own emotions are a mystery to us because we are so out of touch with our bodies, our deeply held beliefs, even the very reasons we do certain things to ourselves. Can we balance the stressors outside our bodies and the pleas from within? Can we reach out to be heard in time to prevent a mild depression from changing into a major life-impairing symptom? How do we find the balance between schedules and pressures on the one hand and our internal search for peace of mind and happiness on the other?

I'm fairly confident that most of us would like to reach an equilibrium, to achieve a calmness that allows us to react spontaneously to life's ups and downs without being thrown by them. We want to go through each day with mental agility, not mental anxiety. As we age, one of the greatest fears is that our bodies will keep going but our minds will dead-end. Lifelong learning keeps our minds agile, stimulated, and ever ready for continuing challenges. Supple minds keep stretching. They are less prone to forgetfulness, depression, maybe even dementia.

Reach out for humor to balance life's inevitable realities. Nothing can combat a positive mental attitude. It offers respite from both our private mental battlefields and the large real-world ones.

Investigate yourself. Analyze your emotions—especially anger. Why rage over waiting in line at the airport? It doesn't change or nourish you. Would the line bother you this much if you had left your house early enough? Decide to leave earlier next time. That's a positive mental attitude, and you just learned something new! Practice this kind of positive problem solving whenever you feel stuck in a cycle of anxiety and minor depression. See it as a lifelong learning experience. Consider yourself a player, a student of life, regardless of your age.

When we have peace of mind our bodies are healthier. It's all connected.

MENTAL SPHERE LONGEVITY BUSTERS

❑ Low self-esteem (you tend to think that you are not smart, skilled, strong, or lucky enough to achieve your goals, and don't deserve to succeed)

❑ Boredom (nothing much excites you anymore)

❑ Frequent, easily triggered angry outbursts

❑ Difficulty expressing or at times even recognizing your feelings

❑ Stagnation (you lean toward passive pursuits such as television viewing and may not have done anything outside your ordinary routine for years)

❑ Hostility (you feel that we live in a dangerous, unpredictable world where most people can't be trusted, so you keep your guard up, ready for a fight)

❑ Untreated depression, anxiety, or other psychiatric disorders

MENTAL SPHERE LONGEVITY BOOSTERS

❑ Efficacy (believing that you have the skills, abilities, and stick-to-itiveness to achieve the goals you set for yourself)

❑ Curiosity and enthusiasm (constantly finding new things that interest you and learning what you can about them)

❑ Being assertive (expressing your feelings and asking for what you need in a clear, forthright manner, while ruffling as few feathers as possible)

❑ An urge to understand what makes people, including you, "tick"—and/or a desire not to repeat your past—possibly fulfilled through counseling, reading self-help books, or participating in a support group

❑ No symptoms of depression, anxiety, or other disorders—or relief from them via therapy, self-introspection, and/or prescribed medications

Although there is an enormous body of scientific evidence on our psychological well-being, we do know that people are incredibly bad at predicting how they will feel in the future. Most of us are not very aware of our day-to-day feelings, mostly because we haven't been keeping track of them. It's a problem to plan for the future if you don't know how the past has affected you—like plotting a retirement plan but having no clue about your earnings or expenses.

Most people spend their lives trying to avoid anxiety. You completely organize your life and your time toward this purpose rather than concentrating on working toward what will make you happy.

Happiness is what people say they want—but happiness and the absence of anxiety are not the same thing.

If we view anxiety as just part of a range of emotions, like a learning experience, it's helpful feedback. And if you can ask "What is this going to teach me?" instead of "How do I avoid this particular emotional state ever again?" that leads you to a whole series of considerations. Seeing anxiety as something that is always to be avoided cuts out a whole aspect of your life. It does more than it appears to do, because you have to eliminate all of those things in your life that you think will lead to those feelings. Some of those things may be (1) solving conflicts with people in your life, (2) taking risks when you don't know the outcome, (3) allowing yourself to get into situations that are unfamiliar, and (4) allowing yourself to quiet down and just *be* rather than *do*.

So you restrict further and further what you do, and how you live your life, and whom you see. And that makes you unhappy because you feel alone. Remember, it's all in order to avoid anxiety and depression. You think mostly about where *you* want to go and what *you* do and get very caught up in yourself. These restrictions make you feel that you are in control, and that, of course, is an illusion. (Who's ever in control of everything?)

How can you feel better about yourself and your world? How can you avoid destructive behaviors? How can you get help if you need to and move toward therapy or people or medications that bring you to a safer place in your mind? What can help you to see the big picture—all the ups and downs, the joys and the tears that are part of this life?

SPHERE #3: KINSHIP

Everyone you interact with has some effect on your longevity. The people in your life, other friends or family, can offer you stability. They can offer you support in times of stress or personal sadness. They can laugh with you and remind you to lighten up.

They can also:
- Berate every opinion you offer and make you feel small
- Never let up in telling you their opinions and their agendas
- Discourage you when you want to try something new
- Not do their equal share at home or at work

- Withhold their love to show they disapprove of or disagree with what you are doing
- Criticize you, undermining your confidence
- Talk you out of going white-water rafting or to a local gym
- Cause problems whenever they come to your house despite the welcoming environment you try to create
- Hurt you emotionally or physically
- Bombard you with negative, pessimistic points of view
- Resist resolving conflicts that might be long-standing

We all want to live well, live long, and live happily. We devour every study, every new finding, every hopeful anecdotal report that even remotely promises to net us a longer, healthier, happier life. And what many of us ultimately learn is that programs involving contact and sharing with other people inevitably produce more positive results than efforts where we try to persevere alone. Time and again it is the interaction with others that changes the way things turn out. Think of all the transitions in our lives—childhood, adolescence, adulthood, and elderhood. The significant turning points, the most clearly focused memories, and the strongest pull are attached to the people who were a part of them.

Some of us need to look more broadly at our social community while others may be more in need of examining strengths and deficits in our personal networks, which include our immediate and extended families, our friends, our marriage and lifelong partners, our colleagues at work—all our fellow travelers on this wonderful journey.

Social networks provide an intangible path to longevity and good health. Take the drama of needing exercise. First scene: You want to exercise, but your spouse says you all need more family time. Second scene: The kids want to eat and go to the neighborhood pool. Third scene: You pack a gigantic picnic lunch full of improbable leftovers, then take a walk or bike ride to the pool. Final scene: Have a delicious, silly lunch before you all go swimming. By combining social and physical sphere activities, you not only spend time with the family and get some exercise but also enjoy the sense of accomplishment that comes with getting two for the price of one.

The sense of well-being that comes from doing something with a *friend* or *family* helps relieve the perception that all you do is work. Times together don't have to be long. They can be between schedules of different people. As long as you want to be with each other, whatever you decide to do will be okay. Often, spending time with family and friends gives you time to talk things over in a more casual way. And don't forget that it's just as important to carve out some time to be alone so that your next social encounter is all the more meaningful.

The kinship sphere, which addresses *social wellness,* encompasses any connection shared by two or more people, one of them being you. Friendships, marriages, intimate partnerships, workplace relationships, business networks, mutual support groups, twelve-step programs, and family ties in their many permutations all reside within the kinship sphere. The stronger and more varied those relationships, the longer and more satisfying our lives.

Why? Because bonds with children, parents, friends, and other people improve our outlook and build self-confidence. Those bonds often motivate us to take good physical care of ourselves as well. We want to enjoy our loved ones' company for as long as possible and not be a burden to them by becoming ill. Social support—from individuals or groups, professionals or peers—also serves as a buffer, helping us get through stressful times. Those of us who have it are less prone to heart disease and have a lower overall mortality rate.

Figures from the Human Population Lab show that folks with few or feeble relationships double their risk of dying young. And in the famous Framingham Heart Study, homemakers who reported being bored and lonely were twice as likely to have heart attacks.

When it comes to warding off disease and premature death, involvement in a loving, mutually gratifying, committed marriage or its equivalent appears to be extremely beneficial. Across the board, married people live longer than single, divorced, or widowed folks. The saving grace lies not in the legally binding contract but in the emotional bonds, trust, and interdependence that these couples develop.

Quality outweighs quantity where kinship is concerned. We can thrive with just a few friends and relatives who listen, accept us as we are, offer emotional support or material resources as needed, and provide company we enjoy. Conversely, we can be starving for human understanding and closeness while our Rolodex is overflowing with

---

KINSHIP SPHERE LONGEVITY BUSTERS

❏ Domestic violence

❏ Lots of angry, argumentative, verbally abusive, or humiliating interactions (the more frequent and severe, the more damage)

❏ Transiency (frequent moves challenge close relationships)

❏ Reclusiveness (very little contact with other people or tolerance for them)

❏ Loss of a loved one through death, divorce, or other life transitions

❏ Overcontrol (expecting people to think and behave in a certain way; doing anything you can to make them conform to your expectations)

❏ Super people-pleasing (seeking acceptance or approval even when it means sacrificing your happiness or compromising your values)

❏ Extreme shyness or social anxieties that make interactions sheer torture and keep you from getting close to people

KINSHIP SPHERE LONGEVITY BOOSTERS

❏ A mutually supportive, intimate, long-term, committed relationship with a legal spouse or other life partner

❏ Emotional support from people who will listen without judging you and offer advice, sympathy, or a pep talk, depending on your needs

❏ Tangible support if you need it

❏ The sense of belonging; being part of a group, community, or family

❏ Exposure to people from different races, walks of life, and points of view

❏ Activities that foster cooperation, friendship, fun, and new friends

❏ The ability to accept people more or less as they are, even if you don't fully understand or agree with their behavior or opinions

❏ Being flexible

---

business contacts, drinking buddies, besotted admirers, and dysfunctional family members.

Since many of us live far away from our blood relatives, our close friends often become our unrelated relatives and function in our lives as the traditional extended family once did. We don't have to see or talk to our "kin" often. A sense that people who matter to us will be available when we need them is more life-enhancing than mere frequency of contact. Then again, it's wonderful to spend lots of time with people whom we like, people who can make us laugh and think and get off our duffs to pursue our dreams.

Of course, some of those same people drive us crazy, pressuring us until we're ready to scream, manipulating us into doing things we'd rather not, and raising the tension level in our already tense lives. I'm sure I don't have to tell you that not all relationships are good for you. Just ask a battered wife or the child of an abusive, alcoholic father. Those of us sandwiched between the demands of our growing children, work relations, and the needs of our aging parents might also have a thing or two to say about the healing powers of ties to other people. Sometimes stress is all we seem to be getting for our efforts.

SPHERE #4: SPIRITUAL

Whenever you hear the word *spiritual,* do you:
- Feel this is missing in your life?
- Think that you want nothing to do with this?
- Wonder if the term means more than *religious*?
- Think about your family traditions?
- Think about death?
- Consider volunteering as a spiritual act?
- Associate things spiritual with nature?
- Wonder how you could meet other people with similar interests?
- Think about a living will?

Physicians rarely talk about religion—it's a topic that's almost taboo and seems out of place unless the patient is dying. Yet there is adequate scientific evidence to show that a spiritual or religious path not only gives solace to those who practice it, but also adds to longevity.

Research has consistently shown that people who attend church regularly appear to live longer. And that's not simply due to the social contact. A spiritual path helps many people cope with depression, reduce anger, and relieve stress; a calm attitude helps when life's problems appear. What in fact is hope, if not the belief that the negative circumstances will someday change to positive ones? The mental and the physical spheres join with the spiritual sphere as we take responsibility for effecting those changes by our own actions. Our *beliefs* influence the lifestyle we choose, our attitudes toward illness, and how we cope with individual or family health problems.

What moves you? What inspires you, touches you straight through to your soul? An operatic aria performed in an acoustically perfect concert hall? The prayer service at your place of worship? Staring up at a sky full of stars on a crystal-clear evening? Watching the sun come up over the ocean? Immersing yourself in a museum exhibit of Egyptian artifacts? Sitting in the lotus position, eyes shut, mind uncluttered, chanting? These kinds of experiences can fill us with awe, wonder, peace, or clarity. They can elevate us to a different plane of awareness. They are the essence of the spiritual sphere.

Some of us associate these extraordinarily vibrant moments with an entity above and beyond our own self-interest—a higher power gently

---

SPIRITUAL SPHERE LONGEVITY BUSTERS

- ❑ Denying the existence or value of anything that you cannot perceive or measure with your five senses
- ❑ Very few or no "still and quiet" moments to meditate, contemplate, or simply shut off the worries of the day
- ❑ Rarely stopping to appreciate and/or get a feel for nature (walks in the woods, puttering in a garden, sleeping under the stars, rafting the Grand Canyon holds no interest for you)
- ❑ Believing that there is no rhyme, reason, or deeper meaning to anything that occurs in this life; that it's all random

SPIRITUAL SPHERE LONGEVITY BOOSTERS

- ❑ Believing in a unifying force or "higher power"—whether the traditional all-knowing deity, your own higher self, or another form
- ❑ Belonging to a group with a spiritual purpose
- ❑ An appreciation of art, music, and nature
- ❑ Practicing meditation, yoga, tai chi, or any other spiritually based discipline
- ❑ Recognizing that there is indeed a rhyme, reason, and deeper meaning to life, and that you can actively seek to understand it or sometimes simply allow it to unfold
- ❑ Helping someone in need

guiding us, a God somewhere watching over us. Others connect our at-one-with-the-universe-type experiences with the highest part of ourselves—the concept of a god within each of us. Still others wouldn't dream of linking their peak moments with anything that could even remotely be construed as religious. For a variety of reasons, they reject the notion of a divine being or the possibility that faith might play as meaningful a role in life as science or logic.

Because of the many different, often strongly held beliefs and emotions triggered by anything that moves our souls, the spirit sphere is the most difficult to describe and quantify. It includes anything we do to contemplate the higher meaning and purpose of our lives: meditation, prayer, attending religious services, reading or listening to inspirational material, chanting, sitting quietly in a garden, floating down a river on an inner tube, painting a landscape, or appreciating a painting. And yes, all of this is connected to life expectancy and life quality.

Duke University researchers found that people who attended religious services at least once a week have healthier immune systems. In the Human Population Lab study, the annual death rate of those who shied away from religion was 36 percent higher than that of those who embraced it. The fact that churchgoers develop a support network accounts for part of the benefit. The physical effects of deep muscle relaxation, focused breathing, repeating a mantra, and other accoutrements of meditation may also play a part.

Serenity, a positive outlook, and generally lower stress levels are the hallmarks of a thriving spiritual sphere. Without one, we tend to be pessimistic and cynical. We wonder whether anything in life has meaning or is worth doing, including actively pursuing longevity and the best life has to offer. Something undefinable may be missing from your life.

SPHERE #5: MATERIAL

At the primal level, we suffer if we don't have a job—or an occupation—that pays us enough in money and benefits. The number-one stressor for new couples is, inevitably, money. But a plethora of other material levels also affect us. Are we satisfied with our jobs? Do we like our co-workers? Is our commute onerous? Is our occupation safe? Is time off for vacation adequate? And the biggie: Are we engaged in meaningful work?

The material sphere is where you find all your "stuff"—all the things outside yourself that can affect how you feel about yourself and your future. This sphere includes your job, your house, your bank account, your credit card debt, the brand-new thirty-thousand-dollar sport utility vehicle you just had to have, or the three-thousand-dollar secondhand compact that you settled for after learning that your daughter needed braces on her teeth.

As with the mind and body spheres, this one includes several components. First up is work, both the paid variety and voluntary activities that allow you to feel productive and part of a team, company, or community effort. Both have the potential to enhance or undermine the quality of your life. They can supply you with either a sense of mastery or of utter frustration. Good work allows you to:

- use your skills and obtain recognition (including a commensurate paycheck) for your contributions
- interact amicably with colleagues and superiors, and cooperate to get jobs done
- gain confidence in your ability to accomplish goals and overcome obstacles

Clearly, every job does not enhance our lives. On the contrary, they may prove to be major sources of stress. Some are so demeaning that our confidence and sense of self-worth suffer; others are so dangerous that our lives are actually on the line; and far too many are so demanding that we have no time or energy available for anything else, including taking care of our health. During our productive years, we often spend as much time with coworkers as with family, and conflicts can arise with the mental and kinship spheres if you find that you are happier at work than at home. If, on the other hand, the work environment is toxic, then we suffer. Obviously, the material sphere touches the social and mental spheres. By sidestepping social contact with colleagues, we skirt a realm of potential support. And the mental anguish of a noxious work environment usually takes its toll in depression and anxiety.

But the material sphere also affects the physical sphere. If you lack health benefits and you become sick, the quality of your life and your longevity suffer. As we look at the financial section of your longevity plan, we'll see that how much you earn can affect how long you'll live, at least for some of us. Where money's concerned, the biggest question always seems to be, "Do you have enough?" Enough to meet your immediate needs, enough saved for retirement, your children's educations, with enough available for emergencies, vacations, and other luxuries? Having a huge home, several cars, memberships at exclusive country clubs, diamonds, personal computers, or season tickets to the opera will not, in and of themselves, make your life better or longer-lasting. However, if *not* having those things causes you to feel ashamed, creates conflict between you and your spouse, or instigates jealousy that damages other relationships, then the ripple effect of lacking what you feel you're entitled to will take its toll. Indeed, simply *sensing* insufficiency can lower life expectancy. In one study, working women who felt that their financial status was worse than other women's (whether or not it actually was) were nearly twice as likely to have heart attacks and die from them than women who believed their financial status was the same as most of their peers'.

Health and life expectancy really suffer when insufficiency is not just a perception but a verifiable fact. It's tough to be health-conscious when debt collectors are hounding us. It's difficult to get the rest, exercise, nutrition, or emotional support we need when we're worried "sick" about keeping a roof over our heads. That's why financial matters need to be included in any personal longevity profile. If they're way out of line, it can be impossible to get the other areas of our lives in order. On the other hand, if we place too much emphasis on them, we may postpone a lot of things we already could be doing for ourselves.

That was certainly the case for Ralph. Prior to his motorcycle trip, nearly every waking moment of his life revolved around work and money, money and work. He was more diligent about saving for the future than anyone I'd ever known. His pension plan was fully funded. His IRAs, which he added to annually, had been compounding interest for decades. And his other investments—all solid growth funds—were growing. He saved and saved and saved, all the while ignoring requests from charities that he easily could have helped and postponing personal purchases until after he retired (some time in the distant future).

The final component of the material sphere is your surroundings, including your home, neighborhood, workplace, and the part of the country you live in. How safe are they? How visually pleasing? How is

MATERIAL SPHERE LONGEVITY BUSTERS

❑ Lots of job stress—from real demands that need to be met within tight time frames as well as from perceived gaps between what you're being asked to do and what you think you're capable of doing (the less confidence you have in your ability to cope, the more stress you feel)

❑ Being a workaholic (this condition, which looks like ambition and extra-hard work, is actually an affliction with recognizable symptoms: working more hours but getting less done, constantly thinking about work, and neglecting other spheres)

❑ Boredom/disconnection (feeling like a cog in a machine with no real impact on what the machine is doing)

❑ A hazardous line of work, such as taxicab driving in a big city, law enforcement, firefighting, washing windows on skyscrapers, demolition, or toxic-waste removal

❑ Too little or no time off for relaxation or vacations

❑ Lots of debt

❑ Lots of debt when you're barely earning enough to keep up with minimum monthly payments

❑ Saving little or no money for retirement

❑ Feeling like a "have-not" in a world of "haves"

❑ Living in a high-crime area

❑ Breathing polluted air, drinking poorly filtered water, working in a poorly ventilated building, or being exposed to other environmental threats

MATERIAL SPHERE LONGEVITY BOOSTERS

❑ A job that challenges you but doesn't demand more than you're willing or able to give

❑ Work that maintains your interest and/or feels meaningful

❑ Volunteer activities that allow you to feel useful, productive, and as if you are contributing something of value

❑ Taking at least an hour a day to replenish yourself with relaxation exercises, naps, walks, soothing or energizing music, or anything that relaxes you (your hour-plus can be broken up into 10- or 15-minute time-outs)

❑ Having time off from work to do things that are completely unrelated to your job

❑ Keeping your debts and spending under control as well as money worries to a minimum
❑ A solid financial plan for your future
❑ An aesthetically pleasing, physically comfortable living space
❑ A safe home with working smoke and carbon monoxide detectors in a neighborhood with a relatively low crime rate and no major toxins nearby

the air and water quality, the noise level, the potential for natural disasters? Do you have access to lakes, forests, mountains, or beaches? Your personal environment has an impact on physical health as well as on emotional and spiritual well-being. Pollution, violent crime, toxic waste, and other factors obviously shorten your life span. Fresh air, the beauty of nature, a sense of safety, the serenity of sitting quietly as waves whoosh against the shore or birds warble overhead . . . these are things that make a life worth loving.

How can we invest in the material sphere? By taking time to invest in ourselves. Plan well in advance, and make decisions about little things with the bigger picture in mind. One of the most blatant differences between lower-income and well-to-do families is how far along life's timeline they plan for the future. The lowest-income families plan for the end of the week; the well-to-do plan, on average, five years in the future. Often those of us who feel financially trapped put off making decisions. But that's a decision. Investing in the material sphere means making an action plan.

Cracking *Your* Longevity Code

In this book's first chapter, I promised you the opportunity to uncover the vital elements of your own longevity code. I said you would get a chance to identify the personal assets and deficits, habits and inheritances, attitudes and life circumstances that make you who you are today as well as determine your best route to a longer, sweeter life. Well, here's that opportunity: the first of several sections geared toward making general ideas and suggestions more individually applicable and personally useful to you. Workbook-type exercises such as what you'll find below also appear at the end of each of the next three chapters.

You can make a project out of these sections, working through each pencil-and-paper exercise completely and pulling together your results on the Longevity Code Summary (see pp. 115–16) to consult when you start selecting appropriate action steps. Or you can approach these sections more casually, simply reading over the exercises and making mental notes for future reference. The important thing is to gain enough insight into your personal makeup to create a comfortably fitting, highly effective longevity prescription for yourself.

EXERCISE 1–Your Physical, Mental, Kinship, Spiritual, and Material Debits and Credits
The five spheres of wellness provide a convenient structure for analyzing the personal habits and attitudes that can work for or against your longer, sweeter life. Below, you will find a series of continuums: linear scales with the -10 at one end representing circumstances that do the greatest possible damage to your life expectancy, and the +10 at the other end denoting circumstances that enhance life expectancy the most; the 0 in the middle stands for no movement in either direction. As a guide, I have given an example of each extreme, although none for the zero—just think of zero as a neutral zone where you are neither harming nor helping your chances to live longer.

To assess your current strengths and deficits as well as set some tentative goals for the future, mark your spot on each continuum as follows.

X = where you think you are today.
1 = where you would like to be one year from now.
5 = where you want to be in five years.

YOUR PHYSICAL SPHERE

Physical Health
-10 _____ 0 _____ +10
-10 = Extremely poor health; severe disability
+10 = Healthy and vital with a sense of well-being

Physical fitness

−10 _____ 0 _____ +10

−10 = Completely sedentary; winded on short walks; very low energy

+10 = Peak physical condition for your age (not necessarily for an elite athlete); engaged in a balanced exercise program that includes aerobics, strength training, balance, and flexibility

Nutrition

−10 _____ 0 _____ +10

−10 = Extremely poor nutrition and eating habits; obese or emaciated; not getting the right nutrients

+10 = Following the food pyramid nearly all the time; a low-fat, fiber- and nutrient-rich diet maintaining healthy weight and taking appropriate supplements

Self-Care

−10 _____ 0 _____ +10

−10 = Engaging in numerous unhealthy habits; never making an effort to avoid health hazards; neglecting to obtain regular medical care and screenings

+10 = Never had or has long since abandoned unhealthy habits; always makes an effort to avoid health hazards; gets regular checkups and screenings

YOUR MENTAL SPHERE

Psychological Health

−10 _____ 0 _____ +10

−10 = Extremely poor; major depression, anxiety, or stress; not receiving treatment or it's simply not working; a feeling of hopelessness

+10 = A feeling of well-being; comfortable with what life has given

Emotional Health

−10 _____ 0 _____ +10

−10 = Hostile, angry, overreactor or flat, emotionally numb nonreactor

+10 = Full range of emotions expressed when and as intensely as circumstances call for but never losing temper or out of control

Attitudes

−10 _____ 0 _____ +10

−10 = Rigid, pessimistic, self-degrading

+10 = Flexible, optimistic, positive self-regard

Cognitive Health

−10 _____ 0 _____ +10

−10 = Doing nothing to stay sharp or improve thinking skills

+10 = Actively learning new things and stretching mentally *all the time*

YOUR KINSHIP SPHERE

Marriage (or Other Long-Term, Committed, Intimate Relationship)

−10 _____ 0 _____ +10

−10 = Isolated from or constantly fighting with spouse/partner; at the breaking point

+10 = A loving marriage; a strong relationship

Immediate Family

−10 _____ 0 _____ +10

−10 = They're dysfunctional; simply can't relate to them; upset whenever they're seen

+10 = Have a great time together and support one another in time of need

Social Network

−10 _____ 0 _____ +10

−10 = Don't have any *real* friends to share joys and sorrows; no one to turn to for help or support

+10 = Have great friends, including some very close ones

Community Ties

−10 _____ 0 _____ +10

−10 = No community involvement, don't know next-door neighbor's name

+10 = Active participant; volunteer, attend events, and know quite a few people

YOUR SPIRITUAL SPHERE

Spiritual Path

−10 _____ 0 _____ +10

−10 = Nothing spiritual or religious; it's all hokum

+10 = Spirituality and/or religion are an integral part of life; engage in some sort of spiritual practice or act of loving kindness nearly every day

Spiritual Community

−10 _____ 0 _____ +10

−10 = Never found anyone who thinks similarly about religious or spiritual things

+10 = In a spiritual community or attend church, synagogue, or other place of worship regularly

Nature

−10 _____ 0 _____ +10

−10 = Never outside and really don't like it

+10 = Always feel uplifted and make time for Mother Nature

YOUR MATERIAL SPHERE

Work

−10 _____ 0 _____ +10

−10 = No job or an extremely demanding, demeaning, or dangerous job

+10 = A job or avocation that is meaningful, satisfying, rewarding, and enjoyable

Financial Life

−10 _____ 0 _____ +10

−10 = Have less money than wanted or needed; a source of anxiety and conflict

+10 = Enough for everything needed and much of what's wanted; all financial ducks in a row, including retirement funds

Surroundings

−10 _____ 0 _____ +10

−10 = Living and/or working in a hazardous, high-crime, highly polluted, depressing environment

+10 = Visually pleasing, safe, clean surroundings; access to nature

Now, based on any insights that came to you while working on these
continuums, fill in the following chart.

SPHERE	STRONG POINTS	WEAK SPOTS
PHYSICAL		
MENTAL		
KINSHIP		
SPIRITUAL		
MATERIAL		

3

Life's Givens:

Playing the Hand You're Dealt

WHEN IT COMES TO LONGEVITY, all people are *not* created equal. Some of us are handed the best of circumstances at birth. We are born into well-educated, well-to-do families with marvelous gene pools and impeccable health histories. We have parents who not only give us all the nurturing we need but also serve as terrific models in all five spheres of wellness. If we follow their leads, we are halfway to a longer, sweeter life before it even occurs to us to seek one.

Not so for those of us who are born poor or sickly to parents whose personal problems prevent them from taking the best care of us or whose genes predispose us to life-shortening conditions such as heart disease or high blood pressure. We have no say in the prenatal care we receive, the socioeconomic status of our families, or the toxic substances we're exposed to in our childhood homes. But those items show up in our longevity code nonetheless, creating physical, emotional, social, spiritual, or material deficits that we will have to overcome in order to live fully far into the future.

Then there are those of us who started out in pretty good shape but did a bit of damage to our minds and bodies over the years. We took up smoking or were less than prudent about what we did with whom. We became drug users or inveterate sun worshipers. Even if we no longer engage in these longevity-busting behaviors, their impact persists, usually in the form of an increased risk of developing certain diseases.

The longevity boosters and busters dealt to us by circumstances beyond our control, and those we're responsible for but can't go back in time to undo, I call "life's givens." They come with the territory of who we are. They are woven into the fabric of our being, and no personal longevity profile could be complete without them. These factors don't just add to the debits and credits in our longevity codes. They also provide crucial information for us to consider when we're deciding which controllable boosters and busters to tackle first and which lifestyle changes to give priority to.

Forewarned is forearmed, the saying goes. And the givens in our lives often serve as red flags. They point out potential threats to our longevity and happiness. They also show us where our previously hidden strengths lie, so that we can use them to our advantage.

Givens Are Guideposts—Not Guarantees

Matt Devereaux, a forty-nine-year-old math teacher, and his thirty-four-year-old wife, Elaine, both adore their only child, Darren, who is eight. But they are worlds apart on the subject of having more children. Elaine desperately wants to expand their family—and the sooner the better. "Neither of us is getting any younger," she says.

Matt knows this. In fact, it's the basis for *his* argument against bringing another son or a daughter into the world. "Don't get me wrong," he says. "It's not that I'm too old to be changing diapers, or too set in my ways to adjust to an infant's schedule, or even too close to retirement to be sinking money into diaper services and preschool tuition. I've loved every minute of raising Darren, and I swear, I would raise a whole houseful of kids—if I thought I'd live long enough to see them grow up." Unfortunately, Matt pegs his personal life expectancy at "another ten years, fifteen tops."

Why such a pessimistic projection? "Family history," Matt explains. "My dad dropped dead from a heart attack at fifty-seven." His mother, despite living quite a bit longer, also succumbed to a heart-related problem. When she expired during bypass surgery several years ago, Matt assumed his fate was sealed. Sure that the genetic deck was stacked against him, dooming him to die prematurely, Matt couldn't justify having more children "just to leave them behind."

It's tough to argue with that logic. But I will, because I'm far from convinced that an early death from heart disease is Matt's destiny. For one thing, his dad had been a heavy smoker and a problem drinker with dangerously high blood pressure—which probably had as much, if not more, to do with his midlife heart attack than his genes did. Likewise, the rampant atherosclerosis in his mother's coronary arteries was probably a by-product of her lifelong aversion to exercise and love of deep-fried food. Even if genetics had played a role, it hadn't hampered her longevity: Mrs. Devereaux died at eighty-two, having remained alert and active until the day she went into the hospital.

Matt also has more healthy habits than his parents did at his age. He is an avid bike rider and hiker who works out with weights twice weekly, maintains a reasonably low-fat/high-fiber diet, and has not smoked in over twenty years. He probably has nearly as many years of active living left as any other illness-free forty-nine-year-old— and that's surely long enough to see any new offspring through puberty, adolescence, and young adulthood, at least. Of course, Matt could take additional steps to reduce his heart disease risk, such as taking an aspirin a day, making sure there's enough folic acid in his diet, and having his blood pressure and cholesterol checked regularly. (I would not recommend a daily glass of wine because his Dad had a drinking problem.)

Looking at the matter from the perspective of Matt's mind and kinship spheres, having at least one more child might actually add years to his life. A child's energy and enthusiasm, curiosity and innocence can rub off on parents, keeping them young at heart and convincing them to take the best possible care of themselves—for their kids' sake. What's more, by agreeing to expand his family—which he actually wanted to do all along—Matt would remove a long-standing source of conflict from his marriage, bringing him closer to his wife, with all the life-extending benefits that would bring.

Now don't get me wrong. I am not recommending procreation as a method for prolonging and invigorating our lives. But I do believe that in Matt's case, choosing not to have more children based solely on what he thought was an inherited predisposition to die prematurely would have been a mistake. His case illustrates a point I hope you'll keep in mind while reading the rest of this chapter: *Taken alone, very few givens actually predict premature death, and none dictates precisely the amount of satisfaction we'll get out of life.* They are guideposts that tip us off to actions we can take to extend and enhance our lives, not guarantees for an early demise—or excuses not to adopt longevity-boosting measures.

What's Shaking in Your Family Tree?

Centenarians are rarely the only long-lived members of their families. Their siblings or first cousins often match them year for year, and their parents or grandparents may have survived into their nineties (a truly extraordinary feat considering the fact that average life expectancy at the time of their births was well under fifty). Remember Jeanne Calumet, the Frenchwoman whose documented 122-year life span is the longest to date? Sociologists found at least three generations of relatives whose lives were exceptionally long compared to selected controls born on the same day in the same part of the world.

Longevity, it seems, was in their genes—not the exact number of years they would live, of course, but rather the propensity to live longer than most. But not genes exclusively. The best data currently available pegs as genetic no more than 50 percent (and perhaps as few as 30 percent) of the factors that influence how long and how well we'll live. The remainder are by-products of our environment or personal lifestyles—and, unlike our genetic makeup, amenable to change.

The famed Framingham Heart Study, now in its fifty-third year and still putting out remarkable findings, identifies heredity as one of the five factors in women most closely associated with surviving from age fifty to age seventy-five or beyond. Once you've made it to midlife, the study reveals, if your parents lived to be seventy-five or older, chances are that you will, too.

Like a minute bit of microfilm, genes are tiny bits of biological information that's passed from generation to generation when sperm and egg unite. Code contributed by your mother may give you her brown eyes or her pear-shaped body type. Data you inherit from your dad may help you become as good a musician as he. Some of the genetic material we get from our parents makes us more vulnerable to heart disease, high blood pressure, diabetes, depression, breast and colon cancers, Alzheimer's disease, or other conditions.

Someday science may have enough information about human genetics to alter troublesome traits, do away with debilitating diseases, or extend our life spans by decades. Right now we can simply recognize, respect, and try to sidestep the longevity-busting traits and tendencies that run in our families—even if we don't know precisely how they got from one generation to the next. But that's a lot. Having a sense of the potential strengths and weaknesses that might have been passed along to you—by example or via DNA—allows you to take a more focused, proactive approach to lengthening your life expectancy.

Let's say that, like Matt, you've had several family members die from heart disease, including a few who were killed by heart attacks when they were young, in their late forties or fifties. That's not irrefutable proof that you'll make a trip to the coronary care unit before you see sixty. It is a red flag, however, a warning that heart trouble *could* lie ahead. And whether it stems from shared genes or common habits, it's a pattern worth paying attention to.

Armed with the knowledge that a propensity for heart disease is one of your life's givens, you can go on to educate yourself about the condition. You can identify the controllable traits or habits that increase your odds of developing it. Then you can choose to change in those areas, filling one part of your personal longevity prescription. The same goes for alcoholism or depression or kidney problems or any other life-limiting conditions. If they appear on your family tree repeatedly, you'll want to minimize or compensate for their impact by devoting some of your longevity-boosting efforts to reducing your risks in those areas.

It's in the Genes

Did you inherit Mom's diabetes or Dad's depression, Grandpa Jim's allergies or Aunt Louise's psoriasis? You don't have to go a genetics lab to figure how your family history influences your potential to live a longer, sweeter life. Just look around at your family members. Pay particular attention to your parents, siblings, and grandparents as well as your parents' siblings and their offspring. What traits do they share? Have any diseases struck repeatedly among you? What other patterns do you see? If any of these close relatives are dead, what did they die of and at what age?

Family histories of heart disease, stroke, cancer, alcoholism, depression/suicide, eating disorders, diabetes, high blood pressure, immune system disorders, and other physical health challenges count as debits in your longevity code. Give yourself credits for the presence of particularly long-lived individuals on your family tree.

EXERCISE 2–Genealogical Chart

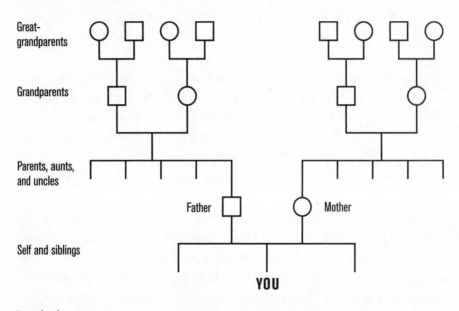

Symbols:
circle = female
square = male
b. = year of birth
d. = age at death (if applicable)
slash through symbol = deceased

Suggested annotations: HD for heart disease; HBP for high blood pressure; C for cancer (specify type); D for diabetes; Dep for depression. You can also indicate habits such as smoking, excessive drinking, and so on.

With a little digging, you can paint a more detailed family portrait.

First, draw up a four-tiered chart like the one on page 58. The top tier will represent your great-grandparents' generation. The second tier should cover your grandparents and their siblings; the third your par-

---

EXERCISE 3–Check All That Apply to You

LONGEVITY DEBITS

❑ Parents who used tobacco and exposed you to secondhand smoke

❑ Childhood illnesses with lingering effects such as asthma, scarlet fever, or polio

❑ Mother had little or no prenatal care

❑ Mother drank during pregnancy

❑ Parents divorced

❑ One or both parents physically, verbally, or sexually abused you

❑ A home life that was unpredictable, inconsistent, or marked by violence

❑ Little nurturing or intellectual stimulation

❑ Inadequate nutrition

❑ Failure to get immunized or receive regular medical care

LONGEVITY CREDITS

❑ Lots of love, nurturing, and opportunities to learn and grow

❑ Parents who modeled positive habits, including healthy eating, regular exercise, dental hygiene, and so on

❑ Few bouts with disease other than the usual childhood ills

❑ Mother had adequate prenatal care

❑ Mother did not drink or smoke during her pregnancy

❑ Growing up in a two-parent family

❑ Parents who provided fair, consistent, nonabusive discipline; taught ethical behavior and values

❑ Family members who treated each other with respect and communicated with openness, so you usually knew what to expect from them

❑ Adequate nutrition

❑ Models of positive "people habits," such as giving, compassion, and social responsibility

ents, aunts, and uncles; and the fourth you, your siblings, and your cousins.

Then fill in as much information as you can find. Possibilities include:

- Each deceased relative's approximate age at and cause of death.
- The incidence and age of onset of any cardiovascular disease (heart attack or stroke).
- The incidence of cancers, and which ones.
- The presence of life-shortening habits such as smoking, excessive drinking, inactivity, domestic violence, and so on. Many of these habits are passed from generation to generation by example, if not genetics.
- The presence of depression or other mental illness.
- Strengths—from lean, athletic body types to a family tradition of prayer and celebration or community service—should be noted, too.

More Givens

Other givens—your health at birth; your gender and age; the highest level of education you attained; and your personal history, including such longevity-busting behaviors such as drug use, indiscriminate and unprotected sex, or alcoholism—also influence your chances for a long, sweet life. Knowing about these givens helps us decide where to concentrate some of our energy.

THE LEGACY OF OUR EARLY YEARS

LIFE EXPECTANCY BY AGE, SEX, AND RACE

Age	ALL RACES		WHITE		BLACK	
	Male	Female	Male	Female	Male	Female
0	73.1	79.1	73.9	79.7	66.1	74.2
45	31.5	36.1	31.9	36.4	27.1	32.8
65	15.7	19	15.8	19.1	13.9	17.2
80	7.3	8.9	7.3	8.9	7	8.5

The information encoded in your genes is not the only longevity-influencing factor that can be counted among life's givens. You did not choose or control your health at birth, for example, or the specifics of your early childhood, but both make an enormous difference in the length and quality of your life.

Robust, full-term babies have higher survival rates than most premature or sickly infants. Almost any baby born to a mother who took good care of herself during pregnancy will fare better than the newborn of a malnourished or addicted mom. The care you receive once you're out of the womb is also critical.

A tremendous amount of crucial activity takes place during your early years. Because you're growing every minute, you must get adequate nutrition. You need proper medical care and immunizations to ward off preventable diseases. You need lots of love and stimulation. There are social and psychological tasks to accomplish as well. Childhood is when we develop our health habits, learn how to cope with frustration or other emotions, and discover how to get along with others. Spending your early years in a safe, stable environment with caregivers who are nurturing, warm, and kind will favorably influence your mental and physical health when you're older.

One of the biggest setbacks we can encounter as children is to have our parents get divorced. According to one study, men whose parents were divorced as children were more likely to die prematurely. As adults they were often more socially isolated and less satisfied with their lives. On the other hand, children raised in a household rife with tension and conflict do better when that conflict is removed. In such cases divorce is most certainly better.

Although an early, solid foundation improves the odds of living an extra-long life, a shaky one does not eliminate that outcome. It simply leaves you, as an adult, with some gaps that may need filling and some ineffective behaviors to replace.

GENDER

Throughout the world, women outlive men. In some countries, there's a gap of as much as ten years. Whether the discrepancy is driven by genetic differences or social conditioning, no one can say with certainty. But we do know that girls seem to have an edge from the start. They survive life in their mother's womb, the birth process, and infancy at greater rates than boy babies. Then they maintain their lead through adolescence and young adulthood, mainly because they don't engage in quite as much outrageous risk-taking behavior as their male counterparts, who tend to suffer from a temporary loss of sensibility sometimes jokingly referred to as "testosterone dementia."

The death-defying feats and occasionally unbelievably dumb moves teenage boys are known for appear to be fueled by copious amounts of the male hormone testosterone. Unfortunately, by the time their hormones stop raging out of control, making life-limiting choices will have become a habit for many men. Males between the ages of thirty-five and fifty-four are less physically active than women, as well as bigger meat and fat eaters. They are less likely to wear seat belts and more likely to drive drunk, less prone to using sunscreen and more prone to develop deadly skin cancers. And they are three times as likely to be alcoholics.

Women do not get off scot-free, however. It appears that their well-fought war for gender equality has proven a bit too successful in the health and longevity department. They have picked up deadly "male" habits such as smoking and heavy drinking and are feeling the impact of job stress on top of the stress of their other roles. As a result, the gap between male and female death rates at midlife has begun to narrow. Women suffer more autoimmune diseases such as multiple sclerosis, lupus, and rheumatoid arthritis. They're also more vulnerable to clinical depression, fibromyalgia, and chronic fatigue syndrome. And when women have heart attacks, they tend to be more severe.

OTHER INFLUENCES ON LONGEVITY AND LIFE QUALITY

- *Race.* In the United States, nonwhites can be expected to live an average of five fewer years than whites. Differences in susceptibility to life-shortening conditions bear much of the blame. African-Americans, for example, are more likely to become infected with HIV and tuberculosis. They are more likely to have hypertension, strokes, and prostate cancer. Diabetes appears at higher rates in Native Americans and Hispanics, while white women have the highest breast cancer rates and are more likely to suffer hip fractures.

  Are these heightened vulnerabilities hereditary? Probably in part, but environment plays a role as well. Racial minorities are disproportionately poor and undereducated, and according to the National Center for Health Statistics, the poor and undereducated die younger and suffer more health problems than people with better bank balances and several years of college. Education alone, or rather a lack of it, creates a glaring gap. High school dropouts die ten to fifteen years earlier than people with two or more years of college.

- *Social class.* Class encompasses education, income, occupation (blue-collar jobs, white-collar jobs, unskilled laborers, CEOs), and other signs of relative status. Let's start with poverty, which definitely puts a damper on life expectancy. Although there have certainly been centenarians who were born poor and lived out their lives under deplorable, deprived conditions, they tend to be the exception. It is simply harder to live a long, long time when you're plagued with money worries. When you're living at the lower end of the socio-economic scale, you're more likely to develop heart disease, diabetes, high blood pressure, and lung cancer. If you happen to get breast cancer or have a heart attack, you're less likely to survive, in part because you have limited or no access to adequate health care.

Many of the same discrepancies have been documented in England, where socialized medicine ensures that everybody has more or less equal access to medical care and prescription drugs. In the now-classic Whitehall study, researchers followed seventeen thousand British civil servants over a ten-year period beginning in the late 1960s and found that men in the lowest employment grade were three times more likely to die from heart disease and other causes than their higher-class, better-paid coworkers were.

It seems that the higher up the social class ladder you go, the more in control you feel. On the job, you make more of your own decisions. You are treated with more respect. You have more confidence and are more optimistic about your ability to influence your own fate.

The Givens We Gave Ourselves

You are more than a compendium of inherited traits and twists of fate. Some of the givens you find yourself living with today are nobody's doing but your own. If you are healthy, energetic, and reasonably content, you can certainly take credit. Perhaps you took up jogging ten years ago and stuck with it, or read up on herb teas and vitamins and now supplement your diet with them. Maybe you quit smoking or never started, bought a car with airbags, or joined a support group to help you cope with the stress of caring for your elderly in-law. Longevity may not have been your prime objective, but it is often the payback for these healthful choices.

Longevity is also what we lose when we make choices and adopt behaviors that threaten our health or safety. Many of us have done this, often unknowingly, and certainly without intending to bring about our own demise. We weren't thinking about life expectancy when we lit up our first cigarette as adolescents, for example. We didn't know that smoking would be implicated in seven of the top ten causes of premature death. An image of ourselves at fifty or sixty with lung cancer or emphysema never crossed our minds. We were concerned with more immediate matters, such as being cool or fitting in or feeling grown-up. Besides, we were going to live forever. Missing sleep or skipping doctor's appointments or having unprotected sex with people we'd just met might harm someone else, but not us.

Even after our imaginary bubbles of invincibility burst, many of us continued down longevity-limiting paths. Sometimes we didn't know any better. Up until the past decade or so, homemade fried chicken, buttery mashed potatoes swimming in gravy, and the other fabulous, fat-laden foods we first encountered on the family dinner table were associated with love, security, and abundance—not high cholesterol, heart attacks, and hardening of the arteries.

Sometimes we believed we had better things to do—careers to pursue, children to raise, college educations to finance, homes to redecorate. Who had time for exercise or balanced meals or walks in the woods or meditation? And sometimes something that started out benignly enough crossed over to dangerous ground before we realized it.

That was the case for Dixie Benton, regional food bank director, school board member, church choir soloist, wife, mother, chauffeur, and more. Dixie was overweight and out of shape and the nicest person you'll ever meet. She had high blood pressure, high cholesterol, questionable blood sugar, and every civic honor awarded to a living resident of her hometown. Dixie was someone you could really depend on. She made time for her kids and her causes, her volunteer work, and the local historical society events her husband organized. Indeed, she was there for everything and everybody but herself. She simply took on too much.

For years the only respite Dixie allowed herself was to "unwind" with a drink, usually at home after the dinner dishes were done and the kids had gone to bed, but sometimes at a local tavern before proceeding to a meeting or choir practice. It started out as "just one or two glasses of wine to take the edge off," Dixie explained. But the number rose steadily until she was stopping for her one or two at the tavern every night plus drinking three or four more at home. Her husband mentioned this once—and only once, because Dixie seemed so hurt by the implication that she might have a drinking problem. Wasn't she entitled to a little relaxation after all she did for everybody else? she asked him. He had to admit that she was. Unfortunately, Dixie started having "a little relaxation" with lunch, and a little more in the basement of the food bank. Finally she got a little too relaxed at a social gathering and was stopped for driving under the influence.

Ordered into a program for problem drinkers, she eventually realized she was an alcoholic, got sober, and got to work on her life. She started with her spiritual sphere, specifically, her need to be kind to herself. Dixie stopped making more commitments than she could comfortably fulfill. She found time to tend to her mind sphere with relaxation techniques that didn't involve alcohol. Then, moving on to the physical, Dixie started taking daily walks through town, which lowered her blood pressure and helped her drop some weight. This got her interested in other measures to reduce her risk of heart disease and diabetes. Both deadly conditions ran in Dixie's family, and her past habits fed right into them.

Dixie can't rewind her life, edit out her alcoholism and other problems, and start over from scratch any more than you or I can go back in time and not pick up our first cigarette or not have those one-night stands or not go on all those outrageous diets. But if she continues to use diet, exercise, meditation, and other measures to keep her weight down, her cholesterol stable, and her blood sugar level under control, she should be able to reduce her risk considerably and have another shot at a longer, sweeter life. But equally important is that Dixie saw the big picture when she discovered how her spheres interacted.

Use the chart on page 66 to jot down specific givens from the hand you were dealt that could be helpful to you in your quest for a long, sweet life. Put them in the Credits column. In the Debits column, note the givens that pose a threat to life expectancy.

EXERCISE 4

CREDITS	DEBITS
1.	1.
2.	2.
3.	3.
4.	4.
5.	5.
6.	6.
1.	7.
8.	8.
9.	9.
10.	10.

Playing the Hand You're Dealt

Life's givens are like the cards you start out with in a poker game. You don't select them. They're dealt to you, and some are better than others. Good genes, a certain gender, adequate education, and economic luck make it easier to survive the fallout of careless living. But taking good care of ourselves is a much better insurance policy.

People squander their genetic and developmental gifts every day. They drink and drive, become drug abusers, stay with spouses who batter them, forget to put batteries in their smoke detectors, and more. Any inherited and cultural leads in the race for longevity we were fortunate enough to start out with are easily eroded.

By the same token, determined, confident individuals armed with good health information can finesse and finagle their way to a long, quality life despite the absence of genetic assistance—or the presence of negative risk factors. This point was driven home by a newspaper story I read, a human-interest article designed to generate enthusiasm for an upcoming event, in this case the 1998 New York City Marathon. The story profiled Sam Gadless, a ninety-one-year-old retired tailor from Boca Raton. He was running in his seventh marathon, after entering his first at age eighty-five. That feat would be amazing enough if Sam had been an elite athlete throughout his life. But he had once been a chain-smoker with an ulcer so severe that more than half his stomach had to be removed. His arthritis got so bad during his seventies that the bones in his big toes had to be replaced with artificial ones. He had high cholesterol, high blood pressure, and blood sugar levels that pegged him as a borderline diabetic. One doctor intimated that he might not have much longer to live, which did not surprise Sam. His father had died at forty-two.

With nowhere to go but up, Sam decided to start over, this time without cigarettes or milk shakes or matzo ball soup glistening with chicken fat. Drawing from books and magazine articles on healthy living, which he read by the droves, Sam built his new diet around fruits, vegetables, grains, selected fish, a glass of red wine now and then, and lots of garlic. He walks up to forty miles per week, swims, and does aerobics, stretching, and light weight lifting. "Age is just numbers," he said. He was the oldest entrant in the New York City marathon. "I'm living my youth now."

What Sam's story said to me that I'm hoping to pass on to you is that we *all* have options to improve our lot in life, regardless of our age. Whether we're thirty-eight with a clean bill of health or sixty with a quadruple bypass, forty-five and living with AIDS, or eighty and still running our own business, we can take steps to circumvent life's givens, undo past damage, and extend our life spans.

If you didn't earlier, go back to page 58 and fill in as much of the genealogical information as you can. These known risk factors will be critical when you begin to plot your own longevity code on page 115, and will help you choose the longevity boosters that will do the most to extend and enhance your life.

4

Longevity Robbers and Quality Thieves
The Conditions That Can Come Between Us and a Long, Sweet Life

WHAT IS THE OPPOSITE OF LONGEVITY? Premature death. And what might that be? Well, you can look at it in terms of age alone. In that case, if the average person in a particular culture is expected to live to a certain age (roughly seventy-five in the United States), then anyone who dies before that age has died prematurely, no matter what they die from. About half of the 2.3 million Americans who die each year fit this description. They are younger than seventy-five at the time of their deaths.

You can also define premature death based on what caused someone to expire. If that condition could have been prevented or screened for and cured following early detection, then anyone of virtually any age who dies from it has died prematurely. In this country, between 60 and 75 percent of all deaths meet that criterion. The ten most common causes of premature death are:

1. Heart disease
2. Cancers

3. Stroke
4. Emphysema and chronic bronchitis
5. Accidents and injuries
6. Pneumonia and influenza
7. Diabetes
8. Suicide
9. Kidney disease
10. Chronic liver disease and cirrhosis

Alzheimer's disease and HIV/AIDS also bear watching, Alzheimer's because it is on the rise and AIDS because the 47 percent drop in its death rate is due to very new drug therapies that may or may not perform as well over the long haul. What's more, the incidence of *new* cases has not gone down.

In this chapter and the next I will profile most of these major killers, placing special emphasis on the factors that can make you more vulnerable to each one. This is valuable information because, unlike infectious diseases, which we had the misfortune to catch and die from in droves during the early part of the twentieth century, most of today's top causes of premature death are at least partially self-inflicted. They are linked to things such as cigarette smoking or stress, high-fat diets or high cholesterol levels, or driving while intoxicated, all of which we can do something about.

Know Your Enemy

Some of your givens as well as some of your changeable habits and attitudes are risk factors for specific causes of premature death (longevity robbers) or disability (quality thieves). The more risk factors you have for a particular condition, the greater your vulnerability to that condition—and the slimmer your chances of living a long, sweet life, unless you lower your risk.

By narrowing your focus to encompass one or several of the causes of premature death, rather than addressing risk factors or adopting longevity boosters at random, you'll be able to take preemptive actions in areas where they will do you the most good.

To find out where you may need the most work, review the risk factors that follow the discussion of each major longevity robber in this chapter. Count up the risk factors you checked—more checks equal more risk. Based on your totals (with some extra weight for big-time factors such as smoking or a first-degree relative with breast cancer), identify the causes of premature death and disability for which you seem to be a prime candidate.

Reducing Risk

A risk factor is anything that alters the odds of a particular outcome occurring. By that definition, not setting your alarm clock could be considered a risk factor for oversleeping. It's not much of a risk factor if you typically awaken and get out of bed before your alarm rings. Because you don't really depend on your alarm to avoid oversleeping, setting it is more of a precaution than a form of risk reduction. On the other hand, your alarm may jolt you out of a deep sleep each morning and not truly rouse you until you've hit the snooze button for the third time. In that case, not setting your alarm clock virtually guarantees that you will oversleep—making it a major risk factor for oversleeping.

When it comes to health and longevity, *major risk factors* are behaviors, physical traits, or various givens that are clearly connected to certain medical conditions. Their impact has been demonstrated repeatedly and dramatically in many separate studies conducted over a long period of time. Cigarette smoking is a major risk factor for lung cancer, for example. Hypertension and high cholesterol are intimately linked to heart disease.

Other risk factors are not so clear-cut or so conclusively proven. We don't know the exact role stress plays in heart disease or unintentional injuries, for example. It's possible that drinking coffee exacerbates osteoporosis. And we have a ways to go before we fully understand the impact of free radicals or what to do about them.

But What Can We Do? And How Far Should We Go?

If you want to reduce your risk of dying in a car accident, you can wear a seat belt. To reduce the risk further, you can drive your car less often. Of course, if you stop driving or traveling by car altogether, the likelihood of being involved in a fatal car accident becomes practically nonexistent. But what would become of your life?

If you're currently on a heart-disease-and-cancer-promoting diet—lots of meat and fried or processed foods—you can lower your risk for both killers (plus a half-dozen others) by simply consuming less red meat and eating fewer fried foods. Since there's mounting evidence that vegetarians live longer and escape more deadly diseases than non-vegetarians, if you want to put a really big dent in your risk profile, you could give up meat entirely. But what about becoming a vegan and giving up eggs, fish, and dairy products, too? On the surface, consuming only fruits, vegetables, and grains seems like it would be the next logical step toward better health and a longer life. However, there's some doubt as to whether vegan eating is actually healthier. Moreover, it raises the life-quality question once again. Does a diet that limited fit into your current lifestyle or your mental picture of a long, healthy, and personally satisfying life? Any risk-reduction effort is likely to come with some kind of price tag. However, our efforts to cut the risk of bad things happening in the future should not be so severe or so numerous that they clearly detract from the quality of our lives or send us into emotional, social, spiritual, or material debt.

And remember, we're talking about *risk* here—odds, chances, and possibilities, not sure things or inevitable outcomes. *No matter how carefully you monitor and modify your risk factors, unexpected events, unexplained variables, or plain old luck can still come along to alter any outcome.*

I know that I, like countless other doctors, have had the sobering experience of giving a young, vibrant patient a clean bill of health one day and then having him die from a heart attack soon afterward. There had been absolutely no indication of a heart problem when I examined him, yet a heart problem killed him. I've also treated folks like Ned Allen, a small-town newspaper publisher who smoked up a storm for close to six decades and not only didn't get lung cancer but was never sick for more than a day in his life. His death came peacefully at age seventy-nine. He simply lay down for a nap after a superb game of golf and never woke up.

The best science can't explain these events, or tell you why a total health nut comes down with a terminal illness, or foresee the sudden death of an elite athlete during a low-key training run. It can merely try to steer us away from the habits and habitats, traits and circumstances that clearly influence when we die and from what.

That's when it makes sense to identify longevity-boosting measures aimed at specific risk factors and build them into your longevity prescription. And that's why I've included risk-factor checklists after each of the causes of premature death that I'll be discussing below. The checklists will help you identify conditions that you have a high probability of experiencing. If no clear-cut pattern emerges, you might try building your longevity prescription around:

- *Highly preventable circumstances that can affect almost anyone.* These are often easy steps with big payoffs, including basic safety measures such as wearing bicycle helmets and preparing foods properly.
- *Things that are of personal importance to you.* If working on a particular risk factor merely brings you peace of mind, then your time may be well spent.
- *The most common causes of premature death.* The top ten, which are profiled on the next few pages, affect so many people and are so closely linked to widespread, controllable behaviors that you are probably at risk for at least one and you may not know it.

Heart Disease

- Heart disease is the number-one cause of premature death in this country.
- Twenty-one million Americans suffer from some form of it.
- More than half of those cases are preventable.

Diseases of the heart and arteries, which include heart attacks and congestive heart failure as well as atherosclerosis, are responsible for up to seven hundred thousand deaths each year, many of them premature.

Eugene Harris was a few days shy of fifty-two when his first chest pains hit. They didn't knock him flat or leave him breathless, although they did cause enough discomfort to send him to the medicine chest for some Alka-Seltzer. The busy restaurateur assumed he had indigestion. But later that evening, when he rushed up the stairs in hot pursuit of his visiting three-year-old grandson, Eugene's discomfort turned to agony. As he would later describe it, the crushing pain he experienced at that moment "felt like someone had circled my chest with a steel band and was squeezing it."

Eugene dropped to his knees, sweating profusely. He used what he feared were his last gasps of air to call out for his wife of twenty-six years, who came running, took one look at him, and dialed 911. A quick trip by ambulance to the emergency room was followed by what seemed like an eternity of waiting for answers. Finally Eugene, whose pain had subsided a bit, was admitted to the coronary care unit for observation and testing. His diagnosis? Angina. That's chest pain resulting from the failure of blood to flow freely through blood vessels precariously narrowed by atherosclerosis—the accumulation of waxy yellow plaque along the inside walls of his arteries that caused them to become harder, stiffer, narrower, and less pliable. Found to some degree in 50 percent of Americans over the age of fifty, atherosclerosis is the most common form of this country's number-one killer.

HEART ATTACKS

- More than 1.1 million heart attacks occur each year. That's one every 90 seconds.
- One-third of heart attack victims–roughly one per minute–die within days or months of their attack.
- Every year a quarter of a million people go into cardiac arrest and die less than an hour after their first symptoms appeared.
- One in six heart attacks occur without any warning.

Like all the other organs in our bodies, our hearts require a constant supply of oxygen. When arteries get blocked by blood clots or become so constricted by the buildup of fatty substances, cholesterol, calcium, and other debris (collectively called plaque), the flow gets dammed up, and everything downstream not nourished by other arteries is deprived of oxygen, causing a heart attack.

OTHER HEART AND ARTERY PROBLEMS

Congestive heart failure, which is characterized by a weakened, often enlarged heart that pumps inefficiently, is a common complication of narrowed coronary arteries, high blood pressure, and heart muscles scarred from past heart attacks.

Atherosclerosis, the slow, progressive buildup of plaque along the inner lining of artery walls, causes numerous problems throughout the cardiovascular system. When the buildup occurs in or blocks coronary arteries, you can have a heart attack; when the buildup blocks the brain, you have a stroke. And atherosclerosis in the arteries feeding your legs can cause pain while walking.

WHAT'S YOUR RISK?

Regrettably, we do not have the knowledge or the tools to do away with heart disease completely. However, changes in personal habits—from giving up cigarettes and getting regular exercise to lowering the fat content of our diets—have drastically reduced its incidence and mortality rate. Deaths from heart attacks have dropped by more than 50 percent since their high-water mark in 1963. But the battle's far from won. The number of people suffering needlessly and dying prematurely could fall precipitously if we took steps to reduce the risk factors within our control.

First, the givens.

❑ Are you over sixty-five?

❑ Are you a man? Between the ages of forty-five and sixty-four, men have three times as many heart attacks as women do.

❑ Are you a postmenopausal woman?

❑ Do you have a first-degree relative (brother, father, sister, mother) who was diagnosed with heart disease before age fifty-five?

❑ Other relatives with heart problems? It runs in families.

Now, the risk factors you *can* control.

❑ Do you smoke? Smokers are two and a half times more likely to develop heart disease than nonsmokers.

❑ Is your total cholesterol level above 200?

❑ Is your LDL (known as "bad cholesterol") greater than 130?

❑ Are your triglycerides greater than 250?

❑ Is your HDL (known as "good cholesterol") less than 35?

❑ Is your blood pressure higher than 140/90?

❑ Do you lead a sedentary lifestyle, with little physical activity?

❑ Does your daily intake of fat, especially the kind found in meat and dairy products, exceed 30 percent of your total calories?

❑ Are you a diabetic? More than 80 percent of people with diabetes die from some form of heart or blood vessel disease.

❑ Are you more than 30 percent overweight for your height and age?

❑ Are nutrients, including vitamins C and E and folic acid, in short supply in your diet because you eat less than five servings of fruits and vegetables a day?

❑ Is there a lot of stress in your life?

❑ Do you lose your temper easily or often? Angry outbursts and hostile actions take their toll.

When we add up all the risk factors we know of and can measure or observe in some reliable manner, we find that they account for just half of all premature deaths from heart disease.

Cancer

- Cancer is the number-two cause of premature death.
- It kills 1,500 American men, women, and children every day, for a grim total of 540,000 deaths annually. Half of those deaths are preventable overall.
- About 1.2 million new cases occur each year.
- Fifty-eight percent of the newly diagnosed will survive for five years or more.
- Cancers linked to tobacco smoke (responsible for 175,000 deaths per year) and heavy alcohol use (9,000 deaths annually) are close to 100 percent avoidable.

Quality versus quantity—it's a choice that those of us who are not yet at death's door hope we never have to face. Most of us want to go quickly, preferably in our sleep, and cancer is our worst nightmare.

THE BARE FACTS

Cancer is not one but many diseases, each involving abnormal cells that grow uncontrollably, leaving devastation in their wake. Cancer cells accumulate to form tumors that attack the normal tissue in their immediate vicinity, or they travel through the bloodstream or lymph nodes to start tumor "colonies" in other parts of the body. The entire process is set in motion by exposure to external carcinogens (such as radiation, chemicals, viruses, or tobacco smoke) or by the impact of internal factors (including hormones, immune conditions, or genetic mutations) that may have occurred decades before the altered cells become detectable. The earlier you catch cancer, the greater the chance of beating it.

THE BIG FOUR
Lung Cancer

- Death rate: 160,000 Americans in 1998.
- New cases diagnosed annually: 170,000 in 1998.
- Percentage surviving for five years following diagnosis: 15 percent.
- Percentage dying within one year of diagnosis: 60 percent.

Lung cancer is responsible for 29 percent of all cancer deaths and 14 percent of all new cancer cases. With no useful, easily available way to screen for it, only about 15 percent of new cases are picked up early. As a result, survival rates are quite low. The reason? Cigarette smoking, which is responsible for 95 percent of all lung cancer cases.

Colon Cancer

- Death rate: 48,000 Americans in 1998.
- New cases diagnosed annually: 95,500 in 1998 (down from 150,000 in the early 1990s).
- Five-year survival rates: 92 percent if diagnosed in noninvasive stages, 80 percent after invading colon walls, 50 percent if abdominal lymph nodes involved.

Cancer of the colon and rectum retained its standing as the second leading cause of cancer death in the United States. Routine screening and preemptive surgeries, especially the removal of benign (noncancerous) polyps have improved survival dramatically.

Breast Cancer

- New cases diagnosed annually: 177,000.
- Deaths per year: 44,000. Roughly 4,700 of the women who die are in their forties.
- Five-year survival rate: 90 percent if detected while the cancer is still localized.
- One in eight women alive today can expect to develop breast cancer at some point.

Each year breast cancer strikes almost twice as many women as lung cancer does, but its death rate is much lower. Public awareness campaigns, earlier surgery, and improved chemotherapy with drugs like tamoxifen are all responsible.

Your odds of developing breast cancer double if your mother, sister, or daughter has had it. If *both* a mother and a sister had it, your risk goes up a whopping sixteen times. But heredity is only one factor influencing the actual incidence of this cancer. Others include advancing age, early menstruation, late menopause, late or no pregnancies, alcohol consumption, longtime estrogen use, and excess body fat.

Prostate Cancer

- New cases diagnosed annually: 185,000 in the United States, mostly in men over sixty-five.
- Deaths: 40,000 American men per year.
- Five-year survival rate: 89 percent. Up to 63 percent pass the ten-year mark.

The second most common cause of cancer death in men, cancer of the prostate grows very, very slowly. Dietary fat is considered a significant risk factor for prostate cancer, which American men are fifteen times more likely to develop than Japanese men, whose diets are much lower in fats and processed foods. African-American men are particularly at risk for this disease. As with many other cancers, cigarette smoking appears to increase risk.

WHAT'S YOUR RISK?

Will you be one of the lucky bunch who doesn't get cancer—or one of the sizable crowd who does? There's a good deal of fate and fortune involved here, but that's all the more reason to actively improve your odds by managing risks where you can.

Although individual cancers are best understood by looking at them individually, it is possible to identify a handful of givens that make us more susceptible to cancer in general.

❑ Are you over forty? The four cancers with the highest mortality rates (lung, colon, breast, and prostate) are rarely seen in people younger than that.

❑ Is there cancer in your family?

❑ Does your personal background include exposure to toxic substances such as asbestos or secondhand smoke?

❑ In your youth, did you spend a lot of time in the sun and get one or more severe sunburns?

❑ Did your mother have radiation during her pregnancy?

Although you can't go back and undo the past, you'll want to keep an eye out for the warning signs of cancers that have been associated with any exceptional exposures you know you've experienced.

Controllable risks:

❑ Do you smoke? Smoking increases your chances of getting colon, prostate, throat, breast, mouth, and cervical cancers, to name a few. And there's absolutely no doubt that it causes lung cancer.

❑ Does your diet lack fiber and certain vitamins? Fall short of the crucial five to seven daily servings of fruits and vegetables? Overdo fats, calories, and proteins derived from meat and poultry? Up to one-third of all cancer deaths are nutrition-related.

❑ Are you currently being exposed to carcinogens such as radon or asbestos in your home, workplace, or neighborhood?

❑ Are you physically inactive? Sedentary lifestyles make you one and a half times more likely to develop colon or breast cancer.

❑ Have you taken estrogen in menopause (as hormone replacement therapy)?

❑ Is it difficult for you to obtain adequate medical care, including screening tests? Half the cancers that will occur this year have the potential to be picked up early through routine screening.

Stroke

- Stroke is the number-three cause of premature death in the United States and the number-one cause of disability.
- Six hundred thousand Americans (one every fifty-three seconds) will have a stroke this year.
- Strokes are 50 percent preventable.

Frank Simmons rarely got headaches, but he had a real beauty the first time I met him. His secretary, a regular patient of mine, brought him to me one afternoon. She drove him over in her car because he was in too much pain to open his eyes, much less see the road.

"In my whole life I've only had one other headache like this," the

According to the American Heart Association, the warning signs of a stroke include:

- Sudden weakness or numbness of the face, arm, or leg on one side
- Sudden dimness or loss of vision, particularly in one eye
- Loss of speech, or trouble talking or understanding speech
- Sudden, severe headaches with no known or apparent cause
- Unexplained dizziness, unsteadiness, or sudden falls, especially when you've had other symptoms

If you notice one or more of these signs, don't wait. Call your emergency medical services. Get to a hospital right away!

thirty-eight-year-old CPA said with some difficulty. He had an open hand pressed against each of his temples as if holding them there would keep his head from exploding. "That was ten years ago. A migraine, the doctor I saw then told me. This must be another one."

Although having just two migraines spaced ten years apart is not unheard of, it was also far enough outside the ordinary to make me wonder if something else might be going on. I gave Frank some pain medication, and just to be on the safe side I sent him for an immediate CAT scan. The scan revealed a small subarachnoid hemorrhage that was causing tremendous pain. If the root of the problem wasn't located and remedied quickly, the blood vessels in the brain would be squeezed shut, cutting off the oxygen supply to Frank's brain cells and precipitating a full-blown stroke.

Fortunately that didn't happen. The culprit turned out to be a tiny, leaky aneurysm ballooning out from a weak spot in an artery leading to Frank's brain. And once it had been repaired surgically, Frank was back on track to live a sweet, healthy, and long life.

Frank was lucky. Timely identification of his problem and swift medical intervention saved him from the devastating consequences of a cerebrovascular attack (CVA) or stroke. Like heart attacks, strokes come on suddenly, are often deadly, and do less damage when they receive immediate attention. Their ultimate outcome can range from Frank's best-case scenario—no permanent damage—to serious disability or death.

Our brains are the home of more than ten billion nerve cells. And those nerve cells receive life-sustaining oxygen and nutrients from thousands of blood vessels that branch off from several major arteries and extend into the brain likes roots on a tree. A stroke occurs most often when a blocked artery or a ruptured blood vessel prevents the blood that normally flows through it from reaching its destination. Nerve cells stop working, along with the functions they once controlled. A limb becomes numb or doesn't work when you want it to. You might feel dizzy or fall down. Or you might try to talk but have no coherent words come out of your mouth. Blurred or lost vision, what feels like the world's worst headache, or unsteadiness also can herald a stroke.

On the bright side, far fewer people have strokes or die from them today than in the past. Because of lifestyle changes and effective treatment for hypertension, the number of strokes that occur each year has dropped by 60 percent since 1972, and could be reduced dramatically by managing known risk factors.

WHAT'S YOUR RISK?

Certain givens increase your vulnerability to strokes.

❑ Are you middle-aged or older? The odds of having a stroke double with each decade beginning at age fifty-five.

❑ Are you male? Men are almost twice as likely to have strokes, and the gender gap widens with age.

❑ Are you an African-American? Death rates from strokes are greater.

❑ Have a number of your family members had strokes?

❑ Have you had a stroke? A prior stroke boosts the odds of having a second.

The parallels between heart disease and strokes extend to the controllable factors that make some of us prime targets for those killers.

❑ Do you have high blood pressure?

❑ Are you a diabetic?

❑ Do you smoke?

❑ Do you have high serum cholesterol?

❑ Do you live on a high-fat/low-fiber diet?

❑ Do you get little or no exercise?

❑ Do you average more than two drinks containing alcohol per day or binge-drink on weekends? Excessive alcohol use increases risk.

❑ Do you use cocaine? It can trigger a deadly stroke.

❑ Are you an intravenous drug user?

❑ Could you have an irregular heartbeat? Atrial fibrillation, a condition that causes a quivering of the heart is a stroke risk factor.

❑ Do you know stroke warning signs? Getting to a hospital as soon as possible after they appear could save your life.

Emphysema and Bronchitis (Chronic Obstructive Pulmonary Diseases, or COPD)

- These diseases are the fourth most common cause of premature death in the United States.
- They claimed a hundred thousand lives in 1995 (more than double the 1979 figure).
- Seventeen million Americans currently live with COPD, including fourteen million with chronic bronchitis and three million with emphysema.
- One million new cases are diagnosed annually.
- Ninety percent are preventable.

In her younger days, Roxanne Rogers was the modern Midwest's answer to the tough-talking, hard-drinking cowboys who herded cattle through the area a century earlier. Tall, broad-shouldered, and often dressed from head to toe in black leather, Roxanne in her thirties and forties cut quite an imposing figure. She had a scowl that could stop you dead in your tracks, but also a hearty laugh you couldn't help joining in with. On most weekends you could find her zooming over bone-jarring unpaved trails on her dirt bike, cheering on competitors at motorcycle rallies, or downing shots and beer at a local tavern with her equally rough-and-tumble husband, Bart.

These days Roxanne is not a regular at any of those locations. She can no longer participate in any of the vigorous, outdoorsy activities she loves. At fifty-five, a devastating illness and an oxygen tank that she must be hooked up to continuously dictate where she can go and what she can do. Along with seventeen million other Americans, she suffers from chronic obstructive pulmonary disease (COPD). It has already diminished the quality of her life and ultimately will shorten it.

Currently fourth among causes of premature death, the incidence of emphysema and bronchitis, which are grouped together under the COPD umbrella, has soared over the past twenty-five years. The

COPD death rate has more than doubled since 1979. Airborne irritants are largely to blame, with cigarette smoke leading the way.

WHAT'S YOUR RISK?

Like lung cancer, chronic bronchitis and emphysema are largely man-made diseases; however, several givens leave you more susceptible.

❑ Do you live with a smoker or work in a smoky place?

❑ Do you have a number of relatives with breathing problems, chronic bronchitis, or emphysema? All three seem to run in families, and emphysema has been clearly linked to a genetic deficiency of the enzyme alpha-1 trypsin.

Now the factors you can do something about!

❑ Do you smoke? Ninety percent of all chronic bronchitis and emphysema cases can be attributed to tobacco smoke.

❑ Does your job put you in daily contact with dust, chemicals, or exhaust fumes? Coal miners, grain handlers, metal molders, and demolition crews are prime targets for chronic bronchitis. If you do develop it, you may have to switch jobs in order to stop the disease from progressing to life-threatening levels.

❑ Are you sedentary? Exercising regularly strengthens the lungs and helps keep airways clear.

❑ Do you have asthma? It dramatically increases your chances of developing COPD.

Accidents and Injuries

- Accidents and injuries are the fifth most common cause of death for all age groups.
- They are the number-one cause of death for one- through forty-four-year-olds.
- Accidents and injuries are responsible for ninety-three thousand deaths per year.
- Forty-three thousand of those deaths involve motor vehicles.
- Thirteen to fifteen thousand of the deaths are the result of firearms being discharged accidentally.
- Seventy-five percent of these deaths are preventable.

Accidents happen. People trip over their kids' toys and tumble down the stairs, or slide on area rugs and crash to the floor. Grease fires ignite kitchen curtains and bad batches of burger meat deposit E. coli bacteria in unsuspecting digestive systems. Cars collide on icy highways.

Bicycles hit potholes, sending their riders headfirst over the handlebars onto hard and abrasive pavement. All told, millions of accidents severe enough to limit our activities, require medical care, or even kill us happen each year. We don't intend for them to happen any more than we intend to have heart attacks or develop cancers. But as you will learn from the Longevity Boosters section, there is plenty we can do to prevent them.

Influenza and Pneumonia

- These diseases combined are the sixth most common cause of death.
- They are responsible for eighty-three thousand deaths per year.
- Eighty-nine percent of such deaths are of people over sixty-five.
- Along with other respiratory conditions, influenza and pneumonia lead to the most sick days each year.

Influenza, which most of us know as the flu, is a moderately severe illness caused by an airborne virus. Its all too familiar chills, fever, sore throat, dry cough, and head and body aches strike more than ninety million Americans each year. Pneumonia is a serious infection of the lungs accompanied by a high fever, chest pain, a productive cough, and extreme fatigue. Not just one disease, pneumonia can be triggered by bacteria, viruses, chemicals, and twenty-seven other causes.

Both of these longevity robbers pose the greatest threat to specific populations. Healthy children and adults usually recover from them. But the odds of developing deadly complications are high for people with chronic lung diseases (asthma, emphysema, cystic fibrosis, etc.), heart disease, chronic kidney disease, diabetes, severe anemia, or conditions that depress the immune system. Advanced age is also a risk factor.

The most effective weapon is immunization, which is thoroughly discussed on pages 257–58 of the Longevity Boosters section.

Diabetes

- Diabetes is the seventh most common cause of premature death in the United States.
- Thirty-six million Americans have diabetes; half don't know it.
- Two thousand new cases are diagnosed daily; this could reach five thousand with more diligent testing.

- Diabetes is directly responsible for sixty-two thousand deaths annually and contributes to two hundred thousand more.
- The disease is 40 percent preventable.
- It is the leading cause of leg amputations, blindness, and kidney failure, and is a major risk factor for heart disease and stroke.

Colleen Walker, a forty-two-year-old elementary schoolteacher who had taken a summer position with the Parks and Recreation Commission, came in for her job physical fully expecting to get a clean bill of health. After all, she *felt* fine. And based on the examination I did in my office, she seemed well enough. But her lab test results showed something amiss. Colleen's blood sugar levels were slightly elevated, a sign that she might have diabetes. When follow-up tests confirmed this diagnosis, Colleen was clearly distressed.

"There must be some mistake," she insisted, confused. "If I had diabetes, wouldn't I feel bad or have some kind of symptom or something?"

The answer—for Colleen and countless others in a similar state of confusion and concern—is "not necessarily."

DIABETES IN A NUTSHELL

Diabetes is a chronic, currently incurable, but treatable disorder caused by the body's inability to properly process glucose, or sugar, from the digestive system and move it into cells that need it for nourishment. As a result, excess, unused sugar floats around in the bloodstream, wreaking havoc on blood vessels and various organs and paving the way for heart attacks, strokes, blindness, kidney disease, and other potentially deadly or disabling conditions.

Half of the diabetics in this country are unaware of their condition. But early detection and intervention have the power to save us from early graves, which is why the National Institutes of Health have started pushing for routine screening and preemptive measures for anyone whose blood sugar is consistently higher than normal. This includes the twenty million Americans who once would have been labeled borderline diabetic. What they really have is early diabetes—and an opportunity to make lifestyle changes soon enough to keep the disease from progressing to its most devastating levels.

WHAT'S YOUR RISK?

The givens:

❑ Are you African-American, Hispanic, or Native American? Then you're more prone.
❑ Are you forty-five years of age or older? That's when the risk of developing type II diabetes begins to rise.
❑ Does one or more of your parents or siblings have diabetes?

There are factors within your control, too. The Nurse's Health Study, a long-term health evaluation of 65,000 nurses, all of them women, started in 1986 and continues to scrutinize the connection between numerous health practices and various diseases, including diabetes. Of the participating nurses who were forty-five to sixty-five years old and not diabetic when the study started, 915 had developed diabetes ten years later. By comparing their health profiles and updates with those of nurses who remained nondiabetics, the researchers were able to uncover a number of clear risk factors for the disease.

❑ Are you 20 percent or more above the recommended weight for your height and age? Obesity clearly increases the odds.
❑ Do you lead a largely sedentary life?
❑ Do you smoke?
❑ Is your diet high in fat and refined sugars but low in fiber? This eating pattern seems to increase risk, while one high in fiber and complex carbohydrates seems to lower it.

Suicide

- Suicide is number eight among causes of premature death.
- It results in the death of more than thirty thousand Americans each year.
- Women make ten times more suicide attempts than men, but men's attempts are more lethal.
- For every female who ends her own life, four males do.

What makes back problems debilitating, cancer more terrifying, and burns among the most traumatizing of all injuries? Pain—shooting, searing, constant, blinding, seemingly inescapable pain. The words alone can make us wince. But as anyone who has ever suffered from depression can tell you, physical pain is not the only kind that can torment us. There's also aching emptiness, pangs of regret, and a pervasive sense of sorrow, loss, and despair that makes the start of each new day sheer agony. Emotional pain can be disabling—and deadly.

Sometimes the pain of depression, which I'll discuss in more detail later, is so relentless or becomes so unbearable that people end their own lives to escape it. On an average day, eighty-four Americans commit suicide, and nineteen hundred more attempt it. The vast majority do so while mired in serious depressive episodes. Eighty percent actually mention their intentions ahead of time. And many exhibit one or more of the following behaviors:

- Talking about suicide, sometimes in a joking way, perhaps "critiquing" the way other people did it or pondering out loud about the best way to go
- Communicating feelings of hopelessness, helplessness, or worthlessness with comments like "Everyone would be better off without me," "Nothing matters anymore. I have nothing to live for," or "I wish I could just disappear"
- Showing no interest in things they previously cared about, including being well groomed and nicely dressed
- Engaging in increasingly self-destructive behavior such as extreme alcohol or drug abuse, cutting or burning their skin, or promiscuity
- Repeatedly taking foolish risks—driving recklessly, climbing to the edge of cliffs, walking between lanes of traffic
- Giving away possessions, getting one's affairs in order

Overall, these signs, especially when coupled with a history of previous suicide attempts or other risk factors, should certainly be taken seriously.

WHAT'S YOUR RISK?

Contrary to the impression you may have received, suicide is not the exclusive domain of disaffected adolescents. Its incidence actually *increases* with age, especially among men. White men over the age of sixty-five are more likely to kill themselves than any other single segment of the population. Other givens play a role, too:

❑ Are you a Native American or of Asian descent? Both groups have disproportionately high suicide rates.

❑ Has a member of your family committed or attempted to commit suicide?

❑ Do you have a personal history of depression or previous suicide attempts? People who have attempted suicide often try again. And depressive episodes, even when they are properly treated, have a tendency to recur.

You can exert a bit more influence over the following risk factors:

❑ Are you reluctant to seek out or accept help for emotional upsets?

❑ Is it difficult for you to find or pay for the kind of help you require? Without that help, many of us will suffer needlessly for extended periods of time.

❑ Do you sometimes use alcohol or drugs to create a comfortable numbness or offer a brief euphoric respite from the dreariness that engulfs you? This "self-medicating" seems to work at first, but once the initial effect wears off, the depression is often worse. In addition, the impaired judgment and tendency to act on impulse can be all depressed individuals need to push them to take their own lives.

Kidney Disease

- Kidney disease is ninth among causes of premature death.
- It kills more than fifty thousand people per year.
- Kidney problems affect thirteen million Americans (5 percent of the population).
- There were 182,000 Americans on dialysis in 1996.
- In 1996, there were twelve thousand kidney transplants from a waiting list of thirty-five thousand.

Healthy kidneys cleanse our blood supply by filtering out waste materials and excess fluid. They also produce hormones needed for building red blood cells, strengthening bones, and regulating blood pressure. When the kidneys are *not* working properly or fail completely, the body retains fluid, blood pressure rises, and our red blood cell supply diminishes. Ultimately, a dialysis machine or transplant may be needed.

While kidney disease is a noteworthy longevity robber and a quality thief, it is nearly always the result of other deadly conditions such as diabetes, hypertension, or arteriosclerosis.

Chronic Liver Diseases and Cirrhosis

- Liver disease is number ten among causes of premature death.
- These diseases are 75 percent preventable.
- Each year twenty-five thousand Americans die from these diseases.
- Over 125,000 new cases of hepatitis B are diagnosed annually.
- Today, two to four million Americans have hepatitis C; 5 percent will develop cirrhosis or liver cancer.

In 1983 Molly Caldwell was badly injured in an automobile accident. During lengthy emergency surgery, a blood transfusion helped save her life. Today she is dying because of it. The blood Mary received sixteen years ago was contaminated with the hepatitis C virus, which has been slowly damaging her liver ever since, completely unnoticed by her.

Aldo Pinelli used to work nights at his brother's restaurant and would start drinking as soon as the last customer was gone. He would polish off a bottle of wine before the cleanup was done and then go right on drinking until he passed out, sometimes in his own bed, but just as often in his car or on the floor of the restaurant's storeroom. I had warned him that such heavy drinking would do serious damage to his liver. His wife begged him to give up the grape. But our pleas went unheeded, and Aldo developed cirrhosis.

Patti Grey contracted hepatitis B from a man she became intimately involved with while working overseas. The virus, which is often spread by bodily fluids, including blood, semen, and vaginal fluids, is actually more contagious than HIV. People can carry it (and pass it on to others) without getting sick themselves. And 5 percent of the folks who do get it never shake it. Regrettably, Patti fell into that category. Hepatitis B had ravaged her liver to the point where a liver transplant would be needed to save her life.

Deaths from liver diseases such as Molly's, Aldo's, and Patti's have decreased significantly over the past few decades. Tests to detect hepatitis in the blood of potential donors contributed to that decline. They have practically eliminated infections caused by transfusions. A vaccine to prevent the spread of hepatitis B has started bringing its incidence and death rate down as well. But they're still high enough for ailments affecting the liver, mainly chronic hepatitis and cirrhosis, to be counted among the top ten causes of premature death.

LIVER DISEASE IN A NUTSHELL

Like a complex chemical factory, the liver produces enzymes that aid in digestion. It processes cholesterol, stores nutrients, helps maintain blood sugar levels, regulates hormones, and keeps toxic substances from reaching other parts of the body. If enough liver cells are destroyed by viruses, alcohol, drugs, or toxic chemicals, usually over a significant stretch of time, the liver stops functioning properly and death ensues.

One of the deadliest diseases to attack the liver is chronic hepatitis, which causes prolonged inflammation and ongoing injury. This illness often, but not always, follows on the heels of an acute infection involving hepatitis B or C.

Hepatitis A is spread directly (by coming in contact with infected feces) or indirectly (from water, shellfish, other food, utensils, or food handlers contaminated with the virus). If you travel often to developing countries, where it is more common, taking the vaccine is prudent.

Hepatitis B is a killer when it chronically lingers in our systems. The virus is usually transmitted through sexual intercourse, blood transfusions, and sharing needles. Fortunately, fewer people are spreading it these days thanks to a safe, effective vaccine.

Hepatitis C was identified in 1989, and an antibody test was developed one year later. Unfortunately, that test didn't find its way into common use until thousands had already contracted the infection from blood transfusions. Like hepatitis B, hepatitis C can become a chronic condition.

Cirrhosis is a condition that occurs when normal liver cells are damaged and replaced by scar tissue, leaving fewer and fewer normal cells to perform the organ's vital functions. By far the most common cause is excessive alcohol consumption, especially when combined with poor nutritional habits. Cirrhosis can also stem from chronic viral hepatitis (HepB or HepC), other viruses, inherited or congenital disorders, an abnormal accumulation of iron in the blood, or exposure to toxic chemicals, including some prescription or over-the-counter medicines. Regardless of the source, much of the scarring that characterizes cirrhosis occurs without our awareness. We can destroy up to 80 percent of the liver before seeing symptoms.

If you have chronic hepatitis or cirrhosis in its early stages, you can help yourself by:

- *Avoiding alcohol.* It aggravates an already inflamed liver—and destroys more healthy cells.
- *Cutting the medications you take to a bare minimum.* An ailing liver doesn't detoxify them well.
- *Maintaining a well-balanced diet.* This improves the odds that an adequate supply of nutrients will reach the body even though the liver may not be functioning efficiently.
- *Taking a multivitamin with B complex.*

WHAT'S YOUR RISK?

There are certain givens that make liver disease more likely.

❑ Does your medical history include a blood transfusion before 1989 (before tests to detect hepatitis C)?

❑ Does your personal history include drug use? Have you ever shared hypodermic needles?

❑ Do you work in a field such as health care or law enforcement, where you're likely to come in contact with contaminated body fluids?

Of course, there are also factors under your control:

❑ Do you consistently drink more than two or three shots of hard liquor, beers, or five-ounce glasses of wine per day?

❑ Do you take more than 4 g of acetaminophen (the equivalent of eight extra-strength Tylenol) daily? You could be damaging your liver. More than 2 g a day can pose a threat to alcoholics or heavy drinkers. Research has linked the combination of alcohol and high doses of acetaminophen to liver failure.

❑ Do you mix medications or take medication you could do without?

❑ Do you work with or around chemicals without taking adequate safety precautions?

❑ Do you have unsafe sex?

HIV/AIDS

- The first U.S. AIDS case was reported in 1981.
- Since then, one million Americans have been infected with HIV and half a million have developed full-blown AIDS.

- New cases per year number between forty thousand and sixty thousand.
- Fatalities in 1997 totaled 22,527.
- The death rate is down by 47 percent, although the rate of new infection remains the same.

HIV/AIDS is caused by the HIV virus, which destroys the immune system. When C. Everett Koop started mainstreaming AIDS education and awareness, the prevalence of AIDS began to drop. Unfortunately, surveys today show that many young men and women, straight and gay, are not taking precautions. This complacency seems to be caused by the development of better pharmaceuticals that have moved AIDS out of the top ten causes of death and created a false sense of security. But in fact we don't know how long these drugs will keep AIDS at bay. HIV remains one of the most serious infectious diseases around. New infections continue to occur at the alarming rate of as many as sixty thousand per year in the United States (five per minute throughout the world), in spite of the fact that HIV is almost 100 percent preventable.

THE BARE FACTS

- Everyone with AIDS tests positive for HIV, but many HIV-positive individuals will go ten years or longer without developing AIDS. Some people, including 5 percent of HIV-positive men in one twenty-year study, have been able to fend off AIDS for more than two decades.

Spread from one person to another when infected blood, semen, vaginal fluids, or breast milk actually enters the bloodstream, HIV invades cells in the immune system, the very system that exists to fight it.

Most HIV-positive individuals start out with few or no symptoms other than a flulike episode that passes after several days or weeks. However, having no overt signs of the illness doesn't mean that HIV is lying dormant. It is taking every opportunity to outproduce antibodies, destroy the white blood cells that bolster the immune system, and kill off T4 cells, which help fight infection.

WHAT'S THE RISK?

Certain givens make it statistically more likely that you will become infected with HIV.

As viruses go, HIV is actually pretty fragile. It can survive only in blood and other internal bodily fluids. Outside the body it is destroyed rapidly by heat, drying, and ordinary household bleach. You *can't* get it from:

• Casual social contact, such as visiting, working, or going to school with someone who has HIV/AIDS.

• Airborne water droplets. Sneezes and coughs do not spread HIV.

• Close personal contact. Neither perspiration nor saliva spreads the virus.

• Doorknobs, bed linens, clothing, towels, or toilets.

• Telephones, showers, swimming pools, eating utensils, or glasses.

• Mosquitoes or other insects that may have bitten someone with HIV before they bit you.

Consider this good news. Can you imagine the state the world would be in right now if a virus as deadly as HIV was as contagious as the common cold?

Passing AIDS from one person to another requires an exchange of bodily fluids, specifically blood, semen, vaginal fluids, or breast milk. This exchange can occur if you:

• Receive transfusions of blood products donated by someone who has the virus. This is a rare occurrence now that blood is tested for the virus.

• Get HIV-infected blood, semen, or vaginal secretions into open wounds or sores.

• Receive tissue or organs transplanted from a donor with the virus.

• Are artificially inseminated by a man who has the virus.

• Have a needle or surgical instrument contaminated with HIV puncture or cut your skin.

A woman with HIV can pass the virus to a fetus during pregnancy or to an infant she is breast-feeding.

❏ Are you African-American or Hispanic? Compared to Caucasians, your rates of HIV infection are six times and three times higher, respectively.

❏ Are you under forty-five? Three-quarters of all AIDS patients are. Even with the overall drop in death rate, HIV/AIDS is number three among premature killers of men thirty-five through fifty-four.

Controllable risk factors have the largest influence on your vulnerability to HIV infection.

❏ Do you have unprotected (condomless) vaginal or anal intercourse with anyone whose HIV status you are not absolutely certain of?

❏ Could your sexual partner (or partners) be having unprotected intercourse with other people or engaging in high-risk pursuits such as IV drug use?

❏ Do you use intravenous drugs and share needles?

❏ Do you get high on alcohol, marijuana, cocaine, or other intoxicants? They lower inhibitions and stimulate feelings of invincibility, increasing the odds that you'll abandon caution and indulge in unsafe sex.

❏ Do you work in a setting where you could be exposed to HIV through needle sticks, violent confrontations, or any other means?

Alzheimer's Disease and Dementia

- Alzheimer's is responsible for twenty-three thousand deaths per year, most among the oldest old.
- It currently affects four million Americans, half over the age of eighty-five.

Nine out of ten forgetful seventy-year-olds just forget stuff a little more often than the average forty-, fifty-, or sixty-year-old and only a tad more than we all did in our twenties. That's all. And even when things do slip our minds, for the most part our ability to think, synthesize, draw conclusions, and make decisions is not affected. We know who we are, where we live, that parkas and not swimsuits are appropriate winter wear, and so on. The same cannot be said for someone who suffers from the relentless destruction of brain cells and erosion of memories, thoughts, and emotions brought on by Alzheimer's disease and other forms of dementia.

Dementia is the umbrella term for conditions characterized by a diminished capacity to reason, remember, recognize the realities of your life in the present, or respond appropriately to everyday situations. And Alzheimer's disease accounts for roughly half of all dementia cases. Its signature symptoms include:

- Frequent forgetfulness or unexplainable confusion that goes beyond occasionally forgetting a deadline or an appointment.
- Difficulty completing familiar tasks such as dressing, for example, but not just getting distracted and accidentally putting on one blue sock and one brown sock.
- Language problems, including substituting inappropriate or nonsensical words for the simple ones we cannot recall.
- Disorientation. Not knowing where we are, the time of year, or whom we live with.
- Poor judgment. Intent on going fishing, for example, the Alzheimer's sufferer might start walking toward the ocean—fifteen miles away—in the middle of a snowstorm.
- Problems with abstract thinking that can render numbers unrecognizable and make performing basic calculations impossible.
- Misplacing things or finding them in odd places such as the refrigerator.
- Rapid mood swings for no apparent reason.
- Drastic changes in personality. Either suddenly or over a period of time, someone who was pretty easygoing may become hostile, suspicious, or extremely anxious.
- Permanent loss of interest and involvement in previously routine or pleasurable pursuits.

These symptoms, which appear in different combinations and to different degrees in each Alzheimer's patient, advance from mild to severely disabling. Average life expectancy from the onset of the illness is eight years, although some patients live as many as twenty.

Of the other forms of dementia, the most common is multi-infarct or vascular dementia, a by-product of ministrokes that briefly cut off the blood and oxygen supply to portions of the brain that control mood, memory, and various intellectual functions. Although the damage can't be undone, multi-infarct dementia can be prevented or stopped from progressing any further by controlling the same elements of your lifestyle that increase your risk of stroke.

WHAT'S YOUR RISK?

Givens:

❑ Are you among the oldest old (those over eighty-five)? Alzheimer's is quite uncommon among the middle-aged, but 57 percent of the over-eighty-five population develops it.

❑ Are you a woman? Recent research suggests that women may be at a greater risk than men.

❑ Have any of your family members suffered from Alzheimer's? Although the disease itself may not be inherited, preliminary research suggests that genetics may exert some influence over who gets it.

To date, science has not identified anything in our lifestyles or environment that makes us more susceptible to Alzheimer's disease. My best advice: Don't ignore symptoms, minimize their impact, or put off seeing your physician for fear of what you'll be told. By doing nothing until your lapses and losses are obvious to everyone around you and seriously limiting your ability to function on your own, you cannot benefit from the few treatments that do exist. They need to be administered early on.

For dementias other than Alzheimer's, there are a number of risk factors you *can* reduce or avoid.

Your chances of developing multi-infarct dementia are elevated by the same factors that make strokes the third most common cause of premature death in this country.

❑ Do you smoke?

❑ Do you suffer from high blood pressure?

❑ Do you have elevated total or LDL cholesterol levels and/or low HDL cholesterol?

❑ Do you consume excessive amounts of alcohol?

Any action that increases your odds of suffering a traumatic head injury or sustaining brain damage because your air supply has been cut off simultaneously increases your risk of developing dementia.

❑ Do you ride a bike, skate, ski, or motorcycle without wearing a helmet?

❑ Do you drive under the influence of alcohol, illicit drugs, or legitimate medications?

❑ Do you live in a residence without carbon monoxide detectors?

These factors cause reversible dementias (or dementia-like symptoms) as well:

❏ Do you suffer from anorexia?

❏ Is your physician sometimes unaware of all the medications you are taking, including over-the-counter drugs or herbal supplements?

5

The Building Blocks of a Longer, Sweeter Life:
Three Elements You Can't Do Without

THINK ABOUT THE MOST EXUBERANT people you know. Are they sixty-five, forty-five, fifteen, or five? Did you think of them because of their accumulated years of educational wisdom or their zest for life? Do their smile and humor just light up a room? When there's a new idea or something to tackle, are they enthusiastic?

The three building blocks of a long, sweet life are not related to age. They are self-fulfilling attitudes and actions that transform our lives:

- Lifelong learning
- Active involvement
- A hopeful outlook

Lifelong Learning

Numerous studies have shown that education is a crucial prerequisite for longevity. Men and women with at least two years of college live ten to fifteen years longer than high school dropouts. Why is this? Because education leads to adaptation, which from a Darwinian point of view makes perfect sense. Suppose you read a study showing that swallowing an aspirin tablet in the morning, or taking modern jazz dance in the evening, reduces the incidence of heart disease. Aspirin keeps your arteries flowing while jazz dance is great exercise for heart and thighs, and nourishes the soul. If you're a *learner* you'll take the data, compare it to other things you know, and make a decision. You'll answer that all-important question, "Is it right for me?"

Luckily, the ability to learn lasts a lifetime. Whenever you need to, you can obtain new knowledge, tools, and skills; become more aware of what can be done to promote wellness; and seek out reliable information on measures for increasing longevity or reducing the incidence of disabilities later in life.

Active Involvement

Not long ago I attended a lecture given by Dr. Robert Butler, author of *Aging in America* and *Sex After Sixty* and founder of the National Institute on Aging. Back when aging was a subject rarely mentioned, he reminded us that how we prepare for aging and treat our older citizens is important to each of us individually and to society as a whole. On the subject of what keeps people going strong through their eighties and nineties or even longer, he notes that the people who live the longest and maintain the most satisfying lives tend to "have a sense of purpose." They are driven to do things, to leave their mark, to engage in pursuits they feel passionate about, and to positively influence people's lives.

People with a sense of purpose like being productive and feeling challenged. These qualities are fundamental ingredients in their formula for a fulfilling life. Everywhere they look they see opportunities to learn, build, and love. They are actively involved in the world around them and convinced that their presence, their contribution, can make a difference.

Senator John Glenn is a case in point. As an astronaut in the 1960s, he became the first American to orbit the earth. But he didn't stop there. He parlayed his fame and—far more important—his self-confident, can-do attitude into an impressive career as a U.S. senator, presidential candidate, and unfailing supporter of space travel. That same attitude no doubt helped him challenge the notion that only the young should go into space. "It's not an old people's thing," he was told. "Just give up," he was advised. But he would not. And as a result, in 1998, when he was seventy-seven years old, John Glenn went on a NASA space shuttle mission.

A sense of purpose can be aimed at world-changing causes such as ending global warming. It can be used to achieve something extraordinary such as becoming a space shuttle astronaut. Planting hydrangeas in window boxes, taking care of disabled folks, seeing grandchildren, being on the local library board can keep all of us feeling young and focused. Anything that captures your imagination and fuels your desire to stick around and stay healthy for lots of tomorrows will do.

A Hopeful Outlook

Folks who live long, rich lives (or seem destined to) don't spend much time worrying about failing to accomplish their goals. They assume they'll succeed. And if they falter, they change their project, their goals, or their perspective. What others might call a failure, they consider a temporary setback. There's always something they can do. And the notion that they might not live long enough or stay well enough to see important projects through to completion rarely crosses their minds.

"I've found that most of the time, most things work out for the best," Alex Hardy once told me. The hope and optimism expressed by many long-lived individuals are more than a reflection of six, seven, or eight decades of life experience. It is an attitude they've possessed throughout their lives, and one that has contributed to their remarkable longevity.

Hope is a life force, optimism a positive motivator. Believing that the eventual outcome of most endeavors will be for the best, optimists are more likely to undertake them and stick with their efforts despite any adversity they might encounter. As a result, they're more likely to achieve their objectives. And each achievement makes them more optimistic. "See, things really do work out for the best," they remind themselves. Then they go on to attempt additional endeavors, explore new subjects, interact more easily with other people, and take a more active role in maintaining their health and well-being—all behaviors that improve their odds of living longer and loving their lives.

IS HOPELESSNESS AS GOOD A PREDICTOR OF PREMATURE DEATH AS CHOLESTEROL? SCIENCE SAYS QUITE POSSIBLY.

How do I know that attitudes of hope and optimism or tendencies toward active involvement increase longevity? There is plenty of anecdotal evidence —the kind you accumulate through surveys, interviews, and word of mouth. In fact, a recent survey of New Jersey residents revealed that feeling "fulfilled in their daily lives" was the factor that played the greatest role in determining overall health. People in the best health reported it more often than any other item on the survey, including not smoking, a balanced diet, and exercise.

The exact impact life fulfillment and optimism have on longevity is difficult to quantify. We can't measure it as easily as serum cholesterol levels or the amount of fiber in your diet, but controlled studies that address the issue are already beginning to bear fruit.

For instance, the Centers for Disease Control and Prevention in Atlanta have been looking into hope's effect on health and longevity as part of their mammoth National Health and Nutrition Education Survey (NHANES). The project, which began in 1971, keeps tabs on the health, exercise, and dietary habits of a representative sample of approximately 15,000 Americans from all walks of life. A subgroup made up of 2,832 adults between the ages of forty-five and seventy-seven also filled out lengthy questionnaires as part of the National Health Examination Follow-up Study (NHEFS).

The NHEFS researchers were looking for one aspect of general well-being that would stand out—a Rosetta stone, if you will, that might predict who would live and who would die during the next decade. So they chose folks who were relatively healthy and free of apparent heart disease or cancer and asked them basic "how ya doing?" questions about their jobs, family life, marital relations, friends, family, and emotions. After the study's coordinators had compiled the data and eliminated variables they knew would influence heart disease and general health, such as smoking, cholesterol levels, education, marital status, blood pressure, and physical exercise, they made several discoveries, one of them involving hope, or more precisely the lack of it.

Participants were asked, "During the past month, have you felt so sad, discouraged, or hopeless or had so many problems that you wondered if anything was worthwhile?" They could select their answer from a six-point scale that ranged from complete agreement ("Extremely so—to the point that I have just about given up") at one end to complete disagreement ("No. Not at all. That's not me") at the other. For those who agreed in the extreme, the chances of dying or suffering a serious heart attack over the next decade were 2.2 times greater than the odds for those who disagreed. This correlation seemed to increase with age, with subjects fifty-five or older who felt the most hopeless having three times the risk. Their counterparts sixty-five or older were nearly *seven* times more likely to have fatal heart attacks. And while we know that treating hypertension and cholesterol undoubtedly increases longevity, it's time to look at hopelessness as a similar factor.

People with hopeful outlooks like the idea of adopting healthy habits at midlife and earlier in order to live longer and better in the future. It puts them in the driver's seat, where their confidence in their own abilities and expectation of positive outcomes make everything seem more manageable, including tasks a pessimist would call impossible. They don't give up hope when unexpected obstacles appear in their path. Even when chronic conditions or terminal illness limits their actual life expectancy, optimists are determined to live fully within the boundaries their disabilities set for them and to make the most of every day of their lives.

Bolstering Longevity's Basic Building Blocks

Clearly attitude counts. Not only have lifelong learning, active involvement, and a hopeful outlook been linked directly to increased life expectancy, but they also greatly influence what we choose to do to lengthen and enrich our lives. If these cornerstones of a long, healthy, high-quality life are part of your longevity code, you have an advantage. If they are not, or if you would describe them as a little shaky, you can gain some ground by developing them.

TO LEARN MORE THROUGHOUT YOUR LIFETIME

- Let curiosity be your guide. What subjects interest, intrigue, or fascinate you? Which diseases or conditions worry you? What kinds of people or historical events inspire you? Make a good long list of topics you wish you knew more about and start investigating them.

- Subscribe to newsletters. They cover almost any topic imaginable: aging, nutrition, financial planning, organic gardening, and nearly anything else that interests you.
- Go on-line often. You'll be able to tap into the vast resources of organizations such as the Centers for Disease Control and Prevention (CDC).
- And don't forget www.longevitycode.com, the longevity code Web site.
- Attend workshops and take courses. In addition to adding to your lifelong learning, classes of any kind provide opportunities to meet people whose interests are similar to your own, adding to your kinship and social spheres.

TO GET MORE ACTIVELY INVOLVED

- Expand your horizons. Go to that theme park. Watch the sun rise over the ocean. Perform your stand-up comedy routine at open-mike night. Skydive (former president George Bush did—on his seventy-fifth birthday). Trace your roots.
- Pursue a passion. Do something that moves and motivates you, excites and engages you, and adds meaning or purpose to your life. Indulge your love of folk dancing or open-water rowing, chamber music or Civil War reenactments. Immerse yourself. Resume an activity you used to love but may have abandoned. Or get involved in a new endeavor, perhaps something you discovered while expanding your horizons. Give it your all.
- Be proactive. On life's merry-go-round, the gold rings of longevity, health, and happiness won't fall into your lap. You have to reach for them. You have to do your part. So listen a little more closely. Speak up a little sooner. Reach out to someone who's in need. If you want to know the answer, ask. By doing a tiny bit extra whenever you get a chance to, you can't help but become more actively involved with life.
- Share the wealth. The wealth of who you are, that is. Offer your services to people who need them. Volunteer your time and talents to organizations whose work you believe in. Participate in fundraisers. Sharpen your skills and pass them on to others by teaching classes or writing articles or mentoring.

TO BUILD A MORE HOPEFUL OUTLOOK

- Accumulate evidence of success. People who are low on hope and optimism tend to focus on their failures, losses, and disappointments and predict more of the same. They did not invent the dark occurrences in their lives. Those things really happened. However, they overlook, forget, or negate the fact that there have been bright spots in their lives as well. They need to readmit that information in order to develop a more balanced and ultimately more positive point of view. One place to start is to list everything in your life that has ever worked out for the best. This includes both the outcomes you were happy about at the time they occurred and those that didn't seem so great initially but ultimately led to better things.

- Halt harmful, hopeless thought processes. How many times have you caught yourself thinking, "This will never work" or "What's the point? Nothing ever turns out the way I want it to"? Few things kill hope and optimism more quickly than this negative self-talk. So the next time similarly self-defeating thoughts start crowding your consciousness, cut them off at the pass. In your mind's eye, picture a stop sign and hold the image until the unwanted thoughts fade. Or imagine an eraser wiping a slate clean of all the offending words.

- Practice positive affirmations. In spare moments—when you're driving alone or vacuuming your carpets or taking a walk—visualize yourself as a lovable, capable person. To reinforce that image, repeat encouraging statements, known as positive affirmations, to yourself. "I am strong and I am well," "I can accomplish what I set out to do," and "I deserve a longer, sweeter life" are just a few examples. If you say them enough, they will take root and become part of your self-perception.

Hold a Picture of the Future You Really Want in Your Mind's Eye

Hope always travels hand in hand with something to hope for—a goal, a dream, a vision of your life as you want it to be five or ten or twenty years down the line. A nice clear picture is most helpful for setting goals and timetables. Fueled by hope, the more you know about where you want to go (or to avoid going), the more likely you'll be to take the right steps to get there. But even a rudimentary sketch may be enough to inspire you and give you something to aspire to.

What should go into your picture? Anything that makes being alive —and striving to stay alive longer—a worthwhile endeavor. And that's a very personal call. There are no hard-and-fast rules when it comes to defining life quality. We each have our own ideas about what drives or delights us; what injects joy, contentment, vitality, and value into our lives; and what is absolutely essential to our overall well-being.

Perhaps the truest test of the sweet life is the genuine joy and contentment it provides. Its ingredients don't leave you feeling guilty or hungover on a regular basis or alone in your king-sized bed while your love sleeps in the guest room. You prize and cherish the behaviors that enhance your life. When you broaden your definitions of the sweet life to include all five spheres, the picture changes.

Although it's harder to come by when you're destitute and distraught over money problems, life's sweetness isn't measured in dollars. And it doesn't demand perfect health. If we all had to be in the same condition as a college or professional athlete in order to consider our lives fulfilling and worthwhile, most of us would be in big trouble.

Likewise, the number of years you've spent on the planet should not dictate your definition of a sweet life. If you're fifty and you want to scuba dive for the first time or enroll in college or start a coffee shop–bookstore, age is no reason not to give it a try. If you can see yourself continuing to kayak or compete in chess tournaments or grow prize-winning orchids until you're ninety, then go ahead, give it your best shot.

Yes, time does change us. It always has. Our aerobic capacity, stamina, vision, hearing, and flexibility may not be what they once were. (Even elite athletes lose a percent or two of muscle mass per year beginning at age thirty.) But we can compensate and adapt.

- We may still be able to run, just not as fast. Or we may choose to give our joints a break and take up fitness walking.
- We can still dance the night away. But instead of bounding out of bed the next morning and heading to the beach to play volleyball, we may need more time to recover. Relaxing on the sofa with the New York Times and a cup of latte is not a bad trade-off.
- We can still concentrate, memorize, and learn new concepts. It may simply take a bit more effort as we age.

If we accept these realities and adapt to normal changes when we notice them, we'll be able to continue cherished pursuits—and explore new ones. Your portrait of an ideal future is always a work in progress anyway.

My friends Howard and Rona, in their thirties, were determined to make lots of money, retire at fifty, and travel the world in high style. They would cruise on luxury liners, play on the world's greatest golf courses, sample the best cuisine any country had to offer, and in short indulge their every whim.

As highly paid professionals who saved religiously, invested brilliantly, and remained childless by choice, it looked as if they would have the financial wherewithal to fulfill their vision. But then both of Rona's parents fell ill, her mother with cancer and her father with multiple sclerosis. Taking care of them was financially and emotionally draining. It not only set Howard and Rona's retirement timetable back a few years but changed the way they viewed life as well. Material things didn't seem to matter as much, while social ties, spirituality, and simplicity meant more. Although an occasional trip in grand style remained in the picture, Howard and Rona's new vision for the future revolved around living with less in a cabin on a lake and having no schedule to stick to and no one depending on their care.

The couple was living out their dream when I met them. But then someone asked for their help raising funds for a local homeless shelter, which somehow led to more charity work and deeper involvement in their community. Now Rona and Howard jointly oversee a community housing organization that builds homes for needy families and runs an emergency shelter. With their schedules tightly packed and countless people depending on them, their golden years aren't quite what they'd expected. Instead, they're better than they ever dreamed.

How's Your Foundation?

Even the most rigorous adoption of the longevity boosters detailed on the pages that follow will be less effective if they are not built on a solid foundation of the three elements I've just discussed: lifelong learning, active involvement, and a hopeful outlook. How do you stack up?

- *Are you committed to lifelong learning?* Knowledge changes us. It shows us how to do things and often motivates us to do them. You might, for example, read a food label, which you had never done before. Perhaps you didn't even intend to read it. This user-friendly information can help you choose your foods wisely. Because you checked the label, you may have decided to eat something with less saturated fat or sugar or salt. And that is a longevity booster.
- *Do you feel fully engaged in your life?* Active involvement means you enjoy things you participate in, and you participate in things you enjoy. You have goals and aspirations.
- *What are you hoping for?* Hopefulness is simply the belief that there is a good life out there for you. After all, if you don't believe that tomorrow can be better than today, why should you quit smoking? Why should you buckle your seat belt? Why should you call your mom and make up after a fight? Why fund your IRA?
- *What's stopping you from taking care of yourself?* From making the positive changes in your life that will bring you more happiness? Is it inertia? Time? Fear? Well, fear is a great motivator, and we can turn it into something positive. But hope feels better.

EXERCISE 5

Think about what you are doing now to keep abreast of information you need to live a longer, sweeter life. It may be reading medical newsletters or learning a new computer program. Anything that exercises your mind counts—*anything*. List your answers in the "Doing Now" column of the chart below. In the "Would Like to Do" column, list things related to longevity and wellness that it would be helpful to know more about or learn how to do. Again, whatever you think constitutes active learning, in any field, counts.

Now think of this another way. Using the chart below, fill in the "Doing Now" column with hobbies, volunteer work, family commitments, paid work, passions, interests, and other activities that you are now actively engaged in.

Do you still get a sense of meaning, purpose, and fulfillment from these activities? Code each item you've listed with a + for things you'd like to do *more* of, a − for things you'd like to do *less* of, and an = sign for those you'd be happy to continue at the same level of involvement.

Then, in the "Would Like to Do" column, list new activities you'd like to try.

DOING NOW	WOULD LIKE TO DO
1.	1.
2.	2.
3.	3.
4.	4.
5.	5.

When most of us think about the years ahead, we hope for health, happiness, self-sufficiency, mobility, closeness, and any number of other features we equate with a sweet life. But what do you see specifically?

Picture yourself two years from now, then five years after that, and again at whatever age you consider really old. Imagine your life as you'd like it to be at each of these milestones. Where are you living? What are you doing with your time? How do you look and feel? With whom are you associating? Do you have support and camaraderie from friends, family, a life partner? Are you living on your own and pursuing activities you've long enjoyed? Have you added new pastimes and passions to your repertoire as well? What are they? How's your health? Are there any habits you've changed or abandoned? Any positive practices you've adopted? What about your finances? Do you have enough money to meet your needs and to afford a few of the extras you want?

EXERCISE 6—My Dreams and Aspirations for the Future

In the space provided here or on a separate sheet of paper, jot down some of the more important images, hopes, dreams, and wishes that come to mind for each period of time.

TWO YEARS FROM NOW	FIVE YEARS FROM NOW	WHEN I'M MUCH OLDER
1.	1.	1.
2.	2.	2.
3.	3.	3.
4.	4.	4.
5.	5.	5.

PART II

Taking Action

Your Personal Longevity Prescription

6

Choosing–and Taking–Your First Steps Toward Longevity

AND NOW THE MOMENT OF TRUTH. You are going to crack your longevity code and set your sights on a sweeter future. I'm sure you have some general ideas about what you can do to get there. The time has come to turn those ideas into actions, to select the measures you want in your personal longevity prescription. The only hurdle remaining is deciding where to start.

Just how *do* you choose the action steps to top your to-do list? If your goal is to live a long, contented, healthy life, the question is which is more worthwhile—taking an aspirin a day or having a healthy marriage? Developing a stronger relationship with your parents or jogging four times a week? What about meditation, or church or synagogue attendance, or having a good laugh? Does one booster have a greater impact than another or make life especially sweet? How can you tell which measures will give you the best return on your investment or not require more time and effort than you're willing to invest?

To answer such questions, you'll need both an understanding of what various longevity-boosting measures entail and a method for judging the relative merits of each—something similar to the Michelin guides that rate restaurants based on the quality of their food, service, and so on. Those brief critiques with their star ratings have saved me from awful dining experiences in unfamiliar cities more than once. Likewise, *Consumer Reports'* reviews of everything from toasters to laptop computers have spared me from weeks or more of arduous research in areas that are not my forte. That's what the system I'm about to describe is designed to do for you.

The System in a Nutshell

From a truly enormous body of information on longevity, I chose seventy-six action steps and divided them into five categories that correspond to the five spheres of wellness. I determined what each booster had to offer as well as what you would need to do to reap those benefits, and I reported on my findings. (Booster summaries start on page 175.) Then I looked for a means of comparing and contrasting those action steps, something that would tell you:

1. Which boosters have the most impact on life expectancy
2. Which ones are most likely to add to life's sweetness
3. Which will take the most (or least) effort to initiate and sustain

Even more important was to find a way to help you determine which of the boosters were the best for you personally.

As I started trying to sequence, compare, and rate longevity boosters, my head was swimming with data. I was faced with a mind-boggling array of information and struggled to organize it by jotting down ideas on Post-it notes and moving them around. This here. That there. The chartreuse more important than the blue . . . and then it struck me. Cards! The entire decision-making, action-planning process would be easier to handle if people could actually handle, study, and sort a deck of cards. You'll find the finished "deck" laid out on pages 135–160.

Each numbered card includes:

• *An impact rating based on a five-star system.* Five stars indicates actions that do the most to increase longevity and life quality (the sweetness factor). Five-star actions also have the most scientific and anecdotal information behind them. A one-star booster would have virtually no impact and no merit in comparison to other boosters. I include only one: annual chest X-rays as a screening test for cancer.

In addition, impact ratings reflect a measure's known risks or reported drawbacks. There are no perfect boosters. Medications have side effects. Screening tests have consequences, from false positive results to dubious treatment options. A booster with positive results in one sphere can have negative repercussions in another. I weighed all of these factors before assigning my star ratings.

- *A list of amplifiers.* These are longevity busters, risk factors, givens, or current life situations that turn up the volume on a longevity booster, increasing its impact level. For instance, a personal history of heart disease, and especially a previous heart attack, amplifies the importance of staying away from cigarettes or controlling blood pressure or taking an aspirin a day. Those are high-impact longevity boosters for anyone, but for someone who has had a heart attack, they are literally matters of life or death. If a booster's amplifier list has one or several of your personal givens, risk factors, or medical conditions on it, that booster will have more impact on you. There's good reason to include it in your personal longevity prescription. You may even want to make it your first step.

- *A thumbnail sketch.* This will give you a rudimentary idea of what the longevity-boosting measure entails. More detailed descriptions appear in the upcoming pages.

- *An action rating.* This lets you know how much effort a particular action step may require. An easy longevity booster is your basic no-brainer. It's quick, uncomplicated, and possibly fun. The only real challenge is getting motivated to do it initially and remembering to do it often enough to form a positive habit. Example: buckling your seat belt.

A booster with a moderate rating is a bit more challenging. You may have to rearrange your schedule, get cooperation from others, locate resources, or overcome fears and preconceived notions. Example: exercising four times a week or meditating for fifteen minutes a day.

Always a challenge, difficult boosters often require major lifestyle changes such as giving up alcohol, switching jobs, or conquering anger. You may have to take a personal risk by going into therapy or giving up something you are physically addicted or emotionally attached to—such as cigarettes.

You will see easy-to-moderate or moderate-to-difficult ratings attached to some boosters, such as "developing skills to cope with stress," because their difficulty depends on which of several specific suggestions you choose to pursue. They also appear where your preferences and/or fears play a role. For instance, getting a Pap test is easy—if you go to your doctor to get one, which is moderately difficult for some women to do.

CREATING YOUR DECK OF LONGEVITY CARDS

- *Start* by getting the materials you'll need to work through this sorting-and-selection process. These include a pen or pencil and notepad or paper to jot down ideas that may occur to you along the way.

- *Next* create your own deck of cards, either by cutting them directly from the book or photocopying them and then cutting. The cards are arranged in numerical order from 1 through 76 (starting on page 135). Take a few minutes to glance through them. If you're curious or intrigued by certain boosters, feel free to skip ahead and read more about them in the cross-referenced booster section (Part III).

- *Finally* set aside a block of time. I recommend an hour, preferably one when you can escape from pressures or distractions. This is very important. There's a certain amount of intuition and insight involved in this process, and both require a calm mind and unhurried time. So try not to pick this up when you are stressed out or in a rush. You may find it helpful to have something to eat, so you're not hungry, and unplug the phone. Take this seriously, because you deserve a long and sweet life.

EXERCISE 7—Your Longevity Code

CRACKING YOUR LONGEVITY CODE IS AS EASY AS 1-2-3

1. Complete *Your Personal Longevity Code Summary.*
2. Fill out and mark up *Your Longevity Buster Questionnaire.*
3. Select the *Longevity Booster Cards* that apply to you and follow the instructions to complete your plan.

STEP 1: YOUR PERSONAL LONGEVITY CODE SUMMARY

Fill in the summary sheet below, turning back to the previous chapters as needed. What have you learned about yourself that might help you put together an effective, palatable prescription for a longer, sweeter life?

Using the space provided below or your own blank sheets of paper, complete the sentences I've started for you. For best results, list at least two but no more than five responses.

Check your vision for the future (Chapter 1).
The goals for my future that are the most important to me include:
1.

2.

3.

Check your wellness sphere summaries (Chapter 2).
My strongest assets in each sphere are:
Physical:

Mental:

Kinship:

Spiritual:

Material:

The deficits in each sphere I'd benefit most from remedying are:

Physical:

Mental:

Kinship:

Spiritual:

Material:

Think about the hand you were dealt (Chapter 3).

The givens that work in my favor include:

The givens I most need to compensate for:

Review your risk factors (Chapter 4).

Based on my givens and habits, the causes of premature death I am most susceptible to are:

The deadly diseases, disabling conditions, and/or effects of aging that I am most concerned about are:

Finally, the actions aimed at increasing longevity that I have already taken are:

STEP 2: YOUR LONGEVITY BUSTER QUESTIONNAIRE

Read through the statements below. They reflect longevity-busting attitudes, behaviors, and circumstances. For each one, ask yourself, "Does this describe me?" When your answer is yes, place a check mark beside the buster. When your answer is no, you can either draw a line through the item to denote that it does not apply to you or simply not check it and move on.

Note: The boosters you see on the questionnaire will be used to develop your longevity plan. How to use them is explained in Step 3 (page 129). The boosters themselves are explained in detail in Part III.

Physical

❑ I smoke cigarettes, cigars, a pipe, or use snuff.
> Booster 1: Stay Away from Tobacco
> Booster 26: Get a Chest X-ray to Screen for Lung Cancer
> Booster 72: Minimize Your Debt

❑ I have more than one drink per day (for women) or two drinks per day (for men).
> Booster 2: Don't Overdo Alcohol
> Booster 72: Minimize Your Debt

❑ I have a significant illness or chronic condition.
> Booster 38: Have a Good Relationship with Your Doctor
> Booster 40: Use Effective Medications Effectively
> Booster 41: Consider Complementary and Alternative Medicine
> Booster 56: Build a Strong Social Network
> Booster 61: Explore the Spiritual Within You
> Booster 62: Get Involved in a Spiritual Community

❑ It's been too long since I've seen a doctor for a routine checkup.
> Booster 37: Get Periodic Tune-ups
> Booster 38: Have a Good Relationship with Your Doctor

❑ I have a sedentary lifestyle and simply don't exercise enough.
> Booster 13: Get Your Muscles Moving

❑ I do not always take precautions to avoid contracting a sexually transmitted disease.
> Booster 2: Don't Overdo Alcohol
> Booster 20: Have Safer Sex to Stop Sexually Transmitted Diseases
> Booster 21: Have Pap Tests to Screen for Cervical Cancer

❑ I have high blood pressure—higher than 130/85.
> Booster 2: Don't Overdo Alcohol
> Booster 5: Eat More Fruits and Veggies–Five to Seven Servings per Day
> Booster 6: Go for the Healthiest Quality and Quantity of Food
> Booster 11: Limit Your Salt Intake
> Booster 27: Monitor Blood Pressure and Control Hypertension
> Booster 40: Use Effective Medications Effectively
> Booster 47: Develop More and Better Skills for Coping with Stress

❑ My total cholesterol level is greater than 200 mg/dl.

> Booster 5: Eat More Fruits and Veggies–Five to Seven Servings per Day
>
> Booster 6: Go for the Healthiest Quality and Quantity of Food
>
> Booster 7: Cut the Fat
>
> Booster 8: Eat More Fiber
>
> Booster 28: Measure Your HDL, LDL, and Total Cholesterol Levels as a Guide to Heart Health
>
> Booster 40: Use Effective Medications Effectively

❑ I am not up-to-date on my immunizations (including influenza and pneumonia).

> Booster 39: Get Immunized

❑ I don't drink the equivalent of eight glasses of water each day.

> Booster 42: Drink Plenty of Water

❑ I am more than 30 percent above my healthiest weight.

> Booster 6: Go for the Healthiest Quality and Quantity of Food
>
> Booster 7: Cut the Fat
>
> Booster 9: Eat Breakfast
>
> Booster 10: Reduce Your Sugar Intake
>
> Booster 12: Limit Snacking
>
> Booster 13: Get Your Muscles Moving

❑ I don't eat enough fiber.

> Booster 8: Eat More Fiber
>
> Booster 22: Screen for Colon and Rectal Cancer

❑ I do *not* take a daily aspirin (when I could do so safely).

> Booster 31: Add an Aspirin Every Day

❑ I do *not* get enough calcium from food or supplements (1.5 grams/day).

> Booster 30: Have Your Bone Density Tested for Signs of Osteoporosis
>
> Booster 36: Make Room for Calcium and Vitamin D

❑ I do *not* have a daily glass of wine.

> Booster 32: Drink a Little Wine

❑ I do not take a multivitamin, vitamin E, or vitamin C daily.

> Booster 34: Take a Multivitamin
>
> Booster 35: Take Advantage of Antioxidants: Vitamins C and E, Beta-carotene, Selenium

❑ I am exposed to significant amounts of secondhand smoke.

> Booster 1: Stay Away from Tobacco
>
> Booster 68: Ensure Job Safety
>
> Booster 75: Nurture Your Home

Booster 76: Reduce Air Pollution, Radon, and Indoor Toxins

❑ I do *not* consume five to seven servings of fruits and vegetables a day.

Booster 5: Eat More Fruits and Veggies—Five to Seven Servings per Day

Booster 22: Screen for Colon and Rectal Cancer

❑ When I am on a boat I do not wear a life preserver.

Booster 19: Practice Water Safety

❑ I use marijuana frequently.

Booster 4: Curtail Illicit Drug Use, Part II—Marijuana

❑ I rarely wear seat belts.

Booster 15: Fasten Seat Belts

Booster 16: Drive Safely

❑ I don't use sunscreen when I am outdoors.

Booster 14: Limit Sun Exposure

❑ When given prescription drugs I do *not* always take them precisely as directed by my doctor or pharmacist. I often don't know the side effects of the medications I take.

Booster 38: Have a Good Relationship with Your Doctor

Booster 40: Use Effective Medications Effectively

❑ I use cocaine, crack, or heroin (even occasionally).

Booster 3: Curtail Illicit Drug Use, Part I—Heroin, Cocaine, Crack, and Other Hard Drugs

Booster 45: Treat Depression

Booster 46: Manage Anger

Booster 56: Build a Strong Social Network

Booster 61: Explore the Spiritual Within You

❑ I don't wear a helmet when riding a bike, boarding, or blading.

Booster 17: Wear a Helmet

❑ I could be a safer driver.

Booster 15: Fasten Seat Belts

Booster 16: Drive Sanely

❑ I do *not* have a good relationship with my doctor.

Booster 37: Get Periodic Tune-ups

Booster 38: Have a Good Relationship with Your Doctor

❑ I do not adequately brush, floss, and take care of my teeth.

Booster 44: Take Care of Your Teeth and Gums

❑ I get less than seven or more than nine hours of sleep per day.

Booster 43: Get Enough Sleep

Booster 45: Treat Depression

❑ I do *not* take estrogen when I could.
>   Booster 33: Take Estrogen

❑ I have not seen a dentist in the last twelve months.
>   Booster 44: Take Care of Your Teeth and Gums

❑ More than 30 percent of my calories come from high-fat foods.
>   Booster 5: Eat More Fruits and Veggies–Five to Seven Servings per Day
>   Booster 6: Go for the Healthiest Quality and Quantity of Food
>   Booster 7: Cut the Fat
>   Booster 8: Eat More Fiber

❑ I have *not* been screened recently for high blood pressure, cancer, heart disease, or diabetes.
>   Booster 37: Get Periodic Tune-ups

Mental

❑ I could be suffering from depression.
>   Booster 45: Treat Depression
>   Booster 47: Develop More and Better Skills for Coping with Stress
>   Booster 51: Cultivate a Resilient, Optimistic, Can-do Attitude

❑ I am worried about my health or safety but *not* doing anything about it.
>   Booster 47: Develop More and Better Skills for Coping with Stress
>   Booster 48: Stop Worrying Yourself to Death
>   Booster 50: Commit to Lifelong Learning

❑ I am too anxious.
>   Booster 47: Develop More and Better Skills for Coping with Stress
>   Booster 48: Stop Worrying Yourself to Death
>   Booster 52: Hang on to Your Sense of Humor

❑ At times I am abusive, destructive, or mean.
>   Booster 45: Treat Depression
>   Booster 46: Manage Anger

> If appropriate, see:
>   Booster 2: Don't Overdo Alcohol
>   Booster 3: Curtail Illicit Drug Use, Part I–Heroin, Cocaine, Crack, and Other Hard Drugs

❑ I get angry easily or often.
>   Booster 45: Treat Depression
>   Booster 46: Manage Anger

If appropriate see:

    Booster 2: Don't Overdo Alcohol

    Booster 3: Curtail Illicit Drug Use, Part I—Heroin, Cocaine, Crack, and Other Hard Drugs

❑ I often feel overwhelmed by demands and responsibilities.

    Booster 47: Develop More and Better Skills for Coping with Stress

    Booster 51: Cultivate a Resilient, Optimistic, Can-do Attitude

    Booster 52: Hang on to Your Sense of Humor

❑ I am stressed out.

    Booster 47: Develop More and Better Skills for Coping with Stress

    Booster 51: Cultivate a Resilient, Optimistic, Can-do Attitude

    Booster 52: Hang on to Your Sense of Humor

    Booster 67: Pursue Job Satisfaction

❑ I am bored or *not* getting enough intellectual stimulation.

    Booster 50: Commit to Lifelong Learning

    Booster 51: Cultivate a Resilient, Optimistic, Can-do Attitude

    Booster 56: Build a Strong Social Network

    Booster 58: Build Good Relationships with Friends

    Booster 61: Explore the Spiritual Within You

❑ I am grieving.

    Booster 56: Build a Strong Social Network

    Booster 61: Explore the Spiritual Within You

    Booster 62: Get Involved in a Spiritual Community

❑ I don't take time to relax and enjoy life. I don't do things that make me happy often enough.

    Booster 47: Develop More and Better Skills for Coping with Stress

    Booster 52: Hang on to Your Sense of Humor

    Booster 56: Build a Strong Social Network

    Booster 61: Explore the Spiritual Within You

    Booster 63: Take Time with Mother Nature

    Booster 66: Volunteer Service to Others

    Booster 67: Pursue Job Satisfaction

    Booster 71: Calculate How Much Is Enough

❑ I lack a vision of where I wish to be five or ten years from now.

    Booster 61: Explore the Spiritual Within You

    Booster 64: Don't Avoid Thinking About Death

    Booster 67: Pursue Job Satisfaction

    Booster 71: Calculate How Much Is Enough

❏ I am afraid and anxious about trying new things.

    Booster 48: Stop Worrying Yourself to Death

    Booster 50: Commit to Lifelong Learning

    Booster 51: Cultivate a Resilient, Optimistic, Can-do Attitude

❏ I rarely read and learn about health, wellness, and fitness.

    Booster 50: Commit to Lifelong Learning

    Booster 64: Don't Avoid Thinking About Death

❏ I don't laugh enough.

    Booster 47: Develop More and Better Skills for Coping with Stress

    Booster 52: Hang on to Your Sense of Humor

    Booster 67: Pursue Job Satisfaction

❏ I don't do enough to keep my memory sharp.

    Booster 49: Address Alzheimer's, Senility, and Dementia

    Booster 50: Commit to Lifelong Learning

    Booster 53: Fight Forgetfulness

❏ I rarely pay attention to my feelings.

    Booster 45: Treat Depression

    Booster 47: Develop More and Better Skills for Coping with Stress

    Booster 51: Cultivate a Resilient, Optimistic, Can-do Attitude

  If appropriate see:

    Booster 2: Don't Overdo Alcohol

    Booster 3: Curtail Illicit Drug Use, Part I–Heroin, Cocaine, Crack, and Other Hard Drugs

    Booster 54: Extract Yourself from Abusive Relationships

Kinship

❏ I am lonely.

    Booster 55: Have a Satisfying, Long-term, Committed Marriage or its Equivalent

    Booster 56: Build a Strong Social Network

    Booster 60: Own a Pet

    Booster 62: Get Involved in a Spiritual Community

    Booster 66: Volunteer Service to Others

❏ I would like to have children.

    Booster 55: Have a Satisfying, Long-term, Committed Marriage or Its Equivalent

❏ I am physically or verbally abused at home or at work.

    Booster 54: Extract Yourself from Abusive Relationships

    Booster 67: Pursue Job Satisfaction

If appropriate see:

Booster 2: Don't Overdo Alcohol

Booster 3: Curtail Illicit Drug Use, Part I—Heroin, Cocaine, Crack, and Other Hard Drugs

❑ I am not married or in a loving relationship.

Booster 55: Have a Satisfying, Long-term, Committed Marriage or Its Equivalent

❑ My relationship with my partner is distant and unsatisfying, or rife with conflict.

Booster 55: Have a Satisfying, Long-term, Committed Marriage or Its Equivalent

Booster 57: Build Good Relationships with Your Family

Booster 59: Savor Sex and Intimacy

❑ I have a distant and unsatisfying relationship with my siblings, parents, or children.

Booster 57: Build Good Relationships with Your Family

❑ I do not feel part of the community where I live.

Booster 56: Build a Strong Social Network

Booster 58: Build Good Relationships with Friends

Booster 71: Calculate How Much Is Enough

❑ I would like to have one good friend, but I do *not*.

Booster 58: Build Good Relationships with Friends

Booster 66: Volunteer Service to Others

❑ I lack a social support system—people I can count on.

Booster 56: Build a Strong Social Network

Booster 57: Build Good Relationships with Your Family

Booster 58: Build Good Relationships with Friends

Booster 75: Nurture Your Home

❑ My sex life is unsatisfying.

Booster 59: Savor Sex and Intimacy

❑ I regularly come in contact with angry, abusive, or difficult people.

Booster 54: Extract Yourself from Abusive Relationships

Booster 67: Pursue Job Satisfaction

❑ I find it difficult to assert myself.

Booster 47: Develop More and Better Skills for Coping with Stress

Booster 50: Commit to Lifelong Learning

Booster 51: Cultivate a Resilient, Optimistic, Can-do Attitude

Booster 52: Hang on to Your Sense of Humor

Booster 54: Extract Yourself from Abusive Relationships

Booster 67: Pursue Job Satisfaction

Spiritual

❑ I would like to expand my spiritual horizons, meditate, practice yoga, or return to my spiritual roots.

    Booster 61: Explore the Spiritual Within You

    Booster 62: Get Involved in a Spiritual Community

❑ I rarely take the time to experience beauty, nourish my soul with art, music, or books, or take time to be with Mother Nature.

    Booster 50: Commit to Lifelong Learning

    Booster 61: Explore the Spiritual Within You

    Booster 63: Take Time with Mother Nature

❑ I haven't thought about dying.

    Booster 64: Don't Avoid Thinking About Death

❑ I do *not* have a living will.

    Booster 65: Prepare Your Living Will and Advance Directives

❑ I don't consider myself a spiritual person.

    Booster 61: Explore the Spiritual Within You

    Booster 63: Take Time with Mother Nature

    Booster 66: Volunteer Service to Others

❑ I rarely volunteer service or donate money to charities or causes in which I believe.

    Booster 56: Build a Strong Social Network

    Booster 66: Volunteer Service to Others

    Booster 71: Calculate How Much Is Enough

Material

❑ I owe too much money.

    Booster 71: Calculate How Much Is Enough

    Booster 72: Minimize Your Debt

❑ I do not budget well. I do not have enough savings.

    Booster 69: Procure Adequate Job Benefits

    Booster 72: Minimize Your Debt

    Booster 73: Maximize Your Savings and Retirement Income

❑ I am in a dangerous line of work

    Booster 68: Ensure Job Safety

❑ I lack sufficient funds to pay for necessities.

    Booster 69: Procure Adequate Job Benefits

Booster 71: Calculate How Much Is Enough
Booster 72: Minimize Your Debt

❑ I don't think I am as well off as I should be at this point in my life.
Booster 67: Pursue Job Satisfaction
Booster 69: Procure Adequate Job Benefits
Booster 70: Make Your Workplace Fun
Booster 75: Nurture Your Home

❑ I am not actively saving money or making adequate preparations for my retirement.
Booster 69: Procure Adequate Job Benefits
Booster 73: Maximize Your Savings and Retirement Income

❑ I am unhappy with my present career.
Booster 67: Pursue Job Satisfaction
Booster 69: Procure Adequate Job Benefits
Booster 70: Make Your Workplace Fun

❑ I do not have adequate health care, disability, and other insurance coverage.
Booster 69: Procure Adequate Job Benefits

❑ My neighborhood is unsafe.
Booster 74: Don't Live in a Violent Environment
Booster 75: Nurture Your Home

❑ I have not taken a vacation recently.
Booster 69: Procure Adequate Job Benefits
Booster 71: Calculate How Much Is Enough

❑ I would rather live in a different town, neighborhood, or part of the country.
Booster 67: Pursue Job Satisfaction
Booster 75: Nurture Your Home

❑ I have a gun or dangerous equipment in my house that is not safe and secure.
Booster 18: Reduce Hazards in Your Home

❑ I work in a dangerous or unhealthy environment.
Booster 74: Don't Live in a Violent Environment
Booster 75: Nurture Your Home

❑ The air where I live is polluted.
Booster 76: Reduce Air Pollution, Radon, and Indoor Toxins

❑ My house has not been tested for lead, radon, carbon monoxide, or other toxins.

    Booster 18: Reduce Hazards in Your Home

    Booster 76: Reduce Air Pollution, Radon, and Indoor Toxins

---

This is a separate longevity questionnaire for those who have a strong family history of heart disease, cancer, stroke, diabetes, depression, suicide, alcoholism, drug abuse, or Alzheimer's. If family history is your overriding concern, then tackle this questionnaire. If not, I recommend that you skip it for now and return to it later. The personal longevity questionnaire that you just completed is more likely to point you in the right direction to crack your longevity code.

❑ I have a strong family history of heart disease.

    Booster 1: Stay Away from Tobacco

    Booster 2: Don't Overdo Alcohol

    Booster 3: Curtail Illicit Drug Use, Part I—Heroin, Cocaine, Crack, and Other Hard Drugs

    Booster 5: Eat More Fruits and Veggies—Five to Seven Servings per Day

    Booster 7: Cut the Fat

    Booster 8: Eat More Fiber

    Booster 13: Get Your Muscles Moving

    Booster 27: Monitor Blood Pressure and Control Hypertension

    Booster 28: Measure Your HDL, LDL, and Total Cholesterol Levels as a Guide to Heart Health

    Booster 29: Have Your Blood Sugar Levels Checked to Detect Diabetes

    Booster 31: Add an Aspirin Every Day

    Booster 32: Drink a Little Wine

    Booster 33: Take Estrogen

    Booster 34: Take a Multivitamin

    Booster 35: Take Advantage of Antioxidants: Vitamins C and E, Beta-carotene, Selenium

    Booster 37: Get Periodic Tune-ups

    Booster 41: Consider Complementary and Alternative Medicine

    Booster 43: Get Enough Sleep

    Booster 44: Take Care of Your Teeth and Gums

    Booster 45: Treat Depression

    Booster 46: Manage Anger

    Booster 47: Develop More and Better Skills for Coping with Stress

    Booster 48: Stop Worrying Yourself to Death

Booster 55: Have a Satisfying, Long-term, Committed Marriage or Its Equivalent

Booster 56: Build a Strong Social Network

Booster 57: Build Good Relationships with Your Family

Booster 58: Build Good Relationships with Friends

Booster 61: Explore the Spiritual Within You

Booster 63: Take Time with Mother Nature

Booster 67: Pursue Job Satisfaction

Booster 71: Calculate How Much Is Enough

❑ I have a strong family history of cancer.

Booster 1: Stay Away from Tobacco

Booster 2: Don't Overdo Alcohol

Booster 3: Curtail Illicit Drug Use, Part I—Heroin, Cocaine, Crack, and Other Hard Drugs

Booster 5: Eat More Fruits and Veggies—Five to Seven Servings per Day

Booster 6: Go for the Healthiest Quality and Quantity of Food

Booster 7: Cut the Fat

Booster 8: Eat More Fiber

Booster 13: Get Your Muscles Moving

Booster 14: Limit Sun Exposure

Booster 20: Have Safer Sex to Stop Sexually Transmitted Diseases

Booster 21: Have Pap Tests to Screen for Cervical Cancer

Booster 23: Screen for Breast Cancer

Booster 24: Screen for Skin Cancer

Booster 25: Screen for Prostate Cancer

Booster 34: Take a Multivitamin

Booster 35: Take Advantage of Antioxidants: Vitamins C and E, Beta-carotene, Selenium

Booster 37: Get Periodic Tune-ups

Booster 41: Consider Complementary and Alternative Medicine

Booster 50: Commit to Lifelong Learning

Booster 76: Reduce Air Pollution, Radon, and Indoor Toxins

❑ I have a strong family history of stroke.
See Heart Disease (page 126)—risk factors are the same, although the most important of these is:

Booster 27: Monitor Blood Pressure and Control Hypertension

❑ I have a strong family history of diabetes.

Booster 5: Eat More Fruits and Veggies—Five to Seven Servings per Day

Booster 6: Go for the Healthiest Quality and Quantity of Food

Booster 7: Cut the Fat

Booster 8: Eat More Fiber

Booster 10: Reduce Your Sugar Intake

Booster 12: Limit Snacking

Booster 13: Get Your Muscles Moving

Booster 29: Have Your Blood Sugar Levels Checked to Detect Diabetes

❏ I have a strong family history of depression.

Booster 2: Don't Overdo Alcohol

Booster 3: Curtail Illicit Drug Use, Part I—Heroin, Cocaine, Crack, and Other Hard Drugs

Booster 4: Curtail Illicit Drug Use, Part II—Marijuana

Booster 41: Consider Complementary and Alternative Medicine

Booster 45: Treat Depression

Booster 47: Develop More and Better Skills for Coping with Stress

Booster 48: Stop Worrying Yourself to Death

Booster 51: Cultivate a Resilient, Optimistic, Can-do Attitude

Booster 52: Hang on to Your Sense of Humor

Booster 54: Extract Yourself from Abusive Relationships

Booster 55: Have a Satisfying, Long-term, Committed Marriage or Its Equivalent

Booster 56: Build a Strong Social Network

Booster 59: Savor Sex and Intimacy

Booster 61: Explore the Spiritual Within You

Booster 62: Get Involved in a Spiritual Community

Booster 66: Volunteer Service to Others

Booster 67: Pursue Job Satisfaction

❏ I have a strong family history of suicide.

See Depression (above)—risk factors are the same.

❏ I have a strong family history of alcoholism.

Booster 2: Don't Overdo Alcohol

Booster 4: Curtail Illicit Drug Use, Part II—Marijuana

Booster 54: Extract Yourself from Abusive Relationships

Booster 55: Have a Satisfying, Long-term, Committed Marriage or Its Equivalent

Booster 56: Build a Strong Social Network

Booster 61: Explore the Spiritual Within You

❏ I have a strong family history of drug abuse.

Booster 2: Don't Overdo Alcohol

Booster 3: Curtail Illicit Drug Use, Part I—Heroin, Cocaine, Crack, and Other Hard Drugs

Booster 4: Curtail Illicit Drug Use, Part II—Marijuana

Booster 54: Extract Yourself from Abusive Relationships

> Booster 55: Have a Satisfying, Long-term, Committed Marriage or Its Equivalent
> Booster 56: Build a Strong Social Network
> Booster 61: Explore the Spiritual Within You

❑ I have a strong family history of Alzheimer's or another form of dementia.

> Booster 1: Stay Away from Tobacco
> Booster 2: Don't Overdo Alcohol
> Booster 3: Curtail Illicit Drug Use, Part I—Heroin, Cocaine, Crack, and Other Hard Drugs
> Booster 4: Curtail Illicit Drug Use, Part II—Marijuana
> Booster 17: Wear a Helmet
> Booster 27: Monitor Blood Pressure and Control Hypertension
> Booster 32: Drink a Little Wine
> Booster 33: Take Estrogen
> Booster 34: Take a Multivitamin
> Booster 35: Take Advantage of Antioxidants: Vitamins C and E, Beta-carotene, Selenium
> Booster 41: Consider Complementary and Alternative Medicine
> Booster 49: Address Alzheimer's, Senility, and Dementia
> Booster 50: Commit to Lifelong Learning
> Booster 53: Fight Forgetfulness
> Booster 68: Ensure Job Safety
> Booster 76: Reduce Air Pollution, Radon, and Indoor Toxins

STEP 3: SELECT THE LONGEVITY BOOSTER CARDS

Now that you have completed the Longevity Buster Questionnaire, pull out the Booster Cards from the deck you created (see page 135) that correspond to the questions you checked. Don't be shy—you'll probably have more boosters than you thought. It's important to pick out any possible boosters that might apply to you. There is no right or wrong number of boosters that you should have, but through the simple exercise described below, you will learn how to cut back your boosters to a manageable number.

1. *Go through* the Booster Cards you have selected and discard any that represent actions you've already adopted (perhaps you are already on a low-fat diet, for instance) or lifestyle changes that simply don't apply. For example, a recovering alcoholic would toss out the card recommending a daily glass of wine *even* if he had heart disease.

2. *Next, add* to your personal stack any other Booster Cards that you think might apply to you, even if you did not choose them the first time. For example, if you're having a stressful relationship with your mom, pull the "Build Good Relationships with Your Family" card.

You should now have in front of you *your own personal* "keeper" pile. This is the group of *Longevity Booster Cards* that you will be using in the final exercise to crack your Longevity Code.

The Final Step in Cracking Your Code

PLAN A: GO WITH YOUR GUT—HOW DO YOU SEE THE CARDS?

With your initial sort completed, spread out your "keeper" cards, sphere by sphere, and just get a general feel for them.

- Do you see any kind of pattern? Is any sphere or category overrepresented—say, diet, job satisfaction, financial matters?
- Are any two or more intertwined in some fashion? You may decide to look for ways to tackle them together. Could you, for instance, reduce your stress levels by working on your marital problems and reducing your debt?

Now reshuffle your cards, mixing all spheres together. You no longer want to keep or think of them separately. That was useful when it came to picking out individual factors you need to work on, but it is counterproductive now. Your longevity prescription should be a reflection of all spheres taken as a whole.

Spread the shuffled cards out in front of you again. Look over them, trusting your intuition. If one card calls to you more than another, listen to it. The cards are like pieces of a puzzle that you put together to take the best possible actions. And sometimes they do just fall into place.

Pick out three to five cards that feel important to you. Move them to one side, and then move them around until you are satisfied that they are sequenced in their order of importance to you.

For some of you, simply playing with the cards is enough. This is especially true if you've started out with just a few cards. You can intuitively see what you need to change and go from there. But for most of you, deciding which step to take first is easier to do using one of the other two plans.

PLAN B: EASY DOES IT

This plan is ideal for those of you who like to tackle the easy things first, saving the more difficult tasks for later.

THE ADVANTAGES

- *It's easy.* Most actions can fit right into your life with very few adjustments required.
- *It's fast-acting.* You can start increasing your life expectancy today.
- *It builds confidence.* Little successes demonstrate that you're capable of tackling bigger challenges.
- *You make progress.* Small, incremental changes eventually add up.
- *You actually go for it.* You're more likely to just do it than you might be if you had to tackle something that requires more effort or planning.

THE DRAWBACKS

- *You may never get going to the big stuff.* Like sorting screws in the garage when you should be doing your taxes or cleaning out the linen closet when an important report is due, the easy boosters need doing, but we sometimes do them to avoid the really important steps.
- *You may think that it exempts you from the big stuff.* All the carrot juice and satisfying sex in the world doesn't counteract a pack-a-day tobacco habit or clinical depression.

PREREQUISITE

- *Be willing to commit to your easy changes.* You have to fasten your seat belt *every* time you're in a car, take an aspirin *every* day, and so on.

With this in mind, shuffle your "keeper" cards.
  1. Separate them into three piles: easy in one pile (on the left), moderate in one pile (the middle), difficult in one pile (right).
  2. Take all the cards in the left-hand pile, which are the easy cards (and possibly some easy-to-moderate cards), and put them in

order based on which are easiest for you personally or which ones you think you would like to begin with. Consider your amplifiers (page 113) when making your choices.

3. Select three that you are willing to start with and sequence them according to your first, second, and third choices to act on.
4. The cards you chose are the first steps of your longevity plan!

PLAN C: THE MOST-BANG-FOR-YOUR-BUCK METHOD

This method works for the person who wants to cover as many longevity bases as possible with one swing of the bat. Feeling a big impact is more important than how difficult or easy it will be to accomplish the booster. For example, giving up cigarettes is the ultimate more-bang-for-your-buck tactic (if you're a smoker). It's certainly one of the most difficult boosters to conquer. Eating five servings of fruits and veggies a day is also a five-star and is easy.

THE ADVANTAGES

- *This method has a high impact.* Many spheres, diseases, and risks can be addressed by a single action.
- *You'll feel a high level of satisfaction when you reach your goal.* It may be tough, but when you get there, you feel as if you can do anything!
- *It builds even more confidence than addressing a lot of little busters.*
- *Usually there are lots of resources and services available to assist you.* Information, medicines, support groups, Internet chat rooms, and other resources can be of significant help with your effort.

THE DRAWBACKS

- *It almost always requires lots of effort.*
- *It may require many adjustments.* You may need to take steps ranging from rearranging your schedule or saying no more often to distancing yourself from certain friends.
- *There is a risk of putting off all other positive steps until this one is completed.* If for some reason you don't succeed or even start, what happens to your chances for a longer, sweeter life?

PREREQUISITES

- *Stamina and stick-to-itiveness are essential.*

With this in mind, shuffle your "keeper" cards and narrow the field to the most important boosters:

1. Separate your cards into three piles based on their impact: five-star boosters in one pile (on the left), four-star boosters in one pile (the middle), and three-star and two-star ones in one pile (right).

2. Start with the five-star pile. (If there are fewer than four cards in it, use your four-star cards and three-star cards as well.) Put them in order based on which are the most important to you. You can base this decision on your instincts, your risk factors, your amplifiers, personal concerns such as a fear of breast cancer, or other incentives such as keeping secondhand smoke away from your kids, money issues, and so on.

3. Select the three boosters that you are willing and able to start with and sequence them according to your first, second, and third choices for action.

4. These are the first three steps of your longevity plan!

Naturally, once you've mastered the first three boosters in your personal longevity prescription, you can choose three more, and more after that. Use the same decision-making method, or switch to another one. And don't forget about your instincts and intuition. As you develop a feel for this longevity-boosting business, both will start playing a bigger role.

Remember . . .

1. *Each of us is unique.* We come into this world with a unique set of genes. We have our own unique combination of experiences and view of the future. This uniqueness will show up in your work with these cards. There is not one correct outcome for all people—each outcome is unique.

2. *There are general rules that apply to all of us.* The impact ratings reflect those rules. No matter who you are, smoking, living in a dangerous neighborhood, and a serious case of depression all tend to shorten your life and steal its sweetness.

3. *You have insight.* You know your circumstances better than anyone else does. You are the most qualified person to create your action prescription. And you *can* do it.

MOVING RIGHT ALONG...

- *Review the appropriate booster descriptions.* Turn to the page referenced on the bottom of your booster card and read about the measure. Familiarize yourself with the specific actions you'll need to take.
- *Make a to-do list.* Record each step for accomplishing your goal.
- *Set a date for taking action—today if possible.* Numerous studies show that people who act on the same day they first think about taking that action are more likely to make lasting changes.

Some Final Words of Advice

You may find it useful to:

- *Combine steps.* In case you wondered, there's no one-change-at-a-time rule. You can take one high-impact, difficult step and some easy steps simultaneously. You might, for instance, give yourself three months to make headway on a high-impact change such as cutting down on alcohol or reducing dietary fat and during those same three months also tackle one easy change every week or so.
- *Arrange for backup.* Change can be tough. It's tougher on some days than others, too. Are there people you can call for pep talks? Tapes you can listen to for inspiration? Less toxic indulgences you can turn to now and then? Sometimes just knowing that these cushions exist can be enough to keep you on track.
- *Build rewards into your plan.* What will you do with all that money you save by not buying cigarettes? How will you celebrate your arrival at a weight-loss goal or getting your blood pressure under control? And what about honoring your ability to maintain a new behavior? These pleasures can tide you over. But they can't compare with the big prize—the joy and fulfillment of a long, sweet life.
- *Remember that amplifiers can make one step more crucial than another.* Take them into consideration when you set your priorities.

Booster 1: Stay Away from Tobacco

Impact ★★★★★

Amplifiers Family history or personal history of heart disease, cancer, diabetes, or asthma

---

Linked to seven of the top ten causes of premature death, smoking snuffs out 350,000 to 400,000, lives per year. Combine that grim total with the toll from passive exposure to tobacco smoke (up to 35,000 deaths annually), the impact of smoking-related medical conditions, and the expense (more than $1,000 a year for a pack-a-day smoker). What you get is a major threat to longevity—and the reason why staying away from tobacco so dramatically improves your chances for a longer, sweeter life. It is the premier five-star longevity booster.

Sphere: Physical   **Page:** 180   **Action rating:** Difficult

---

Booster 2: Don't Overdo Alcohol

Impact ★★★★★

Amplifiers Family or personal history of alcoholism, cirrhosis, or other liver disease; depression

---

Moderate alcohol consumption does little to detract from life expectancy. Indeed, a daily drink, especially a glass of red wine, may even boost longevity. Drinking to excess, on the other hand, will definitely shorten your life span. It is implicated in more than 100,000 premature deaths each year and causes numerous social, occupational, financial, and psychological problems.

Sphere: Physical   **Page:** 183   **Action rating:** Difficult

---

Booster 3: Curtail Illicit Drug Use
Part I—Heroin, Cocaine, Crack, and Other Hard Drugs

Impact ★★★★★

Amplifiers Alcoholism, depression, a previous drug problem, or a family history of addiction or overmedicating.

The life of a hard-drug user is neither long nor sweet. Don't let the numbers fool you. Illicit drugs may be behind just 10,000 to 20,000 deaths in a year (compared to 100,000 for alcohol and 400,000 for tobacco), but even casual, occasional use can compromise your health, abbreviate your life span, and cause you to lose everything you value. Adopting this five-star longevity booster spares you from these devastating long-term consequences.

Sphere: Physical   **Page:** 186   **Action rating:** If addicted, very difficult
                                              If not, easy to moderate

Booster 4: Curtail Illicit Drug Use, Part II—Marijuana

Impact   ★★★

Amplifiers   Alcoholism; depression; family history of alcoholism and/or depression; past or active addictions; risk factors for emphysema, bronchitis, and other smoking-related illnesses

---

Categorized as an illicit drug because its possession and use is illegal in this and other countries, marijuana is actually more like alcohol than hard drugs. It has a milder impact on physical health and life expectancy than either. *Not* smoking pot has several significant benefits. These include sparing your lungs, improving mental functioning, strengthening personal relationships, and enhancing your career.

Sphere: Physical   **Page:** 188   **Action rating:** Easy to moderate

---

Booster 5: Eat More Fruits and Veggies—Five to Seven Servings per Day

Impact   ★★★★★

Amplifiers   Risk factors for heart disease, stroke, or colon, lung, breast, or skin cancer; poor eating habits

---

An apple a day may not keep the doctor away. But an apple plus an orange, a salad, a cup of steamed broccoli, and a glass of grape juice just might. The far-reaching effects of eating five to seven servings of fruits and vegetables daily along with the large body of research supporting it and the relative ease with which it can be accomplished earn this longevity booster a five-star rating. It belongs on everyone's must-do list.

Sphere: Physical   **Page:** 195   **Action rating:** Easy

Booster 6: Go for the Healthiest Quality and Quantity of Food

Impact   ★★★★

Amplifiers   Family or personal history of obesity; poor eating habits, yo-yo dieting; preoccupation with food or weight

---

You can eat your way to a longer, sweeter life. First familiarize yourself with the food pyramid, appropriate portion sizes, and your personal energy requirements. Then use what you've learned to make healthy and satisfying food choices.

Sphere: Physical   **Page:** 197   **Action rating:** Moderate to difficult

Booster 7: Cut the Fat

Impact ★★★★★

Amplifiers Family history, personal history, or other risk factors for heart disease, stroke, and colon or prostate cancer; obesity

If you want to make a major dent in your susceptibility to this country's number-one cause of premature death, this longevity booster is a must-do. By keeping the amount of fat in your diet at no more than 30 percent, you lessen the risk of heart attack, stroke, and angina-precipitating atherosclerosis, combat obesity, and possibly prevent certain cancers.

Sphere: Physical   **Page:** 201   **Action rating:** Moderate to difficult

---

Booster 8: Eat More Fiber

Impact ★★★

Amplifiers Family history, personal history, or other risk factors for heart disease, colon cancer, or irritable bowel syndrome

Have a bowl of oatmeal or a bag of air-popped popcorn. Eat an unpeeled apple or a plate of red beans and rice. Every bite is loaded with cholesterol-lowering, colon-cancer-preventing, longevity-boosting fiber. Try to get 10 to 35 g per day.

Sphere: Physical   **Page:** 204   **Action rating:** Easy

Booster 9: Eat Breakfast

Impact ★★★

Amplifiers Obesity, poor eating habits, nutritional deficiencies

Your mother was right. Starting your day with a good breakfast is good for you. It improves your brainpower, your energy level, even your disposition. And at least one study has linked it to a longer life.

Sphere: Physical   **Page:** 205   **Action rating:** Easy

Booster 10: Reduce Your Sugar Intake

Impact ★★

Amplifiers Age, obesity

Chocolate bars and custard pies, layer cakes, soda and ice cream sundaes—they make life sweeter all right, but not necessarily longer and healthier. Consuming less makes room in our diets for more nutritious foods. It also helps you avoid obesity and tooth decay.

Sphere: Physical **Page:** 205 **Action rating:** Moderate

Booster 11: Limit Your Salt Intake

Impact ★★

Amplifiers Salt sensitivity; fluid retention due to congestive heart failure, kidney disease, or other conditions

---

While there's no point, and possibly some danger, in consuming more salt than our bodies need, severely restricting our intake does very little to boost longevity. For most of us, a few minor modifications will be more than enough.

Sphere: Physical **Page:** 206 **Action rating:** Easy

Booster 12: Limit Snacking

Impact ★★

Amplifiers Obesity; stress

Not to be confused with the nutritional mid morning and afternoon minimeals many dieticians now recommend, snacking every hour or so on sugary or high-fat junk food only clogs your arteries and piles on extra calories

Sphere: Physical **Page:** 207 **Action rating:** Moderate to difficult

Booster 13: Get Your Muscles Moving

Impact ★★★★★

Amplifiers Obesity, arthritis, heart disease, cancer, chronic pain, or other significant medical problems; depression

We are what we eat—and how we exercise. Taken together, these two major activities of the physical sphere have an impact on longevity and life's sweetness that's tough to top. But how much exercise is enough? That depends on you. And it depends on how exercise fits into the balance in your life. Sixty percent of us get hardly any at all.

Sphere: Physical **Page:** 208 **Action rating:** Easy to moderate

---

Booster 14: Limit Sun Exposure

Impact ★★★★

Amplifiers Fair or easily sunburned skin; a family history of melanoma or other skin cancers; an outdoor job or an active outdoor lifestyle; medications that increase sensitivity to sunlight

The harmful effects of the sun's ultraviolet rays have been common knowledge for some time now. Yet many of us are still remiss when it comes to protecting ourselves. If we change our ways and adopt sun-sensible behaviors, including the appropriate use of sunscreens, we may be able to avoid skin cancers, facial wrinkles, and other forms of skin damage.

Sphere: Physical **Page:** 221 **Action rating:** Easy

Booster 15: Fasten Seat Belts

Impact ★★★★

Amplifiers Frequent and/or long car trips; driving for a living; treacherous road conditions

If you're involved in a motor vehicle accident, this measure can make the difference between life and death. This is one of the easiest four-star boosters around.

Sphere: Physical **Page:** 223 **Action rating:** Easy

Booster 16: Drive Sanely

Impact ★★★★

Amplifiers Frequent and/or long car trips; driving for a living; treacherous road conditions

A motor vehicle driven recklessly becomes a deadly weapon. If you drive yours sensibly, you'll not only boost your longevity but other people's as well.

Sphere: Physical   **Page:** 223   **Action rating:** Easy

Booster 17: Wear a Helmet

Impact ★★★★

Amplifiers Children; love of speed, fast bike, in-line skates, skis

Protect your most important organ. Whether you're cruising down the highway on your Harley, tooling around town on your ten-speed, or getting a great workout on in-line skates, a safety helmet is your first line of defense against a fatal or disabling head injury.

Sphere: Physical   **Page:** 224   **Action rating:** Easy

Booster 18: Reduce Hazards in Your Home

Impact ★★★★

Amplifiers An older home; residents who smoke or drink to excess; family members with special safety needs such as children or the elderly

What can happen under our own roofs? Fires, falls, food poisoning, and firearms accidents. They're all big-time longevity busters. And they're all preventable.

Sphere: Physical   **Page:** 224   **Action rating:** Easy

Booster 19: Practice Water Safety

Impact ★★★★

Amplifiers Fear of drowning; not knowing how to swim; being involved in lots of activities on the water (boating, fishing, etc.); drinking during those activities; living on the banks of a lake or river

---

If the only water you immerse yourself in is in your bathtub, you may not have occasion to use this longevity booster. But for the rest of us, bodies of water that can literally swallow us up or wash us away demand our respect.

Sphere: Physical **Page:** 226 **Action rating:** Easy

Booster 20: Have Safer Sex to Stop Sexually Transmitted Diseases

Impact ★★★★

Amplifiers Excessive alcohol consumption, illicit drug use, multiple partners, family history of cervical cancer

---

In the era of HIV/AIDS, sex can be a life-threatening activity. But rather than trying to avoid it completely (who wants to do that indefinitely?), you can take some of the threat out of it by adopting safer sex practices, preferably with one partner whom you know well and trust.

Sphere: Physical **Page:** 227 **Action rating:** Moderate

Booster 21: Have Pap Tests to Screen for Cervical Cancer

Impact ★★★★

Amplifiers Family history of cervical cancer; personal history of cervical cancer, abnormal Pap tests, or sexually transmitted diseases, including human papilloma virus (HPV) infection; becoming sexually active at an early age; multiple partners; low socioeconomic status; smoking

---

An early detection success story. The death rate from cancer of the cervix has dropped 75 percent since women started having simple lab tests known as Pap smears to screen for the disease. Unfortunately, it still kills more than 5,000 women each year, primarily because they failed to have Pap tests or waited too long between tests, which are recommended at intervals of one to three years.

Sphere: Physical **Page:** 229 **Action rating:** Easy to Moderate

Booster 22: Screen for Colon and Rectal Cancer

Impact   ★★★★

Amplifiers   Family or personal history of colon or rectal cancer; a high-calorie diet with lots of meat and little fiber, fruit, or vegetables; excess alcohol consumption; little physical activity; ulcerative colitis

---

Don't allow this slow-growing cancer to shorten your life span. You can reduce your risk through dietary changes, exercise, and vigilance. Screening tests, including an annual fecal occult blood test and a flexible sigmoidoscopy every five years, detect colon and rectal cancer in its earliest, most curable stages.

Sphere: Physical   **Page:** 230   **Action rating:** Easy to Moderate

---

Booster 23: Screen for Breast Cancer

Impact   ★★★★

Amplifiers   A family or personal history of breast cancer, especially a mother or sister who has had the disease; no pregnancies or your first after age thirty-five; early first menstruation; late menopause; advancing age; longtime estrogen use for menopause; possibly a high-fat diet, excessive alcohol consumption, or obesity

---

Death from breast cancer has dropped precipitously since the advent of breast self-examination, breast checks by doctors, and the appropriate use of screening mammography. There is no question that early detection of this frightening and still too often fatal disease can save lives. If more women who stood to benefit from mammograms got them, the breast cancer death rate could drop another 30 to 35 percent.

Sphere: Physical   **Page:** 231   **Action rating:** Moderate

---

Booster 24: Screen for Skin Cancer

Impact   ★★★★

Amplifiers   Family or personal history of skin cancer; history of severe sunburns, especially as a child; sun worshiping as a teenager; outdoor occupation; light complexion (burn easily); a multitude of moles, freckles, and marks

---

Malignant melanoma, the skin cancer that kills, has increased nearly tenfold since the 1940s. Our lifestyle, most notably our penchant for being outside with our skin exposed to direct sunlight, accounts for the difference. But we can also make a difference in the future of the disease. Early detection—by self-examination—could significantly drop the death rate from this cancer that's now on the rise.

Sphere: Physical   **Page:** 233   **Action rating:** Easy

Booster 25: Screen for Prostate Cancer

Impact ★★

Amplifiers Family or personal history of prostate cancer; African-American heritage; age; high-fat/low-fiber diet

Although prostate cancer is the second most common cause of cancer deaths among men, its slow growth rate and the adverse effects of the treatments currently available raise questions about the value of widespread screening efforts. While the controversy is being resolved, your best bet is to explore your options, understand their risks, and determine if (or when) you want testing to be done.

Sphere: Physical   **Page:** 234   **Action rating:** Moderate to Difficult

---

Booster 26: Get a Chest X-ray to Screen for Lung Cancer

Impact ★

Amplifiers Cigarette smoking, regular pipe smoking, frequent exposure to secondhand smoke; exposure to asbestos, outdoor air pollution, and/or indoor radon; diet low in fruit and vegetables

Considering all the people lung cancer strikes (178,000) and kills (160,000) each year, there's no question that some form of screening or early detection could be beneficial. Unfortunately, chest X-rays are not it. CAT scans show promise but aren't ready for widespread use. Our efforts clearly make more impact when they are focused on lung cancer *prevention*, including smoking cessation and protection from environmental carcinogens.

Sphere: Physical   **Page:** 236   **Action rating:** Easy to Moderate

---

Booster 27: Monitor Blood Pressure and Control Hypertension

Impact ★★★★★

Amplifiers Family or personal history of heart disease, stroke, or hypertension; being of African-American descent; diabetes; heavy drinking; obesity; inactivity; stress

High blood pressure, also known as hypertension, doubles your heart disease risk and dramatically increases the odds that you'll have a stroke or experience kidney failure. It's an extraordinary longevity buster that you simply must stop dead in its tracks before it derails your dream of living a long, sweet life.

Sphere: Physical   **Page:** 237   **Action rating:** Easy to Moderate

Booster 28: Measure Your HDL, LDL, and Total Cholesterol Levels

Impact ★★★★★

Amplifiers Family or personal history of high cholesterol, heart disease, or stroke; a diet high in saturated fat

---

Cholesterol is one star in the constellation of factors that contribute to heart disease. But for the last decade or so we've acted as if measuring it and modifying our diets to change it is the whole show. Well, it *is* important to know if your cholesterol has reached risk-raising levels. And it *is* important to use dietary measures or, where indicated, medication to lower that risk. It's just not the whole picture.

Sphere: Physical   **Page:** 239   **Action rating:** Moderate

---

Booster 29: Have Your Blood Sugar Levels Checked to Detect Diabetes

Impact ★★★★

Amplifiers Family history of diabetes; family or personal history of heart disease or stroke; African-American or Native American heritage; sedentary lifestyle; poor eating habits; smoking

---

Diabetes sneaks up on us. Excess glucose roaming through our bloodstreams can do lots of damage to our organs and arteries before we see a single sign that something's amiss. So we can't wait for symptoms to appear. Regular fasting blood tests for glucose can be the impetus for getting our blood sugar under control soon enough to positively influence the length and quality of our lives.

Sphere: Physical   **Page:** 240   **Action rating:** Moderate

---

Booster 30: Have Your Bone Density Tested for Signs of Osteoporosis

Impact ★★★

Amplifiers Family or personal history of osteoporosis; gender (female); race (Caucasian, Asian); age; a diet low in calcium; little weight-bearing exercise; smoking

---

Can you imagine slamming shut the trunk of your car and breaking a bone in your wrist? How about receiving a bear hug from someone you haven't seen in ages and fracturing a vertebra in your spine? Growing shorter? Aching with every step? Osteoporosis turns nightmares like these into everyday reality. If you are at risk for this bone disorder—and twenty-eight million Americans, one in four of them women, are—getting your bone density tested so you can begin to take corrective action can save you years of pain and disability, as well as prolong your life.

Sphere: Physical   **Page:** 242   **Action rating:** Easy to Test, Difficult to Correct

Booster 31: Add an Aspirin Every Day

Impact ★★★★★

Amplifiers Risk factors for heart disease, stroke, or colon cancer, including a family or personal history

---

We all know that aspirin works wonders on pain and inflammation. But it's even more of a wonder drug when taken daily to prevent heart attacks, stroke, and possibly colon cancer.

Sphere: Physical   **Page:** 245   **Action rating:** Easy

(for those who can tolerate it)

Booster 32: Drink a Little Wine

Impact ★★★★

Amplifiers Family or personal history of heart disease or stroke, other risk factors for those conditions

---

Yes, drinking to excess can be deadly. And quite clearly those with a family history of alcoholism or with a predisposition to tip too much should abstain. But for many abstinence is not necessarily the key to a longer, sweeter life. In fact, if you can handle it, a daily drink, preferably of red wine, will help you outlive most teetotalers.

Sphere: Physical   **Page:** 246   **Action rating:** Easy

(if moderation isn't a problem for you)

Booster 33: Take Estrogen

Impact ★★★★

Amplifiers Risk factors for heart disease, stroke, or osteoporosis; hysterectomy

---

A tough call. The list of benefits associated with estrogen replacement at menopause or after a hysterectomy is growing. But the specter of breast and uterine cancer remains and recent research has diminished its role in preventing heart disease. But it's still worth considering. A discussion with your doctor and a close look at your personal longevity profile can help you decide.

Sphere: Physical   **Page:** 247   **Action rating:** Easy

(once you've decided that this is the way you want to go)

Booster 34: Take a Multivitamin

Impact ★★★

Amplifiers Poor eating habits; severely restricted diets; smoking; heavy drinking; getting older; having chronic medical problems (especially digestive disorders)

To remain vital and energetic both physically and mentally, you need the right vitamins and minerals in the right measure. If your daily diet doesn't supply them, taking a daily multivitamin can help.

Sphere: Physical **Page:** 249 **Action rating:** Easy

Booster 35: Take Advantage of Antioxidants: Vitamins C and E, Beta-carotene, Selenium

Impact ★★★

Amplifiers Poor eating habits; severely restricted diets; smoking; heavy drinking; getting older; having chronic medical problems (especially digestive disorders)

Antioxidants may not live up to their advance billing as the answer to aging. But their impact on conditions that seem to come with the territory of getting older makes them worth considering for your inclusion in your personal longevity prescription.

Sphere: Physical **Page:** 250 **Action rating:** Easy

Booster 36: Make Room for Calcium and Vitamin D

Impact ★★★

Amplifiers Osteoporosis or risk factors for it; poor eating habits; lactose intolerance; being older, a smoker, or postmenopausal

Most of us consume roughly half of the calcium we need. Taking in more, along with vitamin D to enhance its effects, is critical for preventing bone loss that can lead to osteoporosis.

Sphere: Physical **Page:** 252 **Action rating:** Easy

Booster 37: Get Periodic Tune-ups

Impact ★★★★

Amplifiers Family or personal history of cancer or heart disease; medical problems; fear of disease

Having a periodic checkup can help you discover problems before they occur. More important, it's a time to reflect on your health habits.

Sphere: Physical   **Page:** 253   **Action rating:** Easy to Moderate

---

Booster 38: Have a Good Relationship with Your Doctor

Impact ★★★

Amplifiers Chronic medical problems; dependent care; HMO limitations

It used to be easy: From earliest recorded history, we trusted some people to give us advice on how to feel better and stay well. From shamans to faith healers, from our grandmother to the neighbor bringing chicken soup, there was always someone who took an interest in our health. And if we believed their advice was good, we took it.

Sphere: Physical   **Page:** 254   **Action rating:** Easy to Moderate

---

Booster 39: Get Immunized

Impact ★★★★

Amplifiers Age; chronic bronchitis, emphysema, or other chronic diseases or disabilities; employment in the health care field or food industry; unsafe sexual activity

Immunization is the most cost-effective way to keep yourself disease free. Most of us think we're set if we were immunized for childhood diseases. We've wiped out polio, diphtheria, and a host of others. But remember, influenza still claims 20,000–40,000 lives annually. Pneumonia, which often invades when we're already ill, has an even worse record—60,000 deaths. If all you need to put these longevity busters (and a couple of others) out of business is a quick shot to the arm or buttock, why miss it?

Sphere: Physical   **Page:** 257   **Action rating:** Easy

Booster 40: Use Medications Effectively

Impact ★★★★

Amplifiers Drug allergies or intolerance; taking multiple medications, medications with adverse side effects, or medications that interact poorly with food or beverages; difficulty communicating with your doctor(s)

We're a pill-popping society. If we're ill or in pain, impotent or upset, we look for a remedy that can be picked up from the local pharmacy. And we often find it. It isn't always the best answer for what ails us, however. What's more, the medications prescribed to make us well sometimes make us sick. This longevity booster helps you get the best results from medications as well as avoid adverse reactions to them—yet another top cause of premature death.

Sphere: Physical   **Page:** 258   **Action rating:** Moderate

---

Booster 41: Consider Complementary and Alternative Medicine

Impact ★★

Amplifier Chronic or acute disease

One of the most controversial topics today between physicians and patients is the role of complementary and alternative medicine. Though consumer-driven and rarely scientifically based, it has a role. Unfortunately, as with standard medicine, promises do not always meet expectations.

Sphere: Physical   **Page:** 260   **Action rating:** Easy

Booster 42: Drink Plenty of Water

Impact ★★

Amplifiers Environment; activities that tend to make us sweat; medications such as diuretics; penchant for taking in dehydrating substances such as alcohol

Plants wilt when they aren't watered. Well, so do we. Keeping your system well hydrated promotes everything from healthy body weight to soft, wrinkle-free skin.

Sphere: Physical   **Page:** 262   **Action rating:** Easy

Booster 43: Get Enough Sleep

Impact   ★★★

Amplifiers   Any illness; high levels of stress, work, or other waking-hours activities that demand clear thinking

With all the things we have to do in a given day, sleep often seems secondary. We skimp on it routinely without realizing how badly we're shortchanging ourselves. When we do get enough sleep, our mood, mental prowess, job performance, and resistance to illness all improve.

Sphere: Physical   **Page:** 263   **Action rating:** Easy to Difficult
(depending on individual circumstances)

Booster 44: Take Care of Your Teeth and Gums

Impact   ★★★★

Amplifiers   Presence of or risk factors for heart disease, stroke, or diabetes; personal history of dental problems or poor dental hygiene

Dental hygiene is one of those pay-a-little-now or a-lot-later longevity boosters. If you take the time to take care of your teeth and gums today, despite the cost or inconvenience, you'll pay much less in the way of pain, poor nutrition, expensive procedures, or illness as you get older.

Sphere: Physical   **Page:** 264   **Action rating:** Easy

Booster 45: Treat Depression

Impact   ★★★★★

Amplifiers   Family or personal history of depression; social isolation; recent loss or life change; excessive alcohol consumption; illicit drug use; stress

Major depression is a medical condition, a treatable illness most likely caused by a chemical imbalance in the brain. Nineteen million Americans suffer from some form of it. On any given day, one in ten women and one in twenty men can fall victim to it. The good news is that they don't have to stay mired in it. This emotionally crippling, physically harmful, longevity-busting condition responds very well to medication with talk therapy or without it. Depressed people, especially those who reach out and receive treatment for their illness, can and do get well.

Sphere: Mental   **Page:** 265   **Action rating:** Moderate to Difficult

Booster 46: Manage Anger

Impact ★★★★★

Amplifiers Family or personal history or other risk factors for heart disease, stroke, or high blood pressure; stress; chronic medical conditions; excessive alcohol consumption; financial, work, or relationship problems

Hissy fits, fistfights and temper tantrums, road rage and shouting matches—take your pick. Anger isn't pretty, and it isn't healthy. Expressing it exacerbates heart problems, raises blood pressure, breeds violence, and cuts us off from people who could care about us. Learning how to stop this emotion from poisoning your life may be one of the very best things you can do for yourself.

Sphere: Mental   Page: 269   Action rating: Moderate to Difficult

Booster 47: Develop More and Better Skills for Coping with Stress

Impact ★★★★★

Amplifiers Personal or family history or other risk factors for heart problems or depression; anxiety; immune system disorders; chronic medical conditions; poor eating or sleep habits; job, family, or money problems

Brought on by anything from a physical malady to a financial faux pas, and implicated in everything from asthma attacks to cardiac arrhythmias, stress is probably the most pervasive of all longevity busters. It can infiltrate and undermine every sphere of our lives. We can't escape stress. It's our body's immediate, indiscriminate response to any demand—good, bad, or indifferent—we face. But we can learn to cope with it more effectively and lower high levels of it.

Sphere: Mental   Page: 272   Action rating: Easy, Moderate, Difficult, depending on the action step you pick

Booster 48: Stop Worrying Yourself to Death

Impact ★★★★

Amplifiers Personal or family history of heart disease, stroke, or hypertension; chronic medical conditions; chronic pain; stress; work, family, or money problems

Worry, worry, worry. Worry that anything capable of going wrong will or that anything you really need to do won't go right. Sometimes referred to as "worry sickness," anxiety is a fear of what *might* happen, a sense of distress or uneasiness in response to our perception that failure, humiliation, pain, or some unavoidable calamity is right around the corner. It drains the sweetness, and possibly some of the longevity, out of life. Treating anxiety disorders with therapy and medication or milder forms of anxiety with time-tested self-help strategies can reverse that outcome and open a door to a whole new world.

Sphere: Mental   Page: 276   Action rating: Moderate to Difficult

Booster 49: Address Alzheimer's, Senility, and Dementia

Impact ★★★

Amplifiers Family history of Alzheimer's, senility, or dementia; family or personal history of stroke; atherosclerosis; excessive alcohol consumption; poor eating habits

When most of us are asked which conditions could convince us to opt for a shorter life, Alzheimer's disease tops the list. It is followed closely by other forms of senility or dementia. And it's not difficult to understand why. These degenerative brain diseases clearly destroy life quality while slowly whittling away at longevity. Although many questions about treatment and prevention remain unanswered, there are some things that we can do to dodge these diseases.

Sphere: Mental   **Page:** 279   **Action rating:** Moderate

Booster 50: Commit to Lifelong Learning

Impact ★★★★★

Amplifiers Any problem in any sphere at any time

Knowledge really is power—the power to make informed decisions, solve problems, explore new horizons, pursue meaningful activities, communicate with our doctors. In other words, it helps us to stay healthier and live longer. To obtain that power all you need to do is open your mind to new ideas, locate resources for investigating your interests, and dive in.

Sphere: Mental   **Page:** 281   **Action rating:** Easy

Booster 51: Cultivate a Resilient, Optimistic, Can-do Attitude

Impact ★★★★★

Amplifiers Stress; anxiety; depression; medical problems; family, job, or financial difficulties

Looking on the bright side of life may sound like naive advice to some of you. But seeking solutions—instead of someone to blame—for your problems, or believing that you can do something rather than whining "I can't," truly makes a difference to your health and longevity.

Sphere: Mental   **Page:** 284   **Action rating:** Easy to Difficult

Booster 52: Hang on to Your Sense of Humor

Impact ★★★★

Amplifiers Stress; anxiety; job dissatisfaction; chronic pain; colds, pneumonia, and other infections

Laughter is great medicine. So turn on some *Cheers* reruns or trade knock-knock jokes with a nine-year-old. Humor, in whatever form tickles your funny bone, is a sure bet to make your life sweeter, and some studies suggest it can make it longer as well.

Sphere: Mental   **Page:** 285   **Action rating:** Easy

Booster 53: Fight Forgetfulness

Impact ★★

Amplifiers Stress, too little sleep, age, inadequate nutrition

More of a quality issue than a threat to longevity, forgetfulness, or "age-associated memory impairment," as psychologists sometimes call it, causes only as much real trouble as you let it. Specific tools and techniques for retrieving and retaining information as well as measures to keep your brain in peak physical condition can make memory loss no more than a minor irritant, and certainly no cause for alarm.

Sphere: Mental   **Page:** 286   **Action rating:** Easy

Booster 54: Extract Yourself from Abusive Relationships

Impact ★★★★★

Amplifiers History of violence in your life; children at home; unemployment, underemployment, or financial dependence; isolation

Personal abuse is a five-star longevity buster, whether the injuries inflicted are physical or mental. Violence wrecks the quality of life, elevating the fear of physical harm or mental anguish to an ever-present reality. It clearly impacts on longevity, while it denies its victims spiritual and emotional freedom. Staying in a long-term abusive relationship cannot be considered an option. Finding a pathway to safety, even in the future, is the only viable alternative.

Sphere: Kinship   **Page:** 288   **Action rating:** Difficult

Booster 55: Have a Satisfying, Long-term, Committed Marriage or Its Equivalent

Impact ★★★★★

Amplifiers Parental divorce or abuse; children at home; financial concerns; self-esteem issues

What's better for you than diet and exercise if you seek a long, healthy life? In a word, marriage. There's no dispute. Study after study shows that married people live happier, longer lives, and with better psychological adjustment. Couples change each other in ways that benefit both partners. That doesn't make marriage a panacea for life's ills. But marriage is clearly a strong social bond if your lifelong partner is a good match for you.

Sphere: Kinship   **Page:** 290   **Action rating:** Easy to Difficult

Booster 56: Build a Strong Social Network

Impact ★★★★★

Amplifiers Any chronic disease, depression, or paranoia; violent neighborhood; poverty; isolation

Social networks enrich life, prevent disease, and promote longevity. With a strong social foundation, your ability to withstand difficult disease increases while the prevalence of simple disease declines dramatically. The corollary is also true: The more isolated you are, the less healthy you will be.

Sphere: Kinship   **Page:** 293   **Action rating:** Easy to Difficult

Booster 57: Build Good Relationships with Your Family

Impact ★★★★

Amplifiers Personal or emotional problems; financial difficulties; residual anger; childhood abuse; illusions of independence

Your immediate family is a subgroup of social relationships that deserves special mention because of its powerful influence. Attending to this important sphere will reduce stress and can greatly sweeten your life.

Sphere: Kinship   **Page:** 295   **Action rating:** Easy to Difficult

Booster 58: Build Good Relationships with Friends

Impact   ★★★★

Amplifiers   Workaholism; poor friendships in childhood; low self-esteem; frequent moving

After marriage, friendship is the most creative and empowering subgroup of social relationships. We pick our friends. We tend to become friends with people who share similar interests, incomes, aspirations, and beliefs. Friends are our playmates in childhood and our companions as adults. Although a past history of having friends is desirable, it doesn't affect our ability to make friends today. This sphere can greatly embellish your life, and when times are troubled and friends are true, our buddies almost always relieve stress and add joy.

Sphere: Mental   **Page:** 298   **Action rating:** Easy to Difficult

Booster 59: Savor Sex and Intimacy

Impact   ★★★

Amplifiers   Marital problems; children; age; heart disease; breast cancer

Lovemaking and intimacy play a vital part in a good relationship with your spouse or life partner. Sexual intimacy is clearly one of life's fondest pleasures, to be enjoyed unhesitatingly. Passion makes us feel young and vital, no matter what our age. Keep this in mind: The most important sex organ in the body is the brain. The attitude that sex is only for the young perished years ago. But intimacy is more than sex. And touch gives us worthwhile comfort throughout our lives.

Sphere: Kinship   **Page:** 300   **Action rating:** Moderate

Booster 60: Own a Pet

Impact   ★★

Amplifiers   Loneliness; death in the family; living in a violent environment

What a joy to add a companion who asks so little. Dogs, cats, birds, and fish can bring us joy and pleasure, especially in times of stress. The care of and responsibility for a dog or cat can prove to be a motivator for physical exercise and a stimulus to socialization. Worth considering if you have the time and inclination.

Sphere: Kinship   **Page:** 302   **Action rating:** Easy

Booster 61: Explore the Spiritual Within You

Impact ★★★★★

Amplifiers Chronic disease; stress; family issues; job problems; fear of death

Every day presents us an opportunity to practice universal tenets of human existence: loving kindness, compassion, and giving. Your life is enhanced when you help others. The secret of inner peace is the practice of compassion, for yourself and those around you. These actions bring a positive benefit to the mental and kinship spheres.

Sphere: Spiritual   **Page:** 302   **Action rating:** Easy to Moderate

Booster 62: Get Involved in a Spiritual Community

Impact ★★★★

Amplifiers Physical or medical problems; family stressors; children

Study after study shows that going to church or synagogue, practicing meditation together, or other group spiritual activities may add years to your life. Whether this is due to the communal aspect of these practices or something else remains to be seen. All we can say now, scientifically, is that it matters.

Sphere: Spiritual   **Page:** 306   **Action rating:** Easy to Moderate

Booster 63: Take Time with Mother Nature

Impact ★★★

Amplifiers Urban environment; stress; little downtime; family commitments; children

For many of us, taking time to be with Mother Nature brings us in touch with our spiritual sphere. Poets have immortalized the beauties of nature for centuries because visual and other sensory environments sing to our soul. Nature reminds us that we are part of a global community created by forces beyond us. When we experience time in nature, our concerns extend beyond our human issues. Every sunset you have seen, every winding path you have walked provided you with the opportunity to reflect on a part of our daily lives that asks nothing from us, only to cherish and protect it as we would do for anything that we love.

Sphere: Spiritual   **Page:** 307   **Action rating:** Easy

Booster 64: Don't Avoid Thinking About Death

Impact ★★★★

Amplifiers Chronic disease; terminal illness; loneliness; spiritual longing; grieving

Death is always with us. It's not optional, although in America we often think that it is. It is one of Americans' taboo topics, coming right after sex and money. You indirectly think about death when you choose not to eat fried chicken, quit smoking, or hit the treadmill. But directly confronting death, thinking about what our last moment on earth would be like, can help us make the right longevity choices. Especially the difficult ones.

Sphere: Spiritual   **Page:** 308   **Action rating:** Difficult

---

Booster 65: Prepare Your Living Will and Advance Directives

Impact ★★★

Amplifiers Older age; deteriorating health; HIV/AIDS; cancer; heart disease; family history of premature death

When it's time to die we all want to go with dignity and without pain. Most when queried say, "Just make it quick." A sudden heart attack perhaps would fit the scene. But far too often the goodbye process is slower. And then our wishes, mitigated by a loved one or perhaps a thoughtful physician who sees life a bit differently than we do, intervenes. Writing out your directives gives you some assurance that if you cannot direct your death process, you can at least be part of it. After all, it is your life.

Sphere: Spiritual   **Page:** 311   **Action rating:** Easy

Booster 66: Volunteer Service to Others

Impact ★★★★

Amplifiers Isolation; recently relocated; depression, anger, or marital discord

Helping others makes you feel good. The world would be a sorry place if none of us volunteered our time for others. Social bonds multiply when you are doing something for someone else. Inevitably the benefit comes back to you.

Sphere: Spiritual   **Page:** 313   **Action rating:** Easy to Moderate

Booster 67: Pursue Job Satisfaction

Impact ★★★★★

Amplifiers Lack of job training or education; excessive financial obligations; dependents; lack of health insurance

In our society job satisfaction ranks as the greatest predictor of personal happiness after family. There are times in your life when you spend more time at your job than at home. Stress, joy, self-worth, financial stability—the list of life's burdens and joys affected by your occupation is endless, making this category worthy of five-star status.

Sphere: Material   **Page:** 315   **Action rating:** Moderate to Difficult

---

Booster 68: Ensure Job Safety

Impact ★★★★★

Amplifier: Dangerous occupation

Workplace safety is the responsibility of the private sector, the government, and the individual. But when it's your job, safety is not an ethereal matter. Safety and improved work conditions are issues equally as important as high blood pressure and cholesterol.

Sphere: Material   **Page:** 318   **Action rating:** Moderate to Difficult

---

Booster 69: Procure Adequate Job Benefits

Impact ★★★★

Amplifiers Any medical problem; pregnancy; family

Whether or not you keep, switch, or quit your job is often intimately tied up with your benefits package. Health insurance is the reason why many people stay in jobs they dislike. But other benefits such as disability clearly affect your longevity and quality of life should you become ill.

Sphere: Material   **Page:** 319   **Action rating:** Easy to Difficult

Booster 70: Make Your Workplace Fun

Impact   ★★★

Amplifiers   Long hours at work, workaholic culture, or excessive demands; marital and other problems at home; financial difficulties; lack of hobbies

After you've looked at job toxicity from the perspective of safety, what about looking at it from the perspective of the other toxic element—the people you work with? Having an occupation where you are respected and liked is gratifying and wonderful. The antithesis is dreadful and leads to multiple stress issues, clearly affecting the other spheres of your life.

Sphere: Material   **Page:** 320   **Action rating:** Easy to Difficult

---

Booster 71: Calculate How Much Is Enough

Impact   ★★★★

Amplifiers   Debt, children, miserable occupation, unpleasant living conditions, lack of savings, or limited education; lack of social supports

An adequate income can affect your life positively. Working harder to make more or cutting back because you don't need as much factor into the picture. Studies show that generally, the more money you earn, the healthier you are and the longer you live, and that's regardless of medical care—up to a point. Does this mean that a Rockefeller will live longer than you do? Not necessarily. But income is clearly a factor that plays a more pivotal role than we would like to admit.

Sphere: Material   **Page:** 322   **Action rating:** Moderate to Difficult

---

Booster 72: Minimize Your Debt

Impact   ★★★

Amplifiers   Past debt, kids in college, too many desires, too many credit cards, or unstable employment; chronic illness; lack of health care; lack of skills

Borrowing for a house to live in or an education that improves your job or enriches your life is most certainly worthwhile. Borrowing for objects you desire, from clothes to vacations to that new SUV, may be more stressful than worthwhile. Your debt load should be balanced by your earning ability.

Sphere: Material   **Page:** 324   **Action rating:** Moderate to Difficult

Booster 73: Maximize Your Savings and Retirement Income

Impact   ★★★

Amplifiers   Past debt, kids in college, or too many desires; job burnout; close to retirement

Whether the kids need college money, you covet that cottage in the country, or you're just looking ahead, money in the bank is key to choice. Perhaps that's easier said than done. Starting and feeding your savings plan is not simple, because purchases seem to ambush you every day. Yet today's transactions may lead you to fewer choices tomorrow.

Sphere: Material   **Page:** 325   **Action rating:** Moderate to Difficult

---

Booster 74: Don't Live in a Violent Environment

Impact   ★★★★★

Amplifiers   Poverty; loneliness; joblessness

Living in a neighborhood that feels unsafe is a frightening thing. If you walk in fear, you worry about muggings, physical assault, street brawls, rape, drug dealers, drive-by shootings. If you live in fear when you are at home, you worry about your safety, robbery, break-ins. Whether violence is random or predictable, with a little foresight you might be able to avoid being hurt.

Sphere: Material   **Page:** 327   **Action rating:** Moderate to Difficult

---

Booster 75: Nurture Your Home

Impact   ★★

Amplifiers   Urban environment; family, medical, or mental problems; stress

All habitats are not created equal. The places that we inhabit create environments that inspire, soothe, stimulate, or annoy us. You're affected by your home and work spaces more than you think. When disease strikes or stress rears its ugly head, it's not only comfort food that helps, it's comfort in your abode.

Sphere: Material   **Page:** 329   **Action rating:** Easy to Moderate

Booster 76: Reduce Air Pollution, Radon, and Indoor Toxins

Impact ★★

Amplifiers Asthma, emphysema, chronic bronchitis, or heart disease

---

Living in a toxic environment can affect your longevity. Anyone who lives in the LA basin or other polluted spaces knows that jogging—even going outside—on the wrong day can be an unhealthy event. What is the real risk of living with polluted air? Should you leave your job? Your neighborhood? Those questions need asking.

Sphere: Material   **Page:** 330   **Action rating:** Moderate to Difficult

7

Making the Commitment

How to Stay on Track

THE NEAT THING ABOUT HAVING a life span longer than a walleye salmon's is the extra time it gives us to correct our mistakes, make up for our oversights, and improve the hand life dealt us. If we don't like where our earlier choices have led us, we can always make different choices and, by doing so, improve our odds of living a longer, sweeter life. But will we?

Two and a half years after a relatively amicable divorce, Kelly Rogers, a thirty-seven-year-old nursing instructor, had gotten back on her feet financially and emotionally. "The fact that we had no kids or custody issues helped a lot," said Kelly. So did the singles group she joined. "We do fun stuff together," Kelly explained. "Outdoor activities mostly, like playing volleyball and kayaking."

More socializing often followed those activities. "After a hike or a softball game, we'll go out for a few beers," Kelly told me. People in the bar, including several members of

Kelly's group, would be smoking. And before she knew it, Kelly, who had given up cigarettes six years earlier, was lighting up, too. "I guess you could call me a social smoker, because I only smoke when I'm out socially," she said. The possible impact on her social life was what was preventing her from quitting again. If she did try, Kelly believed, she would have to avoid the places where she'd been enjoying herself. "I wouldn't be able to resist the urge to smoke in those places, and I'm having too much fun to stop going to them," she asserted. Consequently, she just couldn't see herself quitting cigarettes anytime soon.

"Okay, then," I said when she had finished explaining why she was unwilling to abandon a habit with indisputably adverse effects on health and longevity. "Just for now, let's drop the idea of giving up smoking, and come up with some things you *are* willing to do."

No doubt many members of the American Heart Association or American Cancer Society would be appalled by this response. Some of my fellow physicians would be less than thrilled with it as well. But if my patients can't or won't do this one important thing immediately, then I have them do something else to enhance their longevity or well-being.

You have to start *somewhere.* A crucial element of putting together your personal longevity prescription involves identifying the first step you'll take. If you find the logical place to start but for one reason or another you don't want to start there, start someplace else. Do the second or third or eighth item on your priority list. But do something. Do it even if it isn't the most obvious or most important thing you could do, even if it doesn't directly address a problem you need to remedy or have a half dozen double-blind clinical studies behind it. What seems like nothing could pave the way to something you really need.

But don't kid yourself. If a longer, sweeter life is your goal, you will have to tackle those big changes someday.

The Will Factor

Willingness, a combination of desire and determination, is the spark that sets lifestyle changes in motion, the force that takes us from knowing how something will help or harm us to doing what's necessary to reap those benefits or avoid those consequences. Without willingness, the best data on longevity, the best tools for increasing life expectancy, and the most carefully constructed prescription for a longer, sweeter life are absolutely useless.

Of course, waiting for the mood to strike you isn't the answer either. A better move is to identify, understand, and respect the forces that may be sapping your desire, determination, and discipline.

Locate the Real Impasse

We often say we lack the time, money, or family support to initiate a longevity-boosting effort when something else is actually in our way. More baffling, we sometimes say we want to improve in some area and really mean it, but still can't seem to do it. We adopt healthier eating patterns on Monday morning and abandon them by Thursday night. We purchase exercise equipment and use it faithfully for no more than a month or two before it becomes a convenient place to hang our clothes. Something stopped us, something we didn't anticipate and perhaps could not quite identify because we were looking for it in the wrong sphere.

If you find that your efforts to change a habit or adopt a healthful measure in one sphere are blocked, check the other spheres. Face your fears.

EXERCISE 8—Barriers to Boosters

Drawing from both personal and professional experience, I have identified some of the most common barriers to adopting longevity-boosting behaviors. They're listed below, along with tips for overcoming them. Check the boxes that apply to you.

TIME

❏ I have almost none to spare and can't see how I could possibly find more.

TIP: Look for boosters that you can fit into your existing schedule. The world's busiest person can find time to drink juice or eat a piece of fruit in the morning, walk the stairs once in a while instead of riding the elevator, take vitamin supplements or a daily aspirin, do some deep breathing before a stressful meeting, and so on.

❏ Time for myself is at a premium, but I could probably finagle an extra _____ minutes/hours a week.

TIP: If you can free up time for longevity-boosting activities, schedule them as you would any other appointment. Then keep it!

❏ My schedule is pretty packed but flexible.

TIP: Keep a list of longevity boosters you can do at a moment's notice—things such as meditating or reading inspirational literature, calling a close friend or hiking. Then select something from that list to do when a block of time in your flexible schedule becomes available.

MONEY

❏ My budget is so tight that I couldn't pay for a multivitamin without sacrificing something essential.

TIP: Pick boosters that cost little or nothing. There are lots of them. Try the coin-rolling suggestion I made in Chapter 1.

❏ I have very little to spare, but I'd be willing to fiddle with my budget to find more.

TIP: Make material-sphere longevity boosters a high priority. You'll benefit from getting your finances in order as well as from any measures your newly ordered finances allow you to afford.

❏ I'm willing to devote no more than _____ dollars per year to pay for products and activities designed to increase longevity.

TIP: Good for you. Now choose wisely.

FAMILY

❏ They come first and are very demanding.	**TIP:** See the top item under Time.
❏ They come first, but they're fairly flexible.	**TIP:** Include some boosters that don't require fixed times or locations.
❏ They probably wouldn't care what I did.	**TIP:** A mixed blessing. If their indifference reflects the fact that your family isn't as close and interdependent as you'd like them to be, look over the boosters in the kinship sphere chapter.
❏ They might do some of this healthy stuff with me.	**TIP:** Terrific. This could double as quality family time, a longevity booster in and of itself.
❏ They would be thrilled that I was taking care of myself and support me.	**TIP:** The ideal situation. Think about the kind of support you need most (e.g., someone to do the dinner dishes so you can take a walk in the evening). Then ask for what you need.

WORK

❏ It is my number-one priority at this point, and it's quite stressful and time-consuming.	**TIP:** See the top item under Time. Give some thought to adopting material-sphere longevity boosters.
❏ It takes priority but offers a fair amount of flexibility.	**TIP:** Keep and consult a list like the one I described in the Time section.
❏ It's just a job and wouldn't interfere with anything I'd want to do.	**TIP:** Another mixed blessing. Check the material-sphere section (pages 43–47) to see if there are ways to feel better about what you do or to do something that will make you feel more vital and productive.

SOCIAL LIFE

❏ It's very active and I don't want longevity boosters to interfere with it at all.

TIP: Select measures that fill that bill.

❏ It's very active, but my social circle is pretty health conscious.

TIP: Do what you need to. They'll probably understand.

❏ My social circle gets together for mostly longevity-boosting activities.

TIP: These friends are keepers.

❏ I could use (and I'm ready to look for) a new, healthier, more supportive group of friends.

TIP: Pick a few activities that are done in groups—bicycling, cooking classes, hiking clubs, choir singing, volunteer work. That way you'll be doing something that interests and nourishes you as well as meeting people who share some of your interests. Check out kinship sphere boosters as well (pages 37–41). And why not call an old friend?

COMFORT ZONE

❏ I am nowhere near ready to give up _____ [fill in the name of a habit].

TIP: Focus on other boosters and work on motivating and preparing yourself for the big change. Try one or more of the suggestions found on the following pages.

❏ I'm in the middle of a major life transition or crisis (divorce, new parenthood, retirement, etc.) and think I'll lose my mind completely if I try to change anything else.

TIP: Go for boosters that could ease your transition or improve your mental state.

❏ I need some time to recover from all the things that have gone on in my life over the past few months (or years).

TIP: Start with low-key boosters that might help you meet that need.

❏ I would like to give up certain habits or change certain facets of my lifestyle, but I don't know if I would be able to cope without them.

TIP: Lead up to the big changes with boosters that can build your confidence and strengthen your coping skills. (Try the mental and kinship sphere sections, pages 31–37 and 37–41.)

Sometimes just knowing what's behind an impasse can be enough to get you back on track. Sometimes you'll have to shelve one change effort temporarily while you tackle the obstacle itself. And sometimes you'll just have to build your change muscles by working on other longevity boosters until you're tough and powerful and confident enough to push past the impasse and do what's best for yourself.

In Kelly's case, both her social life and her comfort zone figured prominently in her resistance to giving up cigarettes. She believed that her social life would be negatively affected if she had to avoid places where she'd be tempted to smoke. She also felt that she had changed plenty over the past year or so since her divorce and needed a breather from big self-improvement projects. While these concerns undeniably undermined her willingness to quit smoking, they in no way negated her desire to live a longer, sweeter life. She was perfectly willing to do something toward that end.

"Okay," I told her. "I'd like you to supplement your diet [it had never been ideal] by taking a multivitamin with minerals, plus a calcium tablet and vitamin D—both crucial for warding off osteoporosis, especially in women." I also explained about the importance of fruits and vegetables. A glass of orange juice in the morning and tomato juice in the evening would help her obtain the seven daily servings we all need.

These may seem like feeble gestures when compared with the impact that no longer smoking could have on Kelly's health and longevity. And every step we can take to ward off premature death and make our lives longer and sweeter may not count equally. But they all count.

What's more, good actions are cumulative, just as bad ones are. Once you've succeeded at step one, why not take step two, and after that step succeeds, step three—just like walking, which we all learned to do in exactly this way. By doing some good things for herself while still smoking, there was a chance that Kelly would be in better condition when she did get around to quitting. She definitely would gain more longevity than a smoker who does nothing.

Each step, no matter how small, can create momentum, motivating you to do more, including—eventually—the things you need to do most. As you begin to feel healthier, happier, or more relaxed on one or two fronts, your unhealthy habits in other areas will no longer fit you.

Find Compelling Reasons to Change

I'm happy to report that Kelly finally quit smoking about six months after she started seriously dating a terrific guy. He was a smoker, too, and had two young children who stayed with him on weekends. They played an important role in Kelly's decision to kick the habit.

"We walked into the rec room one Saturday," Kelly told me, "and found the kids playing grown-up. They were sitting at a table pretending to drink coffee when the six-year-old held out a package of crayons and said to his younger sister, 'Cigarette?' She took one, 'lit' it exactly the way I do, and they both did a perfect imitation of their father and me puffing away after a meal." By the following Monday, both she and her new love had signed up for a smoking-cessation course and purchased the nicotine patch.

Kelly became more willing to change once she found a compelling reason to do so—a reason she hadn't even considered when we were discussing quitting. We had covered the physical merits of quitting, the emotional satisfaction she would feel once she had conquered her addiction, even the financial advantages of not spending nearly $1,000 a year on cigarettes. But it had been the social implications of her behavior that had swayed her, once again demonstrating the importance of taking a multisphere approach to longevity.

The reason that compels you to finally make a lifestyle change you've been resisting for ages is not necessarily the most obvious or the most dramatic. It is not the same reason that might compel someone else to make those changes. But it resonates with you. Needless to say, the more reasons you consider, and the more spheres you cover, the more likely you are to find the one that motivates you.

More Will Builders

RECALL YOUR ACCOMPLISHMENTS

There are thousands of things that once were beyond your capabilities but that now come to you as naturally as breathing: walking, talking in complete sentences, pouring just the right amount of milk into your breakfast cereal—you get the gist.

If you look back over your history, you'll also find many things that were different: the first day of school, your first dip in a swimming pool, essays for English class, wearing condoms, getting Pap tests. You didn't want to do these things, but you found enough willingness to get through them, and that experience made it a bit easier to tackle the next task you preferred not to do or felt you couldn't do.

Refreshing your memory can jump-start your motivation. So look back at what you've achieved and even more so at the sense of satisfaction, pride, and optimism you felt in the wake of your accomplishment.

When you're scrambling to cover your monthly expenses or stretched from juggling a job, a family, or maybe college coursework, it's tougher to take the steps that could help you live longer and better somewhere down the line. When your world is topsy-turvy, even drinking a glass of juice, walking a few extra blocks, or meditating for fifteen minutes seems too much to ask. But those simple, positive daily rituals actually can be a source of comfort during periods of stress. They're touchstones. They have the potential to provide predictability and stability under even the most unpredictable and unstable circumstances. There may be nothing else you'll know with certainty on any given day except that you'll drink that juice or write in that journal or walk that mile and a quarter.

PREPARE FOR THE BIG EVENT

There's evidence that taking some time to prepare for a major lifestyle change and taking interim steps toward a larger goal may be the way to go. You might work up to a major change by:
- Investigating a variety of methods for achieving it
- Talking to people who have previously accomplished it
- Joining a support group
- Selecting a change date
- Reordering your schedule
- Announcing your intentions

The key to living a long, sweet life does not lie in warding off every possible threat to longevity. You would never succeed. You could spend every minute of every day trying, only to end up sacrificing just about everything that makes life worth living. That's way too high a price. There is a middle way.

Options, Options, Options

Attaining longevity while maintaining our health does not necessarily require huge sacrifices and a complete lifestyle overhaul. There are dozens and dozens of simple, subtle, enjoyable actions we can take to prevent illness, to promote health.

As we get down to the business of creating personal longevity prescriptions, you'll read about boosters with obvious, immediate benefits: treating depression, for example, or taking a calming walk on the beach. Other options, such as improving your relationship with your parents or learning to manage your anger, offer more long-term rewards. Some are as easy as brushing and flossing your teeth or fastening your seat belt. Others, such as extracting yourself from a destructive relationship, are challenging indeed.

How I Chose the Boosters and Busters

The seventy-six boosters I've chosen from a field crowded with possibilities run the gamut from eating enough fiber and getting enough sleep to fighting forgetfulness and funding a retirement plan. They address all five spheres of wellness.

I stayed away from products or procedures that were much too new and there's not enough data on them. At least two and probably several other items were touted as miraculous and then taken off the market before the ink from my laser printer could dry.

I did not present all boosters as carrying the same weight. Some are clearly more crucial than others. Take managing hypertension, for example. There's no question that high blood pressure is a longevity buster. It starts damaging your heart and arteries even before it's detected. There are very effective treatments for it, with few side effects, and lots of evidence that treating it prolongs life. We also know that *not* treating it increases the risk of stroke. All of this means that if you have high blood pressure, monitoring and managing it is a high-impact longevity booster that you should implement right away.

A different booster—say, supplementing your diet with vitamin C—has no such sense of urgency. While there is some evidence that this micronutrient strengthens the immune system and prolongs life, it is not nearly as extensive or compelling as the data about hypertension. Whether you start it today or two months from now doesn't significantly change your chances of living a longer, sweeter life.

When deciding which boosters to include and judging their potential to increase life expectancy, I drew upon more than two decades of experience reviewing medical information, weighing it, considering its validity, and translating it into practical advice for my patients and radio or television audiences. I looked at what kinds of studies had been done and how good they were, if there were multiple studies, and where they were published. Did the conclusions make sense? Were they provocative, yet still reasonable?

Very, very good studies were reflected in my choices. Little studies published in obscure journals were, too, although they were given less weight. Thus I'll heartily recommend a booster such as taking aspirin to prevent heart attacks, which is backed up by a number of well-constructed, well-executed studies showing significant results. I'll merely point out one such as flossing. Flossing is worth doing for a number of reasons, including the fact that it may prevent heart attacks by cutting down on bacterial invasion through the gums, but the data are much, much weaker. The Web site www.longevitycode.com, will be updated regularly with any data that may influence booster ratings.

Of course, good science (or any science, for that matter) was not available to support every longevity booster. When it wasn't, I relied on anecdotal information, the kind found in personal accounts from people who have used a particular measure successfully.

Any action step will get you somewhere. You could pick longevity boosters at random and still benefit in some way. Doing a little bit of this and a little bit of that with no discernible pattern or goal in mind, you would still drift into some kind of future, even one you might be lucky enough to really love. That outcome is much more likely, however, when you consciously select action steps that directly address your unique needs, strengths, hopes, and habits, as well as other elements of your personal longevity code. With this in mind, shuffle once more through the booster cards you've selected, pick one to start with, and make your first move toward increasing your life expectancy.

Zorba's Guide to the Seventy-six Most Effective Longevity Boosters

Introduction to the Boosters

Now that you've cracked your longevity code you should have a set of cards in front of you. Each card has a number that corresponds to a longevity booster. The card is a thumbnail sketch of the more detailed booster in this section. As you read each, you'll find specific tips and suggestions on how to take action on your longevity plan.

Before you start reading the boosters you might glance at the tables at the beginning of this section. Table 1 organizes the boosters by sphere in numerical order, which is basically a summary of Part III. Note how varied the seventy-six boosters are. Table 2 shows the boosters sorted by impact. The five-star boosters, which give you the most bang for your buck, are listed at the beginning. Be sure to read the introductory sections before many of the boosters. They'll give you additional insight.

TABLE 1 LONGEVITY BOOSTERS BY SPHERE

PHYSICAL	RATING	BOOSTER NUMBER
Toxins		
Stay Away from Tobacco	★★★★★	1
Don't Overdo Alcohol	★★★★★	2
Curtail Illicit Drug Use, Hard Drugs	★★★★★	3
Curtail Illicit Drug Use, Marijuana	★★★	4
Eating Patterns		
Eat More Fruits and Veggies–5 to 7 Servings per Day	★★★★★	5
Go for the Healthiest Quality and Quantity of Food	★★★★	6
Cut the Fat	★★★★★	7
Eat More Fiber	★★★	8
Eat Breakfast	★★★	9
Reduce Your Sugar Intake	★★	10
Limit Your Salt Intake	★★	11
Limit Snacking	★★	12

TABLE 1 LONGEVITY BOOSTERS BY SPHERE (*continued*)

PHYSICAL	RATING	BOOSTER NUMBER
Physical Activity		
Get Your Muscles Moving	★★★★★	13
Accident/Injury Prevention		
Limit Sun Exposure	★★★★	14
Fasten Seat Belts	★★★★	15
Drive Sanely	★★★★	16
Wear a Helmet	★★★★	17
Reduce Hazards in Your Home	★★★★	18
Practice Water Safety	★★★★	19
Preventive Medicine		
Have Safer Sex to Stop Sexually Transmitted Diseases	★★★★	20
Have Pap Tests to Screen for Cervical Cancer	★★★★	21
Screen for Colon and Rectal Cancer	★★★★	22
Screen for Breast Cancer	★★★★	23
Screen for Skin Cancer	★★★★	24
Screen for Prostate Cancer	★★	25
Get a Chest X-ray to Screen for Lung Cancer	★	26
Monitor Blood Pressure and Control Hypertension	★★★★★	27
Measure Your HDL, LDL, and Total Cholesterol Levels	★★★★★	28
Have Your Blood Sugar Checked for Diabetes	★★★★	29
Have Your Bone Density Checked for Osteoporosis	★★★	30
Vitamins and Supplements		
Add an Aspirin Every Day	★★★★★	31
Drink a Little Wine	★★★★	32
Take Estrogen	★★★★	33
Take a Multivitamin	★★★	34
Take Advantage of Antioxidants	★★★	35
Make Room for Calcium and Vitamin D	★★★	36
Regular Medical Visits		
Get Periodic Tune-ups	★★★★	37
Have a Good Relationship with Your Doctor	★★★	38
Get Immunized	★★★★	39
Use Medications Effectively	★★★★	40
Consider Complementary and Alternative Medicine	★★	41

TABLE 1 LONGEVITY BOOSTERS BY SPHERE (*continued*)

PHYSICAL	RATING	BOOSTER NUMBER
Drink Plenty of Water	★★	42
Get Enough Sleep	★★★	43
Take Care of Your Teeth and Gums	★★★★	44

MENTAL		
Detrimental Conditions		
Treat Depression	★★★★★	45
Manage Anger	★★★★★	46
Develop More and Better Skills for Coping with Stress	★★★★★	47
Stop Worrying Yourself to Death	★★★★	48
Address Alzheimer's, Senility, and Dementia	★★★	49
Intellectual Activities		
Commit to Lifelong Learning	★★★★★	50
Cultivate a Resilient, Optimistic, Can-do Attitude	★★★★★	51
Hang on to Your Sense of Humor	★★★★	52
Fight Forgetfulness	★★	53

KINSHIP/SOCIAL		
Extract Yourself from Abusive Relationships	★★★★★	54
Have a Satisfying, Long-term, Committed Marriage or Its Equivalent	★★★★★	55
Build a Strong Social Network	★★★★★	56
Build Good Relationships with Your Family	★★★★	57
Build Good Relationships with Friends	★★★★	58
Savor Sex and Intimacy	★★★	59
Own a Pet	★★	60

SPIRITUAL		
Explore the Spiritual Within You	★★★★★	61
Get Involved in a Spiritual Community	★★★★	62
Take Time with Mother Nature	★★★	63
Don't Avoid Thinking About Death	★★★★	64
Prepare Your Living Will and Advance Directives	★★★	65
Volunteer Service to Others	★★★★	66

MATERIAL		
Work Life		
Pursue Job Satisfaction	★★★★★	67

TABLE 1 LONGEVITY BOOSTERS BY SPHERE (*continued*)

MATERIAL	RATING	BOOSTER NUMBER
Ensure Job Safety	★★★★★	68
Procure Adequate Job Benefits	★★★★	69
Make Your Workplace Fun	★★★	70
Financial Life		
Calculate How Much Is Enough	★★★★	71
Minimize Your Debt	★★★	72
Maximize Your Savings and Retirement Income	★★★	73
Your Surroundings		
Don't Live in a Violent Environment	★★★★★	74
Nurture Your Home	★★	75
Reduce Air Pollution, Radon, and Indoor Toxins	★★	76

TABLE 2 LONGEVITY BOOSTERS BY IMPACT

	RATING	BOOSTER NUMBER
Stay Away from Tobacco	★★★★★	1
Don't Overdo Alcohol	★★★★★	2
Curtail Illicit Drug Use, Hard Drugs	★★★★★	3
Eat More Fruits and Veggies–5 to 7 Servings per Day	★★★★★	5
Treat Depression	★★★★★	45
Manage Anger	★★★★★	46
Develop More and Better Skills for Coping with Stress	★★★★★	47
Commit to Lifelong Learning	★★★★★	50
Cultivate a Resilient, Optimistic, Can-do Attitude	★★★★★	51
Extract Yourself from Abusive Relationships	★★★★★	54
Have a Satisfying, Long-term, Committed Marriage or Its Equivalent	★★★★★	55
Build Strong Social Network	★★★★★	56
Procure Job Satisfaction	★★★★★	67
Don't Live in a Violent Environment	★★★★★	74
Get Your Muscles Moving	★★★★★	13
Explore the Spiritual Within You	★★★★★	61
Add an Aspirin Every Day	★★★★★	31
Cut the Fat	★★★★★	7
Monitor Blood Pressure and Control Hypertension	★★★★★	27
Measure Your HDL, LDL, and Total Cholesterol Levels	★★★★★	28

TABLE 2 LONGEVITY BOOSTERS BY IMPACT (*continued*)

	RATING	BOOSTER NUMBER
Ensure Job Safety	★★★★★	68
Have Safer Sex to Stop Sexually Transmitted Diseases	★★★★	20
Take Estrogen	★★★★	33
Get Immunized	★★★★	39
Calculate How Much Is Enough	★★★★	71
Procure Adequate Job Benefits	★★★★	69
Have Pap Tests to Screen for Cervical Cancer	★★★★	21
Screen for Breast Cancer	★★★★	23
Have Your Blood Sugar Checked for Diabetes	★★★★	29
Screen for Colon and Rectal Cancer	★★★★	22
Take Care of Your Teeth and Gums	★★★★	44
Go for the Healthiest Quality and Quantity of Food	★★★★	6
Fasten Seat Belts	★★★★	15
Drive Sanely	★★★★	16
Wear a Helmet	★★★★	17
Practice Water Safety	★★★★	19
Reduce Hazards in Your Home	★★★★	18
Get Periodic Tune-ups	★★★★	37
Use Medications Effectively	★★★★	40
Drink a Little Wine	★★★★	32
Stop Worrying Yourself to Death	★★★★	48
Hang on to Your Sense of Humor	★★★★	52
Build Good Relationships with Your Family	★★★★	57
Build Good Relationships with Friends	★★★★	58
Get Involved in a Spiritual Community	★★★★	62
Volunteer as a Spiritual Act	★★★★	66
Don't Avoid Thinking About Death	★★★★	64
Screen for Skin Cancer	★★★★	24
Limit Sun Exposure	★★★★	14
Curtail Illicit Drug Use, Marijuana	★★★	4
Have a Good Relationship with Your Doctor	★★★	38
Make Room for Calcium and Vitamin D	★★★	36
Take a Multivitamin	★★★	34
Take Advantage of Antioxidants	★★★	35
Eat More Fiber	★★★	8

TABLE 2 LONGEVITY BOOSTERS BY IMPACT (*continued*)

	RATING	BOOSTER NUMBER
Eat Breakfast	★★★	9
Have Your Bone Density Checked for Osteoporosis	★★★	30
Get Enough Sleep	★★★	43
Address Alzheimer's, Senility, and Dementia	★★★	49
Savor Sex and Intimacy	★★★	59
Take Time with Mother Nature	★★★	63
Prepare Your Living Will and Advance Directives	★★★	65
Make Your Workplace Fun	★★★	70
Minimize Your Debt	★★★	72
Maximize Your Savings and Retirement Income	★★★	73
Fight Forgetfulness	★★	53
Drink Plenty of Water	★★	42
Reduce Your Sugar Intake	★★	10
Limit Your Salt Intake	★★	11
Limit Snacking	★★	12
Screen for Prostate Cancer	★★	25
Consider Complementary and Alternative Medicine	★★	41
Own a Pet	★★	60
Reduce Air Pollution, Radon, and Indoor Toxins	★★	76
Nurture Your Home	★★	75
Get a Chest X-ray to Screen for Lung Cancer	★	26

DR. ZORBA'S SEVENTY-SIX MOST EFFECTIVE LONGEVITY BOOSTERS

Physical Sphere

TOXINS

1. Stay Away from Tobacco — Impact ★★★★★

If you smoke, quit. If you don't smoke, don't start. And whenever possible, avoid being exposed to secondhand smoke.

From a primarily physical perspective, this is probably the single most effective strategy for preserving your quality of life and prolonging your stay on this planet. Why? Because longevity and health have no greater enemy than the toxins found in tobacco smoke.

Smoking kills. That's common knowledge. Yet one in four Americans continues to puff away. If you're one of them, you have your reasons. Maybe you started as a teen. Perhaps you smoke to "calm your nerves" or suppress your appetite. Maybe your social circle is made up of smokers, or your significant other smokes. It's something you share. Then again, you may simply like the sensation of lighting up a cigarette after a sumptuous meal or savoring a cigar with your Corona and lime.

Inhaling tobacco smoke sends a cocktail of toxic chemicals (including forty-three known cancer-causing agents) through your lungs into your bloodstream. The best known is nicotine. Smoking also accelerates the buildup of plaque on the inner lining of artery walls, promoting atherosclerosis. No wonder smokers are two and a half times more likely to develop heart disease than nonsmokers and four times as likely to die suddenly from heart attacks. They are also at least ten times more susceptible to colon, prostate, throat, neck, breast, cervical, and mouth cancers. And there's absolutely no doubt that smoking causes 95 percent of all lung cancer. Smoking also increases your risk of dying from stroke, emphysema, bronchitis, and pneumonia. And don't forget that careless smoking causes half of all household fires. Indeed, tobacco has a hand in one out of three premature deaths in this country, for a total of three to four hundred thousand annually. It is our number-one killer.

The sweet life is also more likely to elude smokers as it increases their risk of diabetes, osteoporosis, dementia, and macular degeneration.

No Way Around It

While the disastrous effects of smoking have the greatest impact on the folks who smoke the most, any amount of tobacco taken into your system can be deadly. And that includes secondhand smoke. But does that mean you're shortening your life each time you have lunch in a smoky restaurant or shoot a few games of pool in a smoky billiards parlor? Probably not. However, working eight hours a day, five days a week, in a smoky room or living with a smoker poses a significant health threat.

Just as there is no safe level of tobacco smoke exposure, there is no safe tobacco product. Chewing tobacco, which is used by some to get off cigarettes, is just as problematic—and equally addicting. And contrary to the impression created by their recent rise in popularity, cigars carry the same risks as other tobacco products. According to a study published in the *New England Journal of Medicine,* smoking one a day is just as deleterious to your health as smoking five to ten cigarettes.

Will Quitting Really Make a Difference?

You bet. After just one year smoke-free, your risk of having a fatal heart attack drops by 50 percent. It will be another ten to fifteen years before your chances of developing any heart disease are the same as a non-smoker's. Your lung cancer risk also drops year by year. After twenty years it equals that of someone who has never smoked.

More than forty-six million Americans already have quit smoking. Don't give up. The average smoker thinks about quitting three or four times a year and even tries once or twice. They may not broadcast their decision or make more than a halfhearted effort, but they do try. And eventually they do succeed, although it takes, on average, four attempts.

You also need the right motivation. In my practice, I probably see ten smokers a day (they tend to get sick and go to the doctor more often than nonsmokers). And I take a couple of minutes to discuss quitting with each of them. At most, one in twenty will go right out and follow my advice. Others will hear the message a few more times before they act. And some will wait until they are diagnosed with lung cancer but then instantly and permanently give up their smokes. Obviously, you don't want to follow their example.

Any reason can work. For me, back in my starving college student days, it was money. At the time, my resources were so limited that I drank powdered milk because I couldn't afford the real stuff. I had to carefully calculate whether I had enough money to buy a tomato for my salad or cookies for dessert. But I always managed to find money for cigarettes. When that dawned on me, and when I realized just how much I spent over the course of a year, I decided I simply couldn't afford the habit, and quit. At a point in my life when the harm I was doing to my body wouldn't have convinced me to stay away from cigarettes, I found something from another sphere—the material sphere —that did. You may want to look around at other spheres for motivation as well.

Five Tips to Help You Quit

1. *Plan ahead.* Giving up tobacco is a big step. You need to prepare yourself for it. This may include making some other changes first. You might want to pick up some stress-management skills or learn some relaxation techniques to use instead of lighting up to calm your nerves. Maybe line up some friends to back you up. The more prepared you are, the less likely you'll be to have your effort derailed by an event you'd normally respond to by lighting a cigarette.

2. *Start by cutting down.* Recent studies show that people who had dropped their nicotine levels several months before their official quit date by cutting back on the number of cigarettes they smoked per day fared much better.

3. *Get yourself through the first day.* No matter what, don't light up. In the same study, smokers who did not have a single cigarette during the first day of their smoking cessation effort were ten times more likely to stay off cigarettes for good.

4. *Consider pharmacological assistance.* There are a number of effective smoking cessation aids available today. For example, Zyban, another form of the antianxiety medication Wellbutrin, seems to control withdrawal symptoms and reduce nicotine cravings. A motivated quitter who uses Zyban has a 50 percent chance of being smoke-free after four months. Nicotine replacement by patch, gum, or inhaler doubles your chances of success.

5. *Mix methods.* All of the pharmacological aids work even better when they are combined with behavior modification. Joining a support group, telling your friends and relatives, having acupuncture, getting hypnotized, or any other adjunct won't hurt. By drawing on more than one sphere of wellness, you can only improve your chances for success.

2. Don't Overdo Alcohol   Impact ★★★★★

Next to milk, beer seems to be the drink of choice in the area of Wisconsin where I live. Many of my patients mark the end of their workday with a brew or two before dinner and another after their meal. Are they putting their lives in jeopardy? Perhaps. Cutting down a bit for some would clearly improve their chances to live longer, sweeter lives.

Excessive alcohol consumption is behind 60 to 90 percent of all deaths from cirrhosis of the liver, 40 to 50 percent of all motor vehicle fatalities, up to 50 percent of all adult drownings, up to 67 percent of household accidents, and a significant number of suicides and murders. And this country's fourteen million alcoholics (one in thirteen adults) are two and a half times more likely to die from almost any cause, from heart disease to pneumonia, than their nonalcoholic counterparts. Their dependence on alcohol, and the erratic, unpredictable, disruptive, aggressive, or abusive behavior that frequently accompanies it, adversely affects millions of spouses, children, employers, and coworkers. It's estimated that 53 percent of Americans know of at least one close friend or family member with a drinking problem.

Moderation Is the Key

Small quantities of alcohol improve appetite, provide a means to unwind at the end of a long and stressful day, put people at ease in social situations, and offer significant protection against heart disease (see page 246). Indeed, it is widely agreed that for most people, drinking in moderation may do some good. But just what does moderate drinking entail? An average of two drinks per day, with a drink being 1.5 ounces of hard liquor, 5 ounces of wine, or a 12-ounce beer, is considered safe for men. Women, who metabolize alcohol more slowly and tend to feel its effects more acutely, can handle half that amount (or the equivalent of one drink per day).

Because the standard of one to two drinks per day is an average, you could conceivably "save up" your daily drinks and have all seven to fourteen on the weekend or even in a single night. But recent information on binge drinking shows that it's super-hazardous.

Physically, when alcohol is used excessively, it irritates the throat and esophagus and damages the lining of the stomach. Alcohol destroys liver cells, leaving behind scar tissue—the hallmark of cirrhosis. The more you drink and the more regularly you drink to excess, the more likely you are to develop this life-shortening illness. Eight out of ten cases of liver disease are alcohol-related. In addition, heavy drinking contributes to weakening of the heart muscle, high blood pressure, stroke, and cancer of the esophagus, mouth, larynx, head, neck, and breast. It's been said that cancer mortality would drop by as much as one-third if more people cut their alcohol consumption to no more than two drinks a day.

As you might suspect, alcohol's adverse effects are not limited to the body. Under alcohol's influence, our thinking becomes more morose and our outlook more devoid of hope.

In the material sphere, heavy drinking is linked to poor job performance, absenteeism, lateness, occupational accidents, and difficulty simply holding on to a job. Finances are often a problem.

And the kinship sphere is also hard hit. Although moderate drinking is a socially acceptable activity, even encouraged in many social circles, heavy alcohol consumption and binges have numerous negative social implications. They disrupt families, contribute to domestic violence, and leave lasting scars on children

Stop Overdoing It—For a Better Shot at a Long, Sweet Life

- Keep little or no alcohol at home, if you have a problem.
- Pace yourself. Drink slowly and alternate alcoholic beverages with soda, water, or juice.
- Learn to say no. Set your limit and don't let others talk you into exceeding it. Stay away from people who give you a hard time about not drinking.
- Ask your family and friends to support your efforts. Perhaps one or more of them would like to cut down with you.
- Recognize when you tend to drink more than you'd like to, and find other, healthier things to do instead.
- Get professional help if you have trouble changing on your own. You may just need a few more suggestions—or there could be more going on than a little bit of extra drinking now and then.

Seek a Program of Recovery to Overcome Alcohol Abuse or Alcoholism

Heavy drinking becomes a drinking problem when drinkers are:

- Neglecting major work, school, or home responsibilities
- Drinking in obviously risky situations, such as while driving a car or operating machinery
- Having legal problems related to drinking
- Continuing to drink even though their drinking is causing or escalating problems in any relationships

Alcoholism is characterized by:

- A powerful craving, or compulsion, to drink
- Often being unable to stop drinking once they've started
- Physical dependence (when alcoholics stop using, their bodies rebel, producing nausea, sweating, shakiness, anxiety, and other withdrawal symptoms)
- Physical tolerance—needing more and more alcohol in order to obtain the same level of intoxication they once got with a smaller amount

How does one overcome an addiction to alcohol? After working with scores of patients who were struggling with alcoholism and other drinking problems, I can state quite emphatically that just using a little willpower isn't the answer. Alcoholism, which tends to run in families, seems to be inherited psychologically (by unconsciously emulating the behavior we observed during our childhood) as well as genetically. It is a complex syndrome, which I recommend you *not* try to fix yourself. The success rate without help is minimal because the road to recovery is not an easy one.

Once alcoholics acknowledge that they have a problem, they need to use every available resource to reach their goal of a long, sweet life. I usually send my patients to a local alcoholism counselor for evaluation. From there, they may:

- Obtain inpatient or outpatient follow-up treatment
- Join a self-help group such as AA
- Practice abstinence on a day-to-day basis every day
- Work with an employee-assistance program

As I said, it isn't easy. There is no pill you can take to overcome alcoholism.

3. Curtail Illicit Drug Use, Part I—Heroin, Cocaine, Crack, and Other Hard Drugs   Impact ★★★★★

Casey Alexander's descent into drug addiction and despair did not begin in the filthy inner-city crack houses where she would one day spend every spare moment of her time. No, Casey took her first hit from a crack pipe in a blue-collar suburb of Chicago during a backyard barbecue given by one of her neighbors. "This was back in the anything-goes, live-for-the-moment eighties," she recalled. "So when someone said, 'Here. You've got to try this,' I did."

The high was "very memorable," Casey noted, and pleasant enough for her to eagerly accept future offers to smoke. "Maybe if it had been a different time in my life," she said wistfully, "a time when I wasn't new to the area or nervous about starting my new teaching job and feeling very insecure, maybe then I could have just taken a little taste and moved on." Instead, she found herself powerfully attracted to crack's euphoric sensations.

"It was a great mental escape. By my fourth or fifth time I was hooked." Soon entire weekends were spent in a crack-induced state. Every penny not earmarked for food or rent went to replenish her drug supply. Even food became expendable after a while. It didn't take long for Casey to tap her savings or start running up credit card bills for cash advances. Naturally, her job performance suffered.

"When I heard rumors that my contract wouldn't be renewed, I asked to be transferred to another school so desperate for teachers that they'd take—and keep—anyone." Eventually the high was all she lived for. Barely functional, Casey made it to work and did "something that passed for teaching," but that was about it.

"I wasn't fooling anyone," she chuckled in retrospect. Her students knew what she did on her lunch hours and where she went at the end of the school day. "Then everyone found out," Casey reported. News of her drug involvement made the local papers after she was attacked and brutally beaten by a fellow crackhead. The six weeks she spent in the hospital recovering from her injuries (and letting the crack clear out of her system) gave her ample time to reflect on her own mortality. "It was a miracle I was still alive," she said. "And I decided to stay that way."

She entered a treatment program and, to date, has been quite successful at staying clean, sane, and sober. Casey may not regain all the years of life expectancy she lost to crack, but she's relatively happy and healthy, gainfully employed, and residing far from her former drug-abusing associates. "I plan to stick around for as long as possible and take the best possible care of myself," she stated.

And that's a statement that people who are as heavily involved in illicit hard drug use as she was often don't live long enough to make.

Smoking crack, snorting coke, shooting heroin or methamphetamine . . . all are totally incompatible with longevity. These drugs are poison. If you used to use them, especially intravenously, get checked for HIV and hepatitis. If you're still using, you need help. You will need a structured program to help you detoxify and fully recover.

Consider the following resources:

- Your family physician
- Members of the clergy
- Employee-assistance programs
- Narcotics Anonymous

4. Curtail Illicit Drug Use, Part II—Marijuana   Impact ★★★

In some circles marijuana is thought of as an innocuous intoxicant—nothing to worry about, except perhaps the possibility of getting caught with it in a state with strict drug-possession laws. In other quarters it is seen as a dangerous gateway to harder drugs. But in my opinion, based on the best available data, this drug falls somewhere between those two extremes. It has some positive, medicinal properties, most notably its ability to control nausea and increase the appetites of patients who have AIDS or are undergoing chemotherapy. And there's not much in the way of science to suggest that occasionally using small amounts of it harms us physiologically. Overall, its impact on longevity and life quality is a lot like alcohol's—it depends on how much you take in, what you do under its influence, and if it interferes with your ability to handle the demands of your daily life.

The risks of causing a fatal automobile accident, starting a kitchen fire, or losing control of your personal watercraft are still there. What's more, if you smoke marijuana late Sunday afternoon, it may still hamper your ability to perform complex or crucial tasks on Monday. In a study conducted a few years back, airline pilots who had smoked pot up to several days earlier were put in flight simulators and asked to handle a number of common flight situations. Their ability to react to those situations was still off-kilter seventy-two hours after they first became intoxicated.

Other drawbacks include:

- *Marijuana's effect on our lungs.* Regular use is associated with chronic bronchitis and emphysema. Some theorize, rightly so, that over time this causes premature heart disease.
- *Marijuana's effect on mental functioning.* Researchers have found that heavy users have trouble remembering recent events or conversations, following complicated thoughts, or solving problems.
- *Marijuana has a potential to exacerbate depression.*

It's my opinion that marijuana intoxication is akin to alcohol intoxication. Becoming inebriated is not an innocuous issue. So if you find yourself toking every day, thinking that this is a harmless activity, you should note that this is similar to the two-martini lunch. It has consequences for the long, sweet life.

EATING PATTERNS

A note to anyone who read the title of this section and thought, "Oh no, not again. Not another doctor telling me I have to lose weight and pitching a diet plan." Actually, this section of longevity boosters is *not* about dieting. It is about making food and behavior choices that increase your chances of living a long, long time with your health, vitality, and mental faculties intact.

Plenty of words have already been written on the perils of obesity. A multitude of diets, diet books, and diet products have found their way into the hands of people who truly need to reduce as well as many others who are merely chasing today's standard of beauty—a superthin, stick-straight body.

Rather than add fuel to this national fascination, I will be concentrating on dietary modifications that preserve health and promote longevity in their own right. Adopt them for their direct benefits, and if you are overweight, there's a good chance you'll drop a few pounds anyway. But whether you do or do not, you will still be making headway toward a longer, sweeter life.

Take a few seconds to complete Exercise 9 (page 191). If you checked one or more of these items, the boosters that follow could be crucial for cracking your personal longevity code.

Eating is a life-giving activity. What we eat nourishes our bodies. How and with whom we eat nourishes our hearts and souls. Food has countless meanings—love, respect, appreciation, tradition, inclusion. Meals bring people together, giving us an opportunity to talk between mouthfuls and laugh and feel close. It provides comfort and security. We have definite emotional attachments to certain foods, and often get quite anxious when faced with the prospect of altering our diets. However, very, *very* few of us will attain a longer, sweeter life without making some changes in our eating habits.

Our diets are intricately linked to longevity. When combined with a sedentary lifestyle, poor ones account for up to an estimated 30 percent of heart attack and stroke deaths, 30 to 50 percent of all fatal cancers (except lung cancer), and one-half to three-quarters of adult-onset diabetes cases. They play a role in more than 550,000 deaths each year.

We've known for more than two hundred years that what we eat determines how healthy we are, and that failing to meet certain dietary requirements leads to specific health problems. Way back in the 1800s British sailors sucked on limes to get vitamin C to prevent scurvy (and it earned them the nickname "limeys"). By the early 1900s we were able to synthesize vitamins and minerals and fortify foods with them to wipe out a number of other diseases caused by dietary deficiencies.

As the twentieth century progressed, so did our knowledge of how our bodies metabolized foods and which ones were best for which functions. This gave birth to the notion of four basic food groups and the advice to have something from each food group at every meal.

These guidelines proved to be a work in progress when the results from Dr. Ancel Keyes's Seven Countries Study started coming in. The landmark study, initiated in the late fifties, looked at the connection between a number of heart-disease risk factors and deaths from heart disease in the United States, Finland, the Netherlands, Italy, Croatia, Serbia, Greece, and Japan. It found, among other things, that diet definitely made a difference, and that the so-called Mediterranean diet, favored by the Greeks and Italians, offered far more protection against heart disease than our own patterns. A direct comparison of Italian and American railroad workers revealed 15 percent higher serum cholesterol levels among the Americans and a 33 percent higher heart disease death rate. When lifestyles were examined, what differed most was diet, with the Italians consuming lots of pasta, greens with olive oil, fresh

---

EXERCISE 9

DO YOU:

❑ Have a family or personal history of or other risk factors for:
   ❑ Heart disease? Stroke?
   ❑ Cancer of the colon: stomach: breast: prostate?
   ❑ Diabetes?
❑ Currently have:
   ❑ High blood pressure?
   ❑ Elevated blood sugar levels?
   ❑ High cholesterol levels?
❑ Rarely manage to make your diet match the recommendations found on the food pyramid?
❑ Worry about your weight? Go on and off diets a lot?
❑ Have physical, emotional, social, or occupational problems related to being obese or overweight?
❑ Eat less than five servings of fruit or vegetables daily?
❑ Often skip breakfast?
❑ Consume more than one-third of your diet in meat, dairy products, and fried food?

---

vegetables, cheese, fruit, and wine. They consumed much less meat than Americans, more fruit, and fewer standard (high-fat) desserts.

These findings, which have been replicated numerous times, led to the development of the food pyramid guide to healthy food choices (see page 200). The portions and proportions it suggests form the foundation for an ideal diet. This optimal way of eating also includes:

- Variety
- Breakfast
- More breads, pastas, and grains than fruit and vegetables; more fruits and vegetables than meats and dairy products; and as little added fat and sugar as possible
- Five to seven servings of fruit and vegetables daily, with a varied selection providing a full complement of nutrients
- More fiber
- No more than 30 percent of daily calories from fats

- Less salt
- Nutritious midmorning and afternoon minimeals instead of sweet snacks that play havoc with our energy levels

Some of you will have to change more than others in order to fit healthy habits like these into your lifestyle. But every step counts, which is why I've broken diet down into eight separate longevity boosters. Their various amplifiers, impact, and action ratings will help you decide where to start.

The Question of Obesity

Marcy Hammond was smart, witty, and compassionate, with a creative flair that made the packages she designed for an advertising and marketing firm award winners. The extra thirty pounds she carried weren't all that noticeable on her five-foot-nine frame, and they didn't seem to be causing any health problems. Yet they dragged her down emotionally and socially like two fifty-pound blocks of cement. She isolated herself because of them, hardly ever going out socially. No matter how nicely she tried to dress, Marcy felt unattractive.

Although she would have made a brilliant art director, Marcy didn't dare try for a promotion. All the women who advanced to that level of the company looked like they just "stepped out of the pages of *Cosmo*," Marcy explained. Trapped at a drafting table in a tiny cubicle by day and exiled to a cluttered apartment at night, Marcy periodically pinned her hopes on some new weight-loss regimen and its promise to make her thin. But whatever she lost, if she lost at all, came back in short order. She soon added "weak-willed failure" to the list of derogatory names she called herself. After a half-dozen dieting ups and downs, Marcy was so depressed that suicide seemed like a reasonable option. Luckily, she checked herself into a hospital instead.

That's where I met her, and together we began to problem-solve. I agreed to put her on a supervised weight-loss plan that I typically recommended to much heavier people with physical health problems. It wasn't going to hurt her, and it might help her recover from the psychological fallout of being heavy in a society that overvalues lightweights. Equally important for Marcy's well-being was encouraging her to look closely at her mental and kinship spheres. A self-help group would access both. Marcy was ready to show herself some compassion.

We make much ado about body weight in this country. We're obsessed with getting thinner, desperate to be as svelte as the models, actors, and marathon runners we see in magazines and movies. Collectively we spend billions of dollars on diet products and programs to lose thousands of pounds that we sometimes gain back. Today, Americans are more overweight than ever before.

Based on body mass index (BMI)—55 percent of Americans exceed the upper limit for healthy weight (a BMI of 25). (The table below gives you the values in pounds and inches.) One in four of us are considered obese (a BMI of 30 or more), which puts us at risk for high blood pressure, adult-onset diabetes, osteoarthritis, heart disease, cancer (breast, colon, prostate, and kidney), gallbladder disease, and sleep apnea. A recently published study from the *New England Journal of Medicine* following more than one million American men and women for more than fourteen years showed that if you were moderately to severely overweight, you were nearly twice as likely to die prematurely.

However, controversial research has shown that obesity's propensity for increasing morbidity declines with each passing year, exerting little influence on the life expectancy of folks over fifty.

As mentioned before, an obese individual's problems aren't limited to the physical sphere. She or he may also suffer social discrimination, financial hardship, and emotional distress. This often extends to moderately overweight and normal-weight individuals who erroneously feel they have failed to attain the size and shape society expects of them. Their inability to lose weight may damage their souls and psyches even more. It's a mistake to underestimate the longevity-busting potential of the cosmetic side of excess body weight. The experience of being ridiculed or overlooked, the perception of yourself as being inadequate and unappealing, and the frustration of starving off pounds and succeeding only to see them all come back take a tremendous toll on the psyche. Marcy taught me that.

If you want to lose weight:

- *Make sure you need to.* Use the table to calculate your body mass index. If it comes out over 30, losing weight may be a good idea, especially if you have weight-related health problems. If it's between 25 and 29.9, you can make the call based on how you feel and whether your weight is interfering with your life.

EXERCISE 10—Determining Body Mass Index from Height and Weight

	BODY MASS INDEX (KG/M^2)				
	18	20	22	23	24
Height (in.)	Body Weight (lb.)				
58	86	96	105	110	115
59	89	99	109	114	119
60	92	102	112	118	123
61	95	106	116	122	127
62	98	109	120	126	131
63	101	113	124	130	135
64	104	116	128	134	140
65	108	120	132	138	144
66	112	124	136	142	148
67	115	127	140	146	153
68	119	131	144	151	158
69	122	135	149	155	162
70	125	139	153	160	167
71	129	143	157	165	172
72	133	147	162	169	177
73	137	151	166	174	182
74	141	155	171	179	186
75	144	160	176	184	192
76	148	164	180	189	197

- *Set a goal.* To date, there is no evidence that dieting down to your presumed ideal weight confers any health or longevity benefits (probably because so few dieters ever get or stay there). We do know that a 10 percent drop for someone who needs to lose brings about a corresponding drop in blood pressure, cholesterol levels, and other health risks. I recommend getting that much off and keeping it off for six months before trying to lose more.
- *Consult a doctor or registered dietician.* A professional can help you put together the food plan that's most likely to work for you.
- *Get more exercise.* The combination is what takes (and, more important, keeps) the weight off.
- *Focus your attention elsewhere.* Get a life and live it. (See the boosters

25	26	27	28	29	30	35
119	124	129	134	138	143	167
124	128	133	138	143	148	173
128	133	138	143	148	153	179
132	137	143	148	153	158	185
136	142	147	153	158	164	191
141	146	152	158	163	169	197
145	151	157	163	169	174	204
150	156	162	168	171	180	210
155	161	167	173	179	186	215
159	166	172	178	185	191	223
164	171	177	184	190	197	230
169	176	182	189	196	203	236
174	181	188	195	202	207	243
179	186	193	200	208	215	250
184	191	199	206	213	221	258
189	197	204	212	219	227	265
194	202	210	218	225	233	272
200	208	216	224	232	240	279
205	213	221	230	238	246	287

in the mental, kinship, spiritual, and material spheres.) Being preoc-cupied with your weight while you're trying to lose it is like wait-ing for a pot of water to boil.

• *Put the diet boosters that follow to use.*

5. Eat More Fruits and Veggies—Five to Seven Servings per Day   Impact ★★★★★

Fresh fruit and vegetables aren't very popular in Scotland. In fact, Scots eat fewer servings per day than folks in most other parts of the world—and their premature death rates are among the highest, especially for women between forty-five and fifty-four. Over in Spain, where fruit and vegetable consumption is four times that of Scotland's, women have a remarkably low midlife death rate. These facts by themselves do not prove that eating plenty of fruit and vegetables boosts longevity. But taken as part of a growing body of data on the subject, they leave little doubt that one of the best things we can do for our health and life expectancy is to consume five to seven servings of fruit and vegetables each and every day.

This practice has been definitively linked to a lower risk of heart disease, stroke, and colon cancer. There's some indication that it prevents lung and non-melanoma skin cancer as well. Eating lots of fruit and vegetables is also an integral part of the diet used to combat hypertension. And in a study of premenopausal women whose mothers or sisters had breast cancer (a major risk factor), those who ate at least five servings of fruit and vegetables a day were 70 percent less likely to develop the disease than women who ate two servings or less. Several Harvard University scientists found that the men and women who consumed the most fruit and vegetables (five or six servings per day) had a 31 percent lower risk than men and women who consumed fewer than three servings.

That's pretty impressive, and it doesn't even address the specific health benefits of particular fruit and vegetables. Take broccoli, carrots, and red peppers. All are high in beta-carotene, which strengthens our immune systems. Broccoli has also been credited with lowering the risk of heart attacks, asthma, and osteoporosis. In addition:

- Tomatoes are loaded with lycopene, instrumental in bringing about a 40 percent reduction in prostate, lung, and stomach cancer risk.
- Spinach is full of folate, or folic acid, which fights cancer, birth defects, heart disease, and mental disorders. It may even have a positive effect on Alzheimer's.
- The equivalent of half a cup of fresh or frozen blueberries may slow or reverse memory failure.

Despite all of this evidence, only 30 percent of men and 50 percent of women actually eat five to seven servings of fruit and vegetables every day. If it weren't for french-fried potatoes dipped in tomato ketchup, those numbers would be lower. Yet meeting the standard is not as difficult as you think. Six ounces of juice with breakfast, an apple at midmorning, a salad with lunch, a sweet potato or a handful of carrot sticks, and you're on your way. Remember:

- *Something is better than nothing.* If you can't eat seven servings, consume at least three, then add a fourth, and when you've grown accustomed to that, add number five. In the Harvard study, every time a fruit was added, the risk of stroke dropped another 6 percent.
- *Variety is as important as quantity.* Different fruits or vegetables provide different nutrients—and you need them all. So try a kiwi or a crenshaw melon, spaghetti squash or Chinese eggplant.
- *Raw is the best way to eat most fruit and vegetables.* The more you cook them, the greater the odds that vital nutrients will be lost.
- *When you do cook your vegetables, frozen are as nutritious as fresh.* Use canned if fresh or frozen aren't available, although most nutrients don't make it through the canning process and canned products tend to be packed with extra salt.

6. Go for the Healthiest Quality and Quantity of Food	Impact ★★★★

When we hear the term *healthy eating,* we think deprivation—no more Big Macs or chocolate bars or Mom's macaroni and cheese. We think boring—meals of bland skinless chicken or flounder broiled without butter five nights a week, with no sauces or dressing or taste, and requiring more time and attention than our jam-packed schedules allow. Wrong!

What healthy eating experts are actually advocating is not the elimination of certain foods or food groups. Be wary of anyone who tells you that you will lose weight and be healthier by eating only protein or just raw fruits and vegetables or as much as you want of any one item so long as you eat nothing else. Whether you hear about healthy eating from the American Heart Association (AHA), your family physician, or your yoga instructor, they do not encourage such drastic reductions in quantity that you're bordering on starvation. (Life *is* too short for that.) And finally, what healthy-eating advocates have to say isn't only appropriate for people with serious weight or health problems.

Anyone who wants to stick around for as long as possible in as healthy, independent, and contented a state as possible will benefit from a diet that is moderate, balanced, and varied. Moderation works because both overeating and undereating can spell serious trouble. Balance works because we need to get the right mix of macronutrients (carbohydrates, proteins, and fats) and micronutrients (vitamins, minerals, and fiber) for our bodies to not just survive but thrive. Variety works for the same reason. Healthy eating loses some of its longevity-boosting power when mealtimes become dull and distasteful. Eating is, after all, an activity that's been giving us pleasure and a number of other social and emotional perks for most of our lives.

Keys to Eating for a Longer, Sweeter Life

Calories Count

This doesn't mean you have to slavishly calculate them, but rather that the fuel (calories) that you put into your body should not exceed the energy you expend on basic life support (breathing, keeping your blood circulating, and so on) and daily activities. If it does, your body gathers up the calories you haven't used and stores them as fat—which is fine up to a point. We all need some body fat to cushion our bones, protect our vital organs, and burn as fuel if we should be forced to go without food for any length of time. Beyond that point, excess fat can adversely affect our appearance and self-confidence, our ability to move about without feeling short of breath, our relationships, and our health.

As I mentioned in the introduction to this section, once we reach the point of obesity, our weight becomes a risk factor for diabetes, high blood pressure, heart disease, and more—perhaps not as great a risk factor as cigarette smoking or genetics, but a risk factor nonetheless.

If we decide to lose some excess fat, calories come into play again. We must create a calorie deficit by taking in less fuel than we need. This forces us to tap into our reservoirs of body fat for energy and can be accomplished by eating less, doing more, or preferably a combination of the two.

How many calories do we actually need? The stock answer would be:

- About 1, 600 for most women and older adults
- About 2,200 for children, adolescent females, active women, and most men
- About 2,800 for teenage boys and active men

However, individuals vary tremendously. If you are fairly muscular, you'll burn more calories than someone who isn't, and therefore you can consume more. Needs also change over time. If you are over forty or forty-five, your metabolism is 5 to 10 percent slower than it was a decade ago, which means you'll use 200 fewer calories per day. Likewise, if you've dieted frequently, yo-yoing up and down the scale, your body may react more slowly the next time you cut back.

If you are clearly obese and starting to suffer in any sphere as a result, you would be well advised to consult a physician or registered dietician to determine your best calorie balance and how to achieve it. Support groups like OA (Overeaters Anonymous) can help. Folks who are simply concerned about their weight can do this as well, although for most of us the general ranges listed above are reasonable targets.

All Calories Are Not Created Equal

If we get our daily allotment from soda, potato chips, and candy bars, we obtain few vitamins, minerals, fiber, or the other nutrients our bodies need to repair and replenish themselves, fight off infections, maintain bone strength, and more. What we need is variety (a diet made up of all different kinds of foods, because each supplies different nutrients) plus balance (the optimal amount of each food in relation to the others and as part of the whole). That's where the Department of Agriculture's food pyramid guide to healthy food choices comes in. The pyramid reflects our understanding that we need more of some foods and less of others to prolong life and stay healthy.

At the base of the pyramid is the bread, cereal, rice, and pasta group. These carbohydrates, which provide us with slow-burning fuel to keep our systems running on an even keel, should be the foundation of our daily diets. Six to eleven servings are suggested for our metabolism and much-needed fiber, vitamins, and minerals.

Up one level, you find both the vegetable group and the fruit group, which were discussed at length in the section that preceded this one. We need five to seven servings from these groups combined.

Next is the milk, yogurt, and cheese group and the meat, poultry, dried beans, eggs, and nuts group. Both are good sources of protein. However, their abundance of fat, much of it the saturated kind, make them less of a mainstay than we need. Two to three servings of each are enough.

Food Guide Pyramid

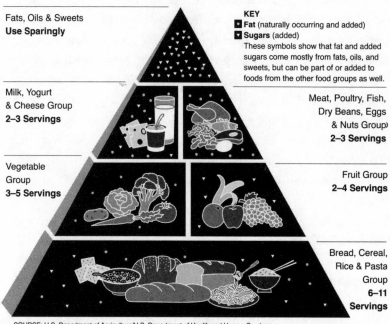

Fats, Oils & Sweets
Use Sparingly

KEY
◼ Fat (naturally occurring and added)
▼ Sugars (added)
These symbols show that fat and added
sugars come mostly from fats, oils, and
sweets, but can be part of or added to
foods from the other food groups as well.

Milk, Yogurt
& Cheese Group
2–3 Servings

Meat, Poultry, Fish,
Dry Beans, Eggs
& Nuts Group)
2–3 Servings

Vegetable
Group
3–5 Servings

Fruit Group
2–4 Servings

Bread, Cereal,
Rice & Pasta
Group
**6–11
Servings**

SOURCE: U.S. Department of Agriculture/U.S. Department of Health and Human Services.

Added fats and sugars, which top the pyramid, could probably be lopped off entirely and never be missed nutritionally. But they do add flavor and make the preparation of our favorite dishes possible. Use them sparingly.

Don't Forget Fish and Seafood

From the Mediterranean to Japan, when people eat fish, they live longer. Research from the mammoth Western Electric Study, which began in the 1950s, and data from the more recent Physicians Health Study show that eating one to two servings per week of fish or seafood may reduce the risk of a premature heart attack by 50 percent.

While some believe that it's the omega-3 fatty acids in fish that protect your heart, others speculate that other fish proteins or micronutrients may be the key. Perhaps that's why there is very little good data to show that taking fish-oil supplements is beneficial.

Vary your seafood selection:

• Tuna, salmon, and mackerel—fish high in omega-3 fatty acids

- Shrimp, oysters, and clams—also high in omega-3s but with differing proteins
- Cod, perch, halibut—low fat

And remember to broil, boil, or poach your fish. The Friday-night fish fries across the country are an example of a good idea gone awry.

Portion Size Matters

America is the home of the Big Gulp, a soft drink so big it has eight times as many calories as the eight-ounce bottles that Coca-Cola originally came in. We have Biggie fries and man-sized frozen dinners, entrées for hearty appetites and giant candy bars. No wonder the vast majority of us don't have a clue about what constitutes a single serving of anything. If we want to eat right and maintain a healthy weight, we have to weigh and measure at first. Here are some sample serving sizes by food group:

- *Dairy*: 1 serving = 1 cup of milk or yogurt; 1.5 oz of natural cheese (the equivalent of a cube with 1-inch sides); 2 oz of processed cheese
- *Protein*: 1 serving = 2 to 3 oz of cooked lean meat, poultry, or fish (roughly the size of a deck of cards); ½ cup cooked beans, 1 egg, or 2 tbsp of peanut butter count as one oz of lean meat
- *Vegetable*: 1 serving = 1 cup raw leafy vegetables; ½ cup of other vegetables, cooked or raw; ½ cup of vegetable juice
- *Fruit*: 1 serving = 1 medium apple; ½ cup of chopped, cooked, or canned fruit; ¾ cup of fruit juice
- *Grains*: 1 serving = 1 slice of bread; 1 ounce of ready-to-eat cereal (may be a cup or ¾ cup, check the package); ½ cup cooked cereal, rice, or pasta.

7. Cut the Fat	Impact ★★★★★

I'm not sure there's any dietary issue that's left the American public as befuddled as the issue of reducing the amount of fat in our diets. First there's all the different kinds of fat (saturated, unsaturated, monounsaturated, polyunsaturated, or partially hydrogenated) and oils (olive, canola, corn, vegetable, or coconut). Then there's the wide range of opinions on how much fat is enough. If 30 percent (the American Heart Association's recommendation) is good, is 25 or 15 or 5 percent even better? Even when we finally accept something—for instance, that margarine, which contains no animal fat, is better than butter, which does—the rug is pulled out from under us, as it now seems that the man-made trans fats in margarine actually raise cholesterol.

Well, let's see if we can sort some of this out, beginning with the bottom line: *Consuming too much fat of any kind is definitely a longevity buster.* The matter has been studied from every imaginable angle, and in practically every instance there has been a close correlation between the fat in people's diets and deaths from coronary artery disease. The higher the percentage of fat, the higher the death rate.

The biggest culprit is saturated fats from meat and dairy products as well as the tropical oils, coconut and palm. Running a close second are the trans fats found in stick margarine and in partially hydrogenated shortenings that are melted down for deep frying, candy snacks, or used in baked goods. Softer margarines in tub or liquid form have very few trans fats, that's why they're safer.

Excessive dietary fat is also a significant risk factor for prostate cancer, which American men are fifteen times more likely to develop than Japanese men, who don't eat nearly as much saturated fat. Colon cancer risk is affected as well. Indeed, if Americans cut their consumption of red meat and other forms of saturated fat by half, we might see a 50 percent drop.

On the other hand, unsaturated fats from plant sources, including the monounsaturated kind supplied by some nuts and olive or canola oils, may even raise good cholesterol and *lower* bad cholesterol. The benefits of the so-called Mediterranean diet—i.e., less heart disease and stroke—may be from its reliance on olive oil.

Likewise, consumption of omega-3 fatty acids, found plentifully in fatty fishes such as salmon, have a positive effect by reducing the risk of heart disease. Eating fish once or twice a week has been shown to be a useful part of a heart-healthy diet.

For health and longevity, most of the fat in your diet should be healthier fat—although not in unlimited amounts. All fats pack an inordinate number of calories into a small quantity of food (100 calories per tablespoon of fat compared to 45 calories per tablespoon of sugar).

So, Just How Much Is Enough but Not Too Much?

You will never hear a reputable scientist or physician recommend a diet completely devoid of fat. For one thing, it would be almost impossible to pull off. For another, we all need some fat to keep our bodies and brains functioning normally. A diet with anything less than 10 percent of its calories from fat might certainly deprive us of vital nutrients. There's some indication that it also might lower good HDL cholesterol, leaving us *more* prone to heart disease.

Okay, then, how about 15 to 20 percent? Some doctors will recommend very low fat diets based on data showing heart disease being reversed. However, the dramatic results were often achieved in only highly controlled inpatient settings. For the average person operating in the real world, limiting your total fat intake to 30 percent of your daily calories is more than adequate. Always keep in mind that monounsaturated and polyunsaturated fats are essential while saturated fats are not.

Since the average American diet is 35 to 40 percent fat, much of it saturated, this may represent a significant drop for many of you, even though it seems small. Your best bet for achieving it is probably not to get caught up in complicated fat-calorie calculations, but rather to make simple but significant modifications wherever you can.

- Switch from whole milk to fat-free, using 2 percent or 1 percent milk to make the transition if necessary.
- Eat less meat. Designate one or several days per week as meatless days. Experiment with vegetarian recipes and experience new tastes. Tofu, anyone?
- Use less butter or margarine. Substitute olive or canola oil for cooking, fruit spreads or fat-free cheeses on your toast or bagel, applesauce or fruit butters when baking.
- Grill and steam foods more. Fry and sauté less.
- Become a spice maven. Sprinkle on the Creole or Cajun spices. Scoop salsa into your baked potato instead of sour cream. Add that cayenne or cumin and you'll hardly notice the missing fat!
- Take advantage of selected reduced-fat or fat-free foods, from dairy products to spaghetti sauces or snack foods. But beware: Low-fat does *not* mean low-calorie. Reduced-fat cookies, cakes, peanut butter, and yogurt all have even more sugar than their higher-fat

counterparts, making them at least as fattening, if not more so. You can't eat unlimited quantities.

8. Eat More Fiber   Impact ★★★

Once considered so expendable—and inedible—that we started processing foods to get rid of it, fiber is now believed to be at least as important as most vitamins and minerals when it comes to maintaining good health. Found only in food from plants, dietary fiber comes in two forms: soluble and insoluble.

Soluble fiber, which dissolves in water, is valuable for keeping diabetics' blood sugar levels stable and reducing the risk of heart disease by lowering serum cholesterol. The best sources are peas, beans of all kinds, oats, barley, apples, oranges, and carrots.

Insoluble fiber absorbs water rather than dissolving in it and is plentiful in whole grains, wheat bran, cauliflower, green beans, potatoes, and many other vegetables. It helps prevent constipation and intestinal disorders such as diverticulitis and irritable bowel syndrome.

Because foods high in either or both of these fibers are relatively low in calories and tend to be filling, eating more of them can be instrumental for maintaining a healthy weight. Better still, whole-grain breads, brown rice, and other fiber-rich foods are packed with more vitamins and minerals than even nutrient-fortified refined or processed plant products such as white bread and white rice can provide.

Clearly, getting enough fiber—the American Dietetic Association recommends 20 to 35 g a day—is a good deal all around. I highly recommend that you gradually increase your daily intake to that level. Most of us are not there yet. The gradual part is important, because adding too much fiber too quickly can cause gas, bloating, and diarrhea.

Your best bets for upping fiber intake?

- Make several of your servings of fruits and vegetables fiber-rich selections. Apples or pears with their skins, oranges, strawberries, raw carrots, cooked broccoli, and Brussels sprouts are all good choices.
- Eat a hearty fiber-filled breakfast.
- Eat baked or roasted potatoes with their well-scrubbed skins on.
- Throw some chickpeas on a salad.
- Eat whole-grain breads and pastas.

- Select soups with legumes in them, such as split pea or lentil.
- And yes, eat more beans (baked beans have 9.8 g of fiber in half a cup).

9. Eat Breakfast   Impact ★★★

Having last eaten the previous evening, we need refueling by the next morning. This condition is easy enough to remedy, but instead of sitting down to breakfast or even grabbing an apple on the run, many of us plunge right into our daily activities without eating anything. This is yet another habit that the Human Population Lab has linked to lower life expectancy.

With no calories to burn, we tend to move, think, and react to stimuli more slowly. In study after study, breakfast skippers turned out to be less productive. In addition, because they tend to succumb to hunger pangs and overeat at lunch or grab a convenient but not necessarily nutritious snack by midmorning, people who miss breakfast have trouble maintaining a healthy weight.

Breakfast is a meal packed with nutrients. We also get an extra longevity boost from vitamin- and mineral-fortified breakfast cereal—which can be an excellent source of fiber as well. Nurse's Health Study subjects whose morning meal included breakfast cereal appeared to lower their heart disease risk considerably and gained a year or two in life expectancy. Why not follow their lead?

For maximum longevity, choose a whole-grain cereal without a lot of added sugar. Breakfast should be your opportunity to stock up on fiber. And don't forget to use low-fat or skim milk and drink a glass of juice or eat a piece of fruit. Other easy morning meals include:
- Whole-wheat toast and jam with a cup of fruit and yogurt
- Fruit with low-fat cheese on a bagel
- Fruit and a turkey, cheese, or peanut butter sandwich on whole-grain bread

10. Reduce Your Sugar Intake   Impact ★★

Most of us have a sweet spot for sweet things—a sweet tooth, if you will. We love our colas and candy kisses, our Oreo cookies and cherry cheesecake. We love them so much that we Americans consume the equivalent of more than 150 pounds of sweeteners—sugar, dextrose, corn syrup—per person per year. It clearly contributes to problems that come between us and a longer, sweeter life.

We know, for example, that people who eat a lot of sweets tend to have dental problems. They're prone to cavities, toothaches, lost teeth, and gum disease. We also know that sweets are calorie dense. What amounts to very little food in ounces packs quite a caloric wallop. It's very easy to take in hundreds of extra calories in no time flat. In addition, sugary foods are famous for creating a surge of energy that dissipates quickly, leaving us sluggish, irritable, and often craving more sweets. Giving in to that craving sets the cycle in motion again.

Some people find that eliminating refined sugars entirely also eliminates their cravings and tendency to overeat. However, I have not seen enough data on the subject to recommend this myself. In fact, you may actually want to eat a bit of chocolate now and then. One and a half ounces of it contains roughly the same amount of antioxidants as a glass of red wine (see page 246) and may prevent bad LDL cholesterol from depositing fat on our artery walls. Although it didn't single out chocolate, in a recent update of the Harvard Alumni Study, it appeared that men who ate candy once or several times per week lived longer than those who ate none.

Of course, that's a far cry from the amount of sugar we both knowingly and unwittingly consume each day. To cut down:

- *Start with soft drinks.* Use water, seltzer, or flavored sparkling waters.
- *Save sugary desserts for once- or twice-a-week treats.*
- *Go with products that are lower in sugar than the ones you have been using.*
- *Switch to unsweetened applesauce or fruits packed in their own juices.*

11. Limit Your Salt Intake   Impact ★★

Salt is essential to maintain the delicate balance of fluids in our body. But the vast majority of us err on the side of overconsumption. Indeed, the average American's diet includes two to three times more sodium than the USDA's daily recommended allotment of 2,400 mg.

Does this pose a serious health threat? It does if you suffer from congestive heart failure or kidney disease, which are complicated by salt's ability to retain water. For years we also believed that taking in extra salt raised blood pressure and that high blood pressure could be lowered significantly by severely restricting our salt intake. We now know its effect is modest and not in everyone.

If we tend to go way over the daily amount of sodium suggested for optimal health, we can bring it down a bit by:

- Tasting food before salting it (many of us automatically reach for the shaker when the dish may not really need it)
- Sticking with fresh or frozen veggies rather than the canned kind, which contain significant salt
- Switching to sauces, soups, and other processed foods that are labeled "low-sodium."

But once you start imposing limits on your salt intake that are stricter than you need, you begin to greatly limit what you can eat, where you can eat (nearly all restaurants are out of bounds), and who will be willing to eat with you. This loss of pleasure and mealtime socializing is actually longevity-busting. (Life only *seems* longer when we're on super-strict diets.) And since there is no clear evidence that such severe restrictions actually benefit the majority of us, I don't recommend them.

12. Limit Snacking   Impact ★★

Back in the seventies, researchers in California, at the Alameda County Human Population Laboratory, identified snacking between meals as one of seven habits that contributed to premature death. But by the mid-nineties most nutritionists and registered dieticians were recommending midmorning and afternoon snacks to keep our metabolism running efficiently. Is it possible to reconcile these seemingly polar opposite points of view? Absolutely—by looking at the foods we snack on.

Snacking frequently on chips or cookies, candy bars, ice cream, doughnuts, or other high-fat, high-calorie, salty, or sugary processed foods gives us a blood sugar rush, a quick burst of energy followed by a letdown that we remedy by reaching for another snack. This cycle can put us way over the top in daily calories and grams of fat, sometimes prompting us to cut back on more nutritious foods at lunch or dinner.

Eating small, nutritionally balanced minimeals at two- to three-hour intervals has the opposite effect. It keeps our blood sugar and overall energy levels on an even keel, making us less likely to overeat throughout the day or at a single sitting. A regimen of breakfast, a mid-morning snack, lunch, an afternoon snack, then dinner may actually be better for us than that old dietary standby, three meals a day with nothing in between. The key is to make healthy snack choices (fruit and cheese, nuts and low-fat yogurt, or half a turkey sandwich).

PHYSICAL ACTIVITY

13. Get Your Muscles Moving   Impact ★★★★

We are designed by nature to exercise. Our ancestors were hunters, gatherers, and farmers. They didn't have the plush, passive life that we have. They did more manual work and walked from place to place to visit or to find food.

A hundred years ago, before the advent of modern transportation, we all got plenty of exercise. We walked, which in my opinion is the absolutely best solitary exercise.

But just look at today's society. When we are young we walk or bike everywhere. When we reach sixteen, though, things change. The automobile, and its cousin public transportation, has made us lazy. It has encouraged us to ride when we could walk, to sit and take a load off instead of moving our muscles.

Studies have shown that people who exercise feel better about themselves. They derive a sense of well-being from exercise itself. This is probably due to the increased level of endorphins (natural neuropeptides in the brain that give us a sense of happiness). The physical reserve that activity gives you often helps you recover from an illness. People who exercise often are back to work sooner following a simple cold or sore throat. And if they fall and fracture anything, exercise is a boon. The rehab and physical therapy you need to recover is easier if you know how to exercise.

We need to broaden the definition of exercise and understand that it includes all of us. We're all capable of movement. It is wonderful and admirable to have a strong exercise program. This section will give you some suggestions on how to put one together. It is also wonderful to redefine exercise so that it includes dancing wildly with your children, hiking a path with your teenager, running the beach with your dog, or gently canoeing on a beautiful river. As long as you get in some sustained movement three or four times a week, you are exercising. Work it up to the point where you sweat and you give yourself more benefit.

Before you determine what exercise is best for you, it's necessary to see what effect exercise has on your longevity and physiology.

Survival and Fitness

Numerous studies, including the Harvard Alumni Study, the Nurse's Health Study, the Physicians Health Study, and the Framingham Study, have shown that those who exercise live longer than those who don't. It's not a panacea. It's not that exercise is a cure for superhigh cholesterol or the antidote for smoking, but study after study shows that it is an independent predictor of longevity.

The classical study published in the *Journal of the American Medical Association* years ago followed more than fifteen thousand people to see how exercise affected longevity. They found that after controlling for smoking, cholesterol, obesity, glucose levels, and family history of heart disease, those who were most fit were least likely to perish early. From heart disease to stroke, diabetes to osteoporosis to depression, exercise helps. And it appears that no matter how old you are when you start exercising, you will receive some benefit. Researchers publishing in the English journal *The Lancet* showed that men and women who begin to exercise in middle age live longer than their slothful counterparts.

So what does this mean to you? If you want to lower your risk of death, then move. A couch-potato lifestyle is a cardiac-disease-prone, cancer-prone lifestyle.

How Much and How Long Must I Exercise to Become Fit?

When we talk about fitness, we're talking about aerobic fitness. The traditional and narrow way of defining that means making sure that your pulse is at 80 percent of its maximal rate for twenty minutes three days a week. To calculate your maximal pulse, simply follow this simple equation:

220 minus your age = maximum pulse

0.8 × maximum pulse

So for years we've had everyone from joggers to aerobic dancers, walkers to swimmers, taking their pulses. If they hit the gold standard of 80 percent of the max, they felt good, and if they didn't, then they assumed the exercise had no value. They were wussing out (as my fourteen-year-old daughter would say). But in fact they may not have been.

Recent research has shown that anything you do will give you value. But we now know that even if you do less, you receive a feeling of well-being plus a significant reduction in premature death.

The best and easiest way to gauge if you're getting some aerobic benefit is to ask yourself whether you're working up a sweat. If the answer is yes, then you are probably exercising aerobically. You can still take your pulse if that is something you like to do and if you would like to know how hard you're working, but it's not necessary in order to know that you're exercising aerobically.

The key is that exercise is additive. You need not do twenty minutes all at one time. You can exercise for five minutes here and ten minutes there to achieve some results.

The problem for many of us is fitting exercise into our daily routine. With work and family duties, many of us discover that finding the time to exercise is as difficult as exercise itself. That's where lifestyle changes come in. A study recently published in the *Journal of the American Medical Association* divided people into two groups. The first group went to aerobics class, hit the treadmill, rode the bike, or swam to the gold standard at least twenty minutes three days a week. This was the traditional aerobics group. The second group was encouraged to incorporate physical activity into their daily routine. So they walked stairs at work, walked around the block at lunch, raked leaves, and when they shopped they parked their car in a space that was far from the door so that they could walk a bit. Every day they tried to incorporate little activities not traditionally called aerobic activity. This was the lifestyle change group.

During the first year the traditional aerobics group had an improved level of fitness over the lifestyle group. But in the second year that began to change. The exercisers began to fall by the wayside, not exercising as much as they originally had. But the lifestyle group never stopped. They continued going strong throughout the entire study.

So who will be the most fit ten years down the line? Those who continue to do something, and that's the issue.

How Many Calories Are You Burning?

Several years ago researchers compiled a list of common activities using a standard measurement called the MET to compare them. A MET is defined as 1 cal/minute. It's a useful measure because it allows you to compare various activities to one another.

Let's take two activities, soccer and brisk walking, and see what sort of calories you'll burn after a thirty-minute workout.

$$\text{Soccer} = 7 \times 30 = 210 \text{ METs} = 210 \text{ cal (of energy used)}$$
$$\text{Brisk walking} = 4 \times 30 = 120 \text{ METs} = 120 \text{ cal (of energy used)}$$

As you can see, soccer is nearly twice as aerobic as brisk walking from a calories = per-minute point of view. But as we've discussed from a longevity point of view, both give you benefit. And there is no evidence to date that you will obtain twice as much benefit in years from soccer than you will from brisk walking.

The chart below gives you an idea of how many METs (calories) some common activities burn.

ENERGY EXPENDITURES FOR EXERCISE

	MET (equivalent to 1 cal/minute of energy expended)
COMPETITIVE EXERCISE	
Basketball	6–8
Biking, competitive	12–16
Biking, mountain	8.5
Carrying groceries upstairs	8
Downhill skiing, vigorous	8
Football	8–9
Handball	12
Jogging	7
Rock climbing	7–10
Rope jumping	8–10
Competitive running	9–12.5
Running	8
Soccer	7–10

ENERGY EXPENDITURES FOR EXERCISE (*continued*)

	MET (equivalent to 1 cal/minute of energy expended)
Swimming	6–12
Tennis, singles	8
MODERATE EXERCISE	
Carpentry	5–6
Cleaning gutters	6
Dancing, aerobic	6
Golf, walking	4–5
Fishing in stream	6
Hunting	6
Mowing lawn, walking	5.5
Walking, fast–paced	5
Weeding	4.5
MILD EXERCISE	
Ballroom dancing	3
Canoeing	3
Cooking + food prep	2.5
Fishing	3–4
Golf, using cart	3
Raking leaves	4.0
Sailing	3–5
Sex (vigorous)	1.5
Sex (passive)	1.0
Washing dishes	2.3

What Aerobic Exercise Is Best for Me?

Anything counts as long as you're consistent and do it every day or so. Making the right choice depends on where you live, what you like, and so on. I generally believe that if you can combine two or more spheres, then you are getting double benefit for your exercise program. That means if you exercise with someone else—a friend, spouse, or child—you're accessing the kinship sphere. If it's outside in

Mother Nature, then your spiritual sphere is activated, too. And if it doesn't cost much money, you'll save on the material sphere as well. Creatively thinking about what will fit into your longevity plan is the key. But of course I do have some general suggestions.

- *Walking.* Time and time again it's been shown that walking does it for us. It's easy. We don't need any special equipment or shoes; we can do it with other people or alone, almost any time of the year. If you're near a mall or a university you can often find a place to walk indoors if the weather is inclement.

- *Swimming and water aerobics.* If your joints aren't what they used to be, adding a little buoyancy to your routine might just make things easier. For anyone with arthritis, swimming can be a boon. It's as aerobic as jogging but without the stress on the joints.

- *Jogging.* If you jog, make sure that your shoes are supple, and fit right, and remember to stretch.

- *Action sports such as soccer, tennis, racquetball, basketball, snowshoeing, skiing, and softball.* Excellent choices for someone who wants excitement and thrill. All accentuate the kinship sphere, which means you're more likely to do it. And the friendships that you develop while you play can be a wonderful buffer for life's stress.

- *Golf.* I mention this as aerobic for the golf walker. If you go in a cart, you're not getting very much play for your heart. My father walked the course twice a week until he was eighty-six.

- *Canoeing and rowing.* A wonderful form of fitness if you like it and if it's available. Rowing teams offer a camaraderie that compares with other team sports and the joy of being with Mother Nature (accenting the spiritual sphere). Competitive rowing teams arise early in the morning, which means your day starts out with energy.

- *Indoor gyms and equipment.* For many of us, indoor exercise has become a way of life. If you're wondering what to purchase, consider this. A recently published article in the *Journal of the American Medical Association* compared exercise bikes, rowing machines, stair steppers, and treadmills. The results showed that at a given level of exercise, the treadmill was perceived as being easier. In other words, folks on the treadmill never felt like they were doing as much as they were really doing. It fooled them. I call that the treadmill advantage, which is why I recommend it as your first choice for exercise equipment.

Other choices include:

- *Spinning.* This is the latest rage in indoor group exercise. It provides wonderful cardiovascular fitness in a social setting.
- *Stair steppers.* These make it easy to push up that heart rate, so your workout need not be as long.
- *Rowing machines.* They're wonderful for all muscle groups, with no pounding. Especially good if you can row during the summer months outside and then use a machine for the winter. There's definitely a big difference in machines, though, and a risk of back injury if you don't know what you're doing.
- *Pilates.* Great stretching and strengthening, done alone or in a group.

Strength and Weight Training

You've seen kids play. They are the perfect exercisers—aerobically running all the time, jumping and climbing. They don't lift weights, but they seem to be strong. Studies have shown that kids who play outside are inevitably fitter than those who spend all of their time passively watching TV or playing on the computer.

When many kids become teens they lift weights. Today this is not just a "boy thing." As any good coach knows, strength conditioning adds stamina and improves performance no matter what activity a teen does.

For most, when the teen years end so does any type of weight exercise. You might see twenty-something people lift weights, but as you age the chances that you'll be pumping iron on a steady basis are less and less. In fact, for many years physicians and trainers were taught that weight lifting should not be done by anyone over forty unless they had had a treadmill test to be sure that they didn't have cardiovascular disease, because the grunting of weight lifting put a stress on the heart that many of us simply couldn't take.

Recent research has shown that that's simply an old doctor's tale. You lose about 1 percent of your muscle mass every year. No matter what you do, you have less muscle tissue at fifty than you did at eighteen. But the muscle tissue you do have will respond to pumping iron just as an eighteen-year-old's will; you just won't meet the same benchmarks.

Let's look at several recent studies of the oldest old. These were men and women who had never done any weight training; all were in their mid-seventies to eighties. They had a personally crafted exercise program in which they pumped iron for thirty minutes three days a week. Their level of fitness and strength was tested before they started the program and eight weeks later. The results were splendid. Their muscles grew in size and were stronger. More than that, the people felt good.

Studies have also shown that people who are strong are less likely to suffer a serious injury during a fall. They recover more quickly if they do fall, and they generally have less pain. Many seniors who start pumping iron start to go out to dances, travel, hike, and do things that they never dreamed that they would do at their age.

Not all of us are seniors, but just as aerobics has a place no matter what your age, so does pumping iron—the trick is how much. I have some suggestions:

- *Do not start on your own.* This is where you do need advice from a trainer or instructor so that you won't get hurt.
- *Use machines rather than free weights.* They're safer.
- *Measure yourself before you start and six weeks later.* Plotting your progress may help you stay on your program.
- *Find the time to do it.* This is exercise that demands a routine of three or more days a week or you may not meet your goals.
- *Add variety.* Don't do the same routine every day.

Agility and Balance

Gladys was a wonderful dancer when she was young. But after three kids and a career in merchandising, she gave it up. She also gave up any form of exercise. Gladys smoked, rarely drank milk, never took calcium tablets or vitamins, and was not an outdoors person. She'd describe herself as a couch potato. She had all the risk factors for osteoporosis.

One day, while carrying some groceries, Gladys slipped on the ice, fracturing her hip. After the artificial one was installed, Gladys went to rehab and succeeded in returning to a normal life. But that wasn't good enough for her. She didn't want it to happen again. So a few months after the surgery she came to my office wondering what she could do to make her body better. She was now on vitamin D, calcium, and an osteoporosis drug called Fosmax, but she wondered about exercise. What was right for her?

Knowing Gladys well, I asked her if she wanted to go to a gym. Her answer was clear: Nobody that she didn't know was going to stare at her, thank you very much. So I suggested that Gladys start with something she liked. That's where dancing came in.

A friend and I both suggested that Gladys join the local dance club and kick up her heels. Eventually she did—and she loved it so much that she started dancing three days a week. It was an aerobic workout with a special flare. And it taught her that agility was part of the key to keeping another fall from happening.

With agility and balance training, you are less likely to fall. As we age, our muscles and joints tend to hurt more. People who learn how to stretch and balance tend to have fewer aches and pains. They also have more confidence when they walk.

The nice thing about balance and agility is that you can exercise at a gym or a health club. Many community centers, schools, and local park districts have programs that are enjoyable and inexpensive.

My recommendations:

- *Choose a form of exercise that you like, such as ballroom dancing.* Maybe even find a friend to do it with you. That way you'll have more incentive to keep doing it—it's your kinship sphere.
- *Consider tai chi.* It's an ancient Chinese form of stretching that anyone can do, especially seniors. And it's good for your spirit.
- *Consider a yoga class.* This would access your spiritual sphere as well as the physical sphere.

Your Exercise Plan—Where to Begin

Step 1: How Fit Are You?

Whether you're fit or a couch potato, you need to take a personal inventory before you start your exercise regime. It's important, because quite a bit of hidden disease lurks in the guise of a healthy-looking person.

George was a decent guy who was a busy psychologist until recently, when he cut back to 50 percent. "Found it easier," he said. About a year later he stopped into my office. George had started a regimen of brisk walking and calisthenics but was fatigued after his workout and throughout the day. He felt he was a bit more exhausted than expected, but then again, since he had never exercised before, he wasn't quite sure what to expect. George had had asthma as a child but not as an adult. He once smoked, but quit a good twenty years ago. He had no chest pain, no discomfort at all.

George's exam, chest X-ray, EKG, lung tests, and echocardiogram were all normal. Finally I decided to put him on the treadmill. The rest was history. His heart disease was so bad that he lasted only twenty seconds. After surgery George resumed his exercise program and is feeling great.

George had absolutely no symptoms except excessive fatigue—no chest pain, no neck pain, no arm pain at all. He had no risk factors for heart disease either, except being a fifty-year-old male.

Step 2: Can I Start My Program Today?

George's story may make you think twice about starting an exercise program without consulting a doctor. But an excellent way to figure your fitness level is to fill out the Physical Activity Readiness Questionnaire (adapted from the British Columbia Ministry of Health as published in *American Family Physician,* August 1995) right here.

EXERCISE 10

❑ Has your doctor ever said you had heart trouble?

❑ Do you frequently suffer from pains in the chest?

❑ Do you often feel faint or have spells of severe dizziness?

❑ Has your doctor ever said your blood pressure was too high?

❑ Has a doctor ever told you that you have a bone or joint problem, such as arthritis? Has this problem ever been aggravated by exercise, or might it be made worse by exercise?

❑ Is there a good physical reason, not mentioned above, why you should not follow an activity program even if you wanted to?

❑ Are you over sixty-five and not accustomed to physical exercise?

If you answered yes to any of the questions above, then you should seek medical clearance before starting your program.

For those of us who answered no to all of them but are still out of shape and a bit leery, there are three exercises that you might start to test the waters. (For many, having a discussion with your doctor may save you problems later on. However, I do think the vast majority of us can start on some programs without medical approval.)

- *Walking.* Nearly all of us can walk. We may not speed-walk, but walking can be safely done by most of us without seeing a doctor.
- *Dancing.* You've done it at weddings without permission, so you can certainly go out on a Saturday night and shake a leg.
- *Biking.* If you can get on the bike without falling off, it's certainly a workout you can do without medical clearance.
- *Swimming.* A gentle and effective way to exercise.
- *Low-impact aerobics.* The classes abound.
- *Yoga, tai chi, pilates.*

Step 3: Integration with Life

Integrate your exercise program with a balanced approach to the rest of your life. The ideal exercise program should have aerobics, agility, and strengthening—and balance. Build a harmony that comes with balancing all the spheres in your own exercise routine. All this leads to making your life sweeter. For some that may mean jogging less so that you can work out with your spouse or kids. For others it may mean joining a gym because you live alone and enjoy company. Balance means thinking about those other aspects of your life that are important.

Put on some old records and move and dance with your kids every day. Or do as our family did years ago: We turned up the volume, but instead of dancing we cleaned like crazy. It was a great, fun fifteen-minute workout that helped with those chores. Be silly. They'll love it; so will you. Motivation is the hardest exercise I know of, at least for myself.

It's terrific if you can combine a couple of kinds of exercise with a couple of other spheres. For example: on Monday, walk with a friend at lunch for half an hour; on Wednesday after work, go to yoga; on Saturday, bike with your family.

Societies have personas. Our society favors relaxation over activity. That is not the same everywhere. Recently my wife, Penelope, and I traveled to Spain to visit our son, who was studying at the University of Madrid. The first thing that hit us in this magnificent city was how thin the people are. After a few days, two things became obvious: Spaniards eat less fat and smaller portions of food than we do in America, and they walk absolutely everywhere. When they go out to eat, to visit friends, to shop, they usually walk. Even when they take the subway, they walk to and from the subway station. The streets at night are alive, magically animated with walkers.

Step 4: Money, Money, Money

Don't join a health club today. And don't buy a treadmill today. It may be a worthless investment. Many of us love buying memberships to health clubs but rarely use them. If you decide to make a purchase, sit down and take a deep breath first. Remember that the sales rep's goal is to have you sign up before you leave the building, because once you're home you may come to your senses and not join. I don't believe in impulse buying of anything. It can wreck your material sphere.

Step 5: So Where Should You Begin?

Make a plan you think you can stick to and try to conquer whatever barriers you've been putting up in the past. Here are the most common examples I hear about on the radio show or in my office.

- *Exercise takes too much time.* Well, it takes time, but usually you get rewards for the time you put in. First of all, most people who exercise sleep better. Most regular exercisers also find they are more productive after they've exercised. Finally, exercise often gives you personal time that can help you decompress.
- *I'm too tired after work to exercise.* Perhaps you might walk at lunch one day. Maybe you can free up time before you shower one morning. And although routine is best, flexibility is the key. How about taking the stairs? Parking farther away?
- *Exercise is too costly.* Spending money on a good pair of shoes is all you really need—and for walking, you may not even need that.
- *I'm too embarrassed to do it.* Choose your environment. If you're too concerned about other people seeing you, then work out at home using a video or workbook. Give yourself credit for wanting to look and feel better.
- *I'll injure myself.* Here are the best ways that I know to avoid injury: Start slowly. Don't forget about warm-ups and cool-downs. They are essential. And if you're doing tai bo, be careful of those beginning stretches. They can be a killer if you haven't warmed up. Take a class. The number one cause of serious injury is not being properly trained.

Give some thought to what you would like to do. Plan some action. It might be taking a yoga course at the local Y or going out to dance tomorrow. But there is something that you could start on today. In fact, I suggest putting down this book now and taking a walk.

EXERCISE 11—More Physical Sphere Boosters

Do you:

- ❑ Spend a lot of time outdoors?
- ❑ Love to sunbathe?
- ❑ Almost never apply the sunscreen you feel compelled to buy?
- ❑ Consider things like seat belts, bike helmets, or life jackets to be more hindrance than help?
- ❑ Eat your lunch, go through your mail, or talk on a cell phone while you're driving?
- ❑ Assume that the smoke detectors and fire extinguishers in your home will work if there's ever a fire?
- ❑ Not know how to swim?
- ❑ Own guns?
- ❑ Like activities that push the envelope?

Then you could use some of the measures profiled in this section.

Not every step toward a longer, sweeter life requires a substantial change in lifestyle. Some longevity-boosting measures are as easy as smearing on sunscreen or fastening your seat belt. This point was illustrated for me in a most personal way by the 1998 recipient of Wisconsin's Saved by the Belt Award—my son Eli.

On a sunny summer afternoon, Eli, then seventeen, left our home in an eight-year-old Ford with four brand-new tires. With his seat belt fastened and his guitar wedged behind the passenger seat, he drove at the posted speed limit along country roads lined with eye-high corn. He did not see the vehicle barreling down the side road he was approaching, and the driver of that vehicle must not have seen him—or the stop sign. He entered the intersection a split second after Eli, broadsiding my son's car at 50 mph.

The Ford spun out of control, leaving a huge C-shaped tire tread mark in the road. Then it flipped and rolled over twice before landing right side up, a mangled mass of metal among the cornstalks. Eli's guitar was squashed. Both the front and rear windshields were shattered. The impact had been so powerful that the car radio had been pushed out of its spot on the dashboard and propelled into the backseat. Yet Eli was fine. Other than bruises and body aches that bothered him for a couple of weeks and nightmares, mostly replays of the accident, that lingered a bit longer, he was basically okay. Considering the extent to which his car was damaged, there was no doubt that had his seat belt and shoulder harness not been fastened, Eli would be dead.

In an instant, sixty or more years of Eli's life expectancy could have been lost. But thanks to the small, simple action of fastening his seat belt, it was not. Most of the measures I'm about to describe promote longevity in that way. They won't increase your life span by a single second if you're lucky enough to never get in an automobile accident, experience a residential fire, or lose control of your bicycle on a steep, rocky trail. But if such twists of fate should befall you, they'll prevent you from cutting your stay on this planet short by decades.

14. Limit Sun Exposure   Impact ★★★★

Sunshine streaming through a window, glistening on the water, parting the clouds after a rainfall, shepherding in a new day . . . ahhh. Synonymous with hope, happiness, and renewal, the sun makes new-fallen snow sparkle, bleak moods brighten, and plants grow. When it's shining, we'll often get an irresistible urge to eat lunch on a park bench, drive a convertible with the top down, or slip into our swimsuits and stretch out on a chaise longue. At those moments, we find it hard to believe that exposing ourselves to the sun's rays could really harm us. Yet the threat to our health and longevity is quite real. Thanks in part to the deteriorating ozone layer, but mostly to our sun-worshiping lifestyles, one American in ninety will get melanoma, the deadliest skin cancer, at some point in their lifetime. By making a few simple changes, you may be able to sidestep that fate.

Sun Facts
The fact that too much sun causes premature wrinkling and raises our risk of developing melanoma and other skin cancers is not news. Ultraviolet B (UVB) radiation is the biggest troublemaker. Overexposure to

it by intensive sunbathing causes sunburn and increases our odds of developing skin cancers.

When it comes to melanoma, the deadliest form of skin cancer, ultraviolet A (UVA) may also play a role. If you hear or read that tanning beds are a "safe" way to get a suntan because they emit UVA radiation rather than UVB, don't believe it.

So what is a longevity-minded person to do? The most obvious answer would be to stay out of the sun altogether. But that option is far too restrictive. Besides, sunshine isn't all bad. It is a source of vitamin D, which our bodies need to absorb calcium and build bone strength. It's a natural antidepressant—many of us feel our moods improve when the sun is out. Our physical, mental, and spiritual health would suffer if we could not jog around the reservoir or take long walks to commune with nature or picnic with our families in the park.

The keys?

- *Wear sun-protective clothing.* Whenever possible wear a lightweight, cool fabric. The less total sun exposure you receive to your arms, legs, and neck, the better off you are.
- *Wear a hat with a brim.* Shading your face can keep away wrinkles.
- *Practice sun-sensible behavior.* The hottest sun is between 11 A.M. and 3 P.M. If you're going to have fun in the sun, consider doing it when the sun isn't at its zenith.
- *Use sunscreen correctly.* .

The Scoop on Sunscreens

Selecting a sunscreen isn't calculus. SPF (sun protection factor) tells us how much longer we can stay in the sun without burning.

Minimum protection	SPF 2–12
Moderate	SPF 12–30
High	SPF 30 or more

The higher the better. No sunscreen offers 100 percent protection against skin damage, and even the best products are effective only when you:

- *Use enough.*
- *Put it on early enough.* Sunscreen should be applied thirty minutes before you go out in the sun.
- *Reapply it often enough.*

15. Fasten Seat Belts   Impact ★★★★

The American Automobile Association estimates that the average driver gets into a motor vehicle accident every seven years—most of them fender benders, but many serious ones as well. Car crashes claim in the neighborhood of forty-five thousand lives annually. When I worked in an ER, I could tell instantly who was buckled up and who wasn't. You can guess how.

Estimates show that fatalities would drop by 45 percent if we all buckled up. I've seen too many parents buckle their kids into place only to drive away without wearing a belt themselves. Asked why, the answer usually is, "It's only a short ride to the store." But in fact those short drives comprise the majority of our driving.

Driving or riding with your belt on improves your odds of surviving a potentially fatal accident sevenfold. And all you've invested are the three to five seconds it took you to fasten your lap and shoulder restraints.

16. Drive Sanely   Impact ★★★★

Okay, you're in your car with your seat belt fastened. What's next?

Well, don't even put your key in the ignition if you've been drinking. Booze is involved in 40 percent of motor vehicle accident deaths. Many drugs, including allergy medications, cold preparations, and certain painkillers, also impair our ability to safely operate our vehicles. So know the side effects of any medication you're on (see page 258).

Once you've determined you're clearheaded enough to drive:

- *Keep unsafe driving practices in check.* Avoid speeding. Don't tailgate. Use your turn signals. Don't cut off other drivers. These driving behaviors cause accidents. They also instigate angry, even violent, responses from rage-prone fellow drivers—a problem of near epidemic proportions in many urban areas. And they can make you angry and hostile, too, elevating your blood pressure and causing your body stress that it doesn't need.
- *Maintain your vehicle.* Don't be done in by faulty brakes, bald tires, or windshields without working wipers.
- *Adapt to changing road conditions.* Rain-soaked or snow-covered pave-

ment can be treacherous. So take your time. Keep your distance. Know what to do if your car starts to skid.

- *Stop when you get sleepy.* If you catch yourself taking lots of long blinks, find a safe place to park for a while and take a little nap.
- *Beware of cell phones.* These modern conveniences appear to quadruple your risk of getting into an accident.

17. Wear a Helmet   Impact ★★★★

Automobiles are not the only source of motor vehicle fatalities. In fact, motorcycles, especially when ridden without protective helmets, result in so much irreversible head trauma or brain death, which make the rider's other organs available for transplant, that we doctors sometimes refer to them as "donorcycles." This doesn't mean that no one should ride them, but rather that those who choose to ride them should respect how risky they are and act to reduce that risk by wearing a helmet.

Helmets can also make a life-or-death difference for bicycle riders of all ages. Seventeen hundred people are hospitalized and eight hundred people die in the United States every year from bicycle-related head injuries. Far too often I see parents strap a helmet on their kids and then neglect to wear a helmet themselves. Find a helmet that feels right to you and be sure that it's certified to meet national safety standards. And don't forget your helmet when you RollerBlade and board.

18. Reduce Hazards in Your Home   Impact ★★★★

Accidents happen. And a good many of them happen in the place where we feel the safest—our homes.

Fire

Every eighteen seconds a fire department responds to a fire. Every two hours someone dies in one of those fires. In 1997 more than three thousand Americans died in household fires alone. To sidestep this fate:

- *Equip your home with smoke detectors and keep them in working order.*
- *Obtain and maintain fire extinguishers.* Put one by the furnace, another in the kitchen, and one on each floor.

- *Have a fire plan.* Decide on the best exits and escape routes in advance. Then have the whole family practice using them.
- *If you smoke, take precautions.*

Falls

Falls—from ladders, off rooftops, down stairs, on icy sidewalks, while getting out of the bathtub, and elsewhere—are the second most common cause of death by accidental injury. They account for fourteen hundred deaths every year. Falls pose the gravest threat to men and women over the age of sixty-five, who often sustain injuries severe enough to stop them from functioning independently. You can reduce your own and your family's risk by:

- Keeping stairs and doorways clear of clutter
- Removing things that could be tripped on
- Forgoing throw rugs, or using double-sided tape to affix them
- Applying nonslip strips to tub and shower floors
- Climbing ladders or taking on precarious tasks only when someone else is around
- Improving the lighting in dimly lit areas

Poisoning

Poisoning has the potential to cut short thousands of lives each year. These incidents most often involve common household products—cleaning preparations, pain relievers, cosmetics, plants, cough and cold preparations, and, increasingly, prescription medications (see page 258). So store them where kids can't get to them, and exercise caution yourself. Read directions carefully. Know toxic side effects. Stick to recommended uses, and don't mix products. It's common sense.

Carbon Monoxide Poisoning

If you heat your home with anything other than electricity, don't forget to have carbon monoxide detectors. Put on the same floor as your bedrooms, they save lives. And while you're at it, why not have that furnace checked once a year when the heat goes on?

Food Poisoning

Researchers estimate that up to five thousand people a year die from contaminated and undercooked food. Young kids, the elderly, or anyone with a chronic medical problem is at risk for the most common bacterial problems, caused by *E. coli* and salmonella. The spread of food-borne illnesses is one of this country's fastest-growing community health problems. Fortunately it's not hard to prevent.

- *Don't leave perishable foods unrefrigerated for more than two hours.* This is especially true for cooked leftovers (whose initial heat promotes bacteria to grow) and for dairy products.
- *Cook foods completely.* Do this especially with eggs and poultry, which can carry salmonella, and ground beef, which can be infected with *E. coli.* Your chicken and your burger should never be pink.
- *Wash raw foods thoroughly.* Use lots of water.
- *Avoid cross-contamination.* Before reusing, wash anything that has come in contact with uncooked meat, poultry, or eggs. This includes dishes, cutting boards, knives, utensils, countertops, and your hands. Use soap and very hot water whenever you can.
- *Also do this with anything anyone eats with or off.* And don't forget the sponge you clean with. Run it through the dishwasher or give it a good soaking.

Firearms Accidents

There are thirty-six thousand firearm deaths each year in the United States. Twenty thousand are suicides, fourteen thousand are homicides, and two thousand are unintentional. There are three nonfatal firearm injuries for each death. Not all of these occur in the home, of course. However, it's been well documented that guns kept in the house for protection are several times more likely to kill a resident than an intruder. Consequently, if you collect guns or own one for self-defense:

- Keep your collection unloaded, in a locked case, with bullets stored elsewhere
- Never leave a loaded weapon where a curious child or despondent family member could find it
- Learn how to properly store, maintain, and discharge guns

19. Practice Water Safety	Impact ★★★★

Drowning ranks third on the accident fatality parade. It causes four thousand deaths each year. Most occur in swimming pools. Half involve alcohol. Boaters and fishermen account for many of these fatalities. Too many go out, party, get drunk, and drown. However, you can also be sober and have a storm come up unexpectedly, a leg cramp incapacitate you, or a riptide incessantly pull you away from the shore. To reduce your risk of drowning under those and other circumstances:

- *If you can't swim, and there's even a slim chance that you'll ever need to, consider learning how.* Most Y's and community pools have classes for adults only. Some even have classes for the terrified, which use standardized methods to get you over your fears.
- *Have and use safety equipment, including life jackets, on boats or personal watercraft and when water-skiing.* If you don't like life vests, consider buying the nonbulky inflatable units that clip on like a fanny pack. When immersed in water, these high-tech life preservers blow up to keep you out of harm's way.
- *Take a boating safety course.*
- *Never mix alcohol with water sports.*

PREVENTIVE MEDICINE

20. Have Safer Sex to Stop Sexually Transmitted Diseases   Impact ★★★★

Jasmine, a lifelong patient of mine, was twenty-five when she came in to be treated for what she thought was a urinary tract infection. Despite her discomfort, she chattered amiably about her new job and her new boyfriend, Michael. She didn't see him nearly enough now that she was working days and he was still managing the night shift at the restaurant where they met. The logical solution would be for them to move in together, she thought. But that plan abruptly lost its allure when I had to inform her that the pressure and burning sensation she was experiencing were symptoms not of a urinary tract infection but of chlamydia, a sexually transmitted disease (STD).

After a round of shocked denials followed by a torrent of tears, Jasmine admitted that her friends had warned her that Michael "slept around." But he claimed he had been given a clean bill of health before he met her. "Either he was lying then or he's cheating now," Jasmine sniffled. Either way, he had "betrayed" her. Worse yet, she was faced with the terrifying prospect that he could have passed other

STDs on to her. She might have AIDS. Even after antibiotics cured the chlamydia and Jasmine learned she was not infected with anything else, the mere idea that she might have been made her shiver with fear and anger. "Why didn't he use condoms when he was with other women?" she asked. "Why didn't I make him wear one when he was with me?"

Much to the dismay of public health officials everywhere, Jasmine's situation is not unique. Many, many American men and women are still allowing their sexual behavior to jeopardize their futures. As a result, sexually transmitted diseases—chlamydia, genital warts, HPV (human papilloma virus), genital herpes, hepatitis B, and even the old standbys syphilis and gonorrhea—are clearly on the rise. And despite widespread awareness of high-risk activities, the deadliest—HIV/AIDS—continues to claim new victims at the same rate as ever. Researchers estimate that as many as one million Americans have the deadly virus.

What Are STDs and Who's Vulnerable to Them?

STDs are diseases caused by viruses, bacteria, or other microorganisms that are passed from one person to another during sexual activity. Any activity, from fellatio to intercourse, can spread an STD, but rectal intercourse is the highest risk activity. STDs directly or indirectly cause well over thirty thousand premature deaths per year. Anyone who has unprotected sex with an infected partner is at risk; the more partners you have, the higher your risk.

Are They Curable?

Drugs take care of STDs caused by bacteria or certain other microorganisms, such as chlamydia, syphilis, or gonorrhea, but of course there are no cures for viral STDs such as genital herpes, chronic hepatitis B, and AIDS. At best, they can be controlled with medications. Prevention is really the key.

Play It Safer

- *If you choose to have sexual intercourse, know your partner.* What's his or her HIV status? Could he or she have hepatitis B or any other STD? Does he or she have other sex partners? Is he or she an IV drug user who might share needles?

- *If you have any reason to suspect that you or your sexual partner(s) have HIV, hepatitis B, or any other sexually transmittable infection (or you don't know a partner well enough to be sure), practice safer sex.* Use a latex condom from start to finish every time you have vaginal or anal intercourse. Be sure not to use oil-based lubricants with latex condoms, as the oil degrades the latex.
- *Be tested and treated as soon as you suspect you may have been exposed to any STD.* Having one may make you more susceptible to others.
- *Stay in charge.* Safer sex requires good judgment and self-control. Alcohol and drugs weaken both. Don't overdo either.

21. Have Pap Tests to Screen for Cervical Cancer   Impact ★★★★

Each year Pap tests pick up over fifty thousand cases of cervical cancer in their very early stages. And virtually 100 percent of them can be cured completely using simple procedures performed right in a gynecologist's office. Cancerous or precancerous cells can be killed with laser surgery or cryosurgery. They also can be removed surgically.

A Pap test isn't foolproof, of course. Some cancers go undiagnosed and untreated. However, when a sample is properly collected and examined, abnormal cells are rarely missed. If they're there, they're identified 90 to 95 percent of the time. And if they aren't picked up on one test, there's a good chance that your next test will detect them in time for successful treatment.

Current screening guidelines call for women to have a Pap test every year beginning at age eighteen or as soon as they become sexually active. They should continue to be tested throughout their lives, but after three consecutive negative tests can consider having them less frequently, perhaps as much as three to five years apart. Nevertheless, women affected by the amplifiers I listed on the longevity card should continue to have Pap tests annually.

To further lower your risk:
- *Practice safer sex.* This cancer appears to be sexually transmitted, possibly in association with the human papilloma virus (HPV), which causes genital warts.
- *Quit smoking.* Smoking is speculated to be a risk.
- *Eat more fruits and vegetables; perhaps take a vitamin C supplement.*

There's some indication that taking in too little vitamin C, folic acid, and beta-carotene raises cervical cancer risk.

22. Screen for Colon and Rectal Cancer   Impact ★★★★

Rarely seen earlier this century, colon and rectal cancer is now the second most common form of cancer in the United States. One in seventeen Americans can expect to get it at some point in their lives. And the older you get, the more vulnerable you are. Each year, close to 120,000 new cases are diagnosed in this country. With early detection and timely treatment, the cure rate for colon and rectal cancers is over 90 percent. In the best-case scenario, where patients' polyps are discovered and removed while they're still small and precancerous, nearly 100 percent survive.

Screening Measures

- Annual Fecal Occult Blood Tests. Get a fecal occult blood test once a year beginning when you turn fifty, earlier if you have a family history of colon cancer. Because growths in the colon, whether cancerous tumors or benign polyps, have a tendency to bleed, one way to detect them is to look for blood in your stool. This is accomplished with a take-home test performed in the privacy of your own bathroom. A positive result—the presence of blood—is followed up with other tests to determine the cause. Other things, such as hemorrhoids, bleed, too. Annual testing for occult blood is estimated to decrease colon and rectal cancer death rates by 40 percent.
- Flexible Sigmoidoscopy. This screening measure, recommended once every five years after age fifty, uses a thin, flexible, lighted tube to examine the lower portion of the colon, where over half of all colon cancers reside. Screening once every three to five years after the age of fifty is credited with cutting death rates by 60 to 80 percent.

COLONOSCOPY

A colonoscopy is recommended if you have had polyps, have blood in your stool, or know that the disease runs in your family. This procedure allows a doctor to examine the inside of your entire colon using an instrument similar to a flexible sigmoidoscope, but longer. While colonoscopy is the gold standard for colon and rectal cancer diagnosis, it is also too costly (at roughly $1,000 per test) and time-intensive, not to mention too invasive, to use for routine screening.

Prevention
The key is to address controllable risk factors. For colon and rectal cancers, these are:

- *Avoid a high-fat, high-calorie, low-fiber diet.* A diet heavy on meat and light on fruit and vegetables puts you at greater risk. Changing your eating habits with boosters such as those described on pages 197–201 can cut your risk by 50 percent.
- *Avoid a sedentary lifestyle and a job that requires a lot of sitting.* You simply must get up from your desk or sofa and move around.
- *Avoid excessive alcohol consumption.* Colon and rectal cancer is one of the areas where having more than one (for women) or two (for men) alcoholic beverages a day takes its toll.
- *Avoid cigarette smoking.*

Heredity and certain medical conditions also play a role. Twenty percent of all colon cancer cases are thought to be genetic. Ulcerative colitis, a disease of the bowel that leads to pain, spasms, and in many cases the eventual removal of the colon, puts you at superhigh risk.

23. Screen for Breast Cancer   Impact ★★★★

The cancer that strikes the most fear in the hearts of women is also the most prevalent among them. One in eight women alive today will get breast cancer at some point in her life, usually later rather than sooner. Close to two hundred thousand new cases are diagnosed every year, with forty-four thousand deaths. Lagging behind both lung and colon cancer totals, the breast cancer death rate is significant but far less astounding than it once was, especially for women whose cancer was spotted in its early, noninvasive stage. They have a 90 to 95 percent survival rate, thanks to early detection. With the lion's share of risk factors for breast cancer falling under the heading of life's (unpreventable) givens, early detection is what we must rely on to prevent this disease from killing us.

Sometimes the potential to diagnose breast cancer very early assuages a woman's fears. That was the case for Atikah Holloway, a long-time patient who came to see me about a year ago absolutely terrified. Her best friend's mother, a woman in her late sixties, had just died from breast cancer, and that had spooked her. Even though she was not a blood relative and knew full well that breast cancer was not contagious, Atikah had worked herself into a frenzy.

Couldn't I *please* order a mammogram for her? she asked. I might not have hesitated if Atikah had been older (she was forty) or if there was a history of breast cancer in her family (there was none). What's more, she had had a mammogram ten months before (many authorities believe that a mammogram every two years for women between the ages of forty and fifty is more than enough).

I explained all of this and warned Atikah that her insurance company probably wouldn't pay for the procedure, but she was more concerned with "finding out one way or another." She would pay for it herself. She just couldn't function with this nagging question hanging over her head. Atikah got her mammogram, which didn't have a single suspicious speck on it, and the reassurance she needed to get on with her life.

Screening by Self-Exam

On the frontline of prevention is the practice of examining your own breasts for lumps on a monthly basis. Volunteers from your local branch of the American Cancer Society can show you the best way to do this. Or hop on the World Wide Web to find illustrated instructions; www.cancer.org is a good place to start. If you should feel a lump or mass or anything out of the ordinary, take action immediately.

Screening by Mammogram

Mammograms are X-rays of the breast. Using them to routinely screen for signs of breast cancer means that one-third fewer women over the age of fifty will die from the disease. Of course, mammography isn't perfect. It can miss up to 10 percent of cancers in women between the ages of fifty and sixty-nine and be off by as much as 25 percent for women in their forties, whose denser breast tissue produces an X-ray that's harder to read.

Despite its shortcomings, every woman between the ages of fifty and sixty-nine should have one every year. I also recommend them annually for women over seventy, even though early detection isn't as important for the slow-growing form of breast cancer they tend to get. One mammogram should probably be taken at age forty to establish a baseline, but how often women should have them after that is debatable. Some authorities favor annual screening. Others feel there's not enough evidence to support screening at all before fifty. Still others believe that every two years is sufficient. I lean toward having individual women and their doctors go over the pros and cons and make their own decisions. Finally, a mammogram is appropriate at any age if a lump has been detected.

24. Screen for Skin Cancer	Impact ★★★★

In terms of sheer number of cases, skin cancer is by far the most prevalent cancer in this country. More than one million people are diagnosed with skin cancer each year. But most aren't very dangerous. Basal cell cancer, which accounts for 75 percent of all cases, grows slowly and usually does not spread to distant parts of the body. Squamous cell cancer, which accounts for 20 percent of skin cancer, is more aggressive and more likely to attack bone, muscle, and other tissue below the skin. In only a small percentage of cases does it metastasize and turn deadly. Malignant melanoma, on the other hand, is much less common than the other two skin cancers but many times more deadly, because it spreads easily to remote areas of the body. Once it has, it is very difficult to successfully treat. Sixty-five hundred Americans die from it annually, although it, too, can be cured if detected early.

The person most likely to detect skin cancer is you. The American Cancer Society has excellent brochures with color photographs that can help you detect it. You need to be familiar with the appearance of your own skin and the moles, freckles, or other dark spots on it. If you are at high risk, you may even want to have your body photographed to aid you in detecting new moles. Then you should examine your own body once a year. This is best done with the assistance of someone else.

What are you looking for? The *ABCD* signs that any mole or brown spot might be cancerous:

A = *Asymmetry.* One half does not match the other half.

B = *Borders* that are irregular, ragged, notched, or blurred.

C = *Color* that varies or is primarily red, black, or pink.

D = *Diameter.* The mole is bigger than a pencil eraser or growing.

Obviously, just looking isn't a highly accurate and reliable way to detect skin cancer. You may miss something. Doctors can, too. Some are better than others at distinguishing between cancerous and noncancerous skin abnormalities. If you're concerned about a particular mole, insist on a biopsy. For tips on preventing skin cancer from developing at all, see page 221.

---

25. Screen for Prostate Cancer   Impact ★★

Prostate cancer is a male disease. It results from the growth of malignant cells in the walnut-sized prostate gland, found in front of the rectum at the base of the bladder. More than 200,000 new cases are diagnosed annually, most of them in men over age sixty-five. It is so prevalent in this age group that one out of six men in their sixties and seventies can expect to develop it at some point. Although prostate cancer accounts for forty thousand deaths in the United States each year, men can and frequently do survive prostate cancer that is diagnosed before it reaches an advanced stage: 89 percent are alive at least five years after diagnosis; 65 percent survive ten years.

Some prostate cancers are detected by a digital rectal exam, but unfortunately this technique misses many cancers. That's where the prostate-specific antigen (PSA) blood test comes in. But the decision whether or not to have the test is actually one of the most controversial topics in medicine today. For starters, the test has some accuracy problems. For every hundred men tested, ten will have an elevated PSA level (more than 4 ng/ml), and of those ten, just three will turn out to actually have prostate cancer. For those men the blood test was not only wrong but also hazardous—they have to go through unnecessary procedures and undue anxiety before ultimately being told they don't have the disease.

But unfortunately there is another error, the so-called false negative. That's where the PSA says there is no cancer but it's wrong. One in four men who actually have prostate cancer has a normal PSA.

Groups opposed to routine PSA testing, including the American Academy of Physicians and the U.S. Preventive Health Services Task Force, also point out that with the exception of very aggressive forms of the disease, which sometimes strike men under fifty, most prostate cancer grows very slowly. Ten, fifteen, even twenty years can pass before it causes symptoms or spreads, if it ever does. Many prominent researchers argue that there is little proof that treatment promotes longevity or cure. And since most of the men who get this disease are sixty-five or older when it's detected, they'll likely die from some other cause before prostate cancer does them any harm. Do they really need an early warning?

The available treatments are anything but benign. Needle biopsy through the rectum is uncomfortable. Radiation and surgery leave many patients impotent. One in five become incontinent. "Watchful waiting," a term that essentially means doing nothing until something gets worse or goes obviously wrong, makes a lot of sense but also causes a lot of anxiety. It's quite a psychological burden to know that cancer cells are hiding in your body and getting ready to pounce. In all of these ways, PSA testing adversely affects life quality. And you have to ask yourself whether gaining at most a few extra months, ten or fifteen years down the line, is worth the loss of quality and the extra agony you'll be experiencing in the meantime.

My best recommendation with regard to prostate cancer screening is for men fifty years of age and older to have an annual digital rectal exam and a PSA test as a follow-up if abnormalities are found. Whether or not to have annual PSA tests beginning at around the same time is a serious matter for you and your doctor to decide together.

The American Cancer Society recently reversed its position on annual PSA testing, recommending that it should be done, but I don't consider their arguments that persuasive.

Prevention

Several studies point out that prostate cancer risk might be lessened by:
- Keeping your weight down (see page 77).

- Increasing the amount of physical activity you get every day (see pages 208–221).
- Drinking eight or more glasses of water a day.
- Tweaking your diet to include less saturated (animal) fat.
- Eating lots of fiber, fruit, and vegetables, especially tomato products, from pasta sauce to salsa. Tomatoes contain lycopene, an antioxidant carotenoid that appears to help protect you from prostate cancer.
- Taking antioxidants such as vitamins C and E and a carotenoid and flavonoid supplement. But the data on the effectiveness of this are very skimpy.

26. Get a Chest X-Ray to Screen for Lung Cancer   Impact ★

The most common cancer, other than skin cancer, striking Americans today is also the deadliest. Sixty percent of lung cancer patients die within a year of their diagnosis. Unfortunately, only 15 percent of all lung cancers are found before they've spread beyond the lungs. There simply is no routine screening program for people prone to this condition and no accurate, reliable method for detecting the disease in its precancerous or very early stages. Some doctors still recommend chest X-rays, especially for heavy smokers or folks exposed to asbestos and other carcinogens, but we rarely pick up early lesions from them. More sophisticated tests are in the works but are not yet accurate, cost-effective, or accessible enough to make a difference. As a result, *you* are apt to be the first one to spot your lung cancer warning signs, so don't ignore things such as:
- A cough that won't go away
- Chest pain
- Hoarseness
- Weight loss and loss of appetite
- Bloody or rust-colored sputum (spit or phlegm)

Bring these symptoms to your doctor's attention as soon as possible. With the help of chest X-rays, a CAT scan, or a sputum cytology study to look for abnormal cells, your doctor may be able to make a reasonably early diagnosis.

Prevention

Tobacco smoke should be avoided at all costs. It's behind 95 percent of all lung cancer cases. Homes should be free of radon and asbestos.

27. Monitor Blood Pressure and Control Hypertension   Impact ★★★★★

According to the American Heart Association (AHA):

- Fifty million Americans have high blood pressure.
- More than a third don't realize they have it.
- Of those who do know, more than half are not doing anything about it.
- Of those receiving treatment, close to 30 percent are not taking the right medication or making the needed lifestyle changes.

Is this a big deal? You bet. Blood pressure is the tension created by the heart pushing blood into our arteries and the artery walls pushing back or resisting the flow. We need some of this pressure to keep our blood moving around our circulatory system, but too much threatens both health and longevity. Hypertension kills directly—up to forty thousand Americans annually—and contributes to the deaths of as many as two hundred thousand more.

Back in the 1960s we thought that elevated blood pressure was a natural function of age. Physicians had formulas to calculate it, and they believed there was a viable reason for its steady rise. As you got older, they theorized, you needed more pressure to help push the blood through your vessels. They were wrong.

Arteries that resist too much while blood is trying to rush through them force our heart to pump harder than it was designed to. Over time that overtaxed organ enlarges and weakens, and when this happens, congestive heart failure is not far behind. High blood pressure also damages blood vessel walls, inviting aneurysms and atherosclerosis. It increases our chances of experiencing a stroke, heart attack, or kidney failure, and becomes even more deadly in the presence of other risk factors, most notably diabetes, obesity, and stress.

The good news is that all of this is well within our control. Indeed, our success at monitoring and managing blood pressure is one of the greatest public health advances in decades. When it comes to preventing needless death and disability, it's right up there with the polio, rabies, and tetanus vaccines. Since 1972, when we began aggressively treating this condition, stroke death rates have dropped nearly 70 percent and heart attacks have been cut by half.

Blood Pressure Monitoring

Hypertension is easily measured and detected.

NORMAL RANGE	SYSTOLIC	DIASTOLIC
Normal	< 130 mm Hg	< 85 mm Hg
High normal	130–139	85–89
HYPERTENSION		
Stage I	140–159	90–99
Stage II	160–179	100–109
Stage III	> 180	> 110

We used to accept slight elevations as "borderline hypertension," which we would watch but not treat. We now know that's wrong. Research has shown that even those with slightly elevated blood pressure (such as the "high normal" group) live longer if they're treated earlier. I recommend that adults over the age of twenty have their blood pressure checked every two years. Once you hit fifty it should be yearly.

Managing Hypertension

In terms of treatment, I agree with the National Institutes of Health: Lifestyle changes should be tried first. A loss of ten pounds will control hypertension in many folks. Reducing alcohol consumption to one drink a day for women and two for men may just do it, too. Although anxiety doesn't make much difference beyond a temporarily elevated reading now and then, relaxation techniques and relaxing activities such as yoga and tai chi, when combined with weight loss, less alcohol, a bit of salt restriction, and more physical activity, can contribute to control without drugs. Improving your social and material spheres might just take away the stress that aggravates hypertension.

However, lifestyle changes alone will help only some, perhaps 10 to

20 percent, of people with hypertension. For the rest, medication is the answer.

28. Measure Your HDL, LDL, and Total Cholesterol Levels   Impact ★★★★★

What Are We Dealing With?

Cholesterol is a soft, waxy substance that your body uses in cell membranes, hormones, and other tissue. Too much of it spells trouble, since the excess often ends up adhering to blood vessel walls—it's a blockage waiting to happen. This is most likely to occur when you also have an abundance of low-density lipoprotein (LDL), which transports fats, proteins, and cholesterol to and from your cells.

Even so, many people who have heart attacks don't have outrageously high cholesterol levels, and others with high total and LDL cholesterol have no signs of heart disease. The explanation lies with a second cholesterol carrier, high-density lipoprotein (HDL), which is sometimes called "good" cholesterol because it carries excess cholesterol away from the arteries, bringing it to the liver for disposal instead. We want lots of it (at least 35 mg/dl), because the more cholesterol it transports, the less there is for LDL to dump in our blood vessels. In fact, some cardiologists believe that for every mg of additional HDL cholesterol in our bloodstream, our risk of fatal heart attack drops by 2 to 3 percent.

There are no hard-and-fast rules about when to start having your cholesterol checked. I recommend every one to three years beginning in your forties. You may want to start earlier or be tested annually if troublesome cholesterol counts or early heart disease run in your family.

Cholesterol matters. Right now it is one of the better ways we have to predict future heart problems and shouldn't be ignored. However, controlling it doesn't cure *everything*. What's more, it is only one risk factor among many that we can work on to avoid dying prematurely from heart disease.

What Can You Do About It?

To have any value, cholesterol levels need to be looked at in conjunction with other major heart disease risk factors, including:

- Age (males over forty-five, females over fifty-five)
- Family history of premature heart disease (specifically, a dad, uncle, or brother who had significant heart problems before age fifty-five; before sixty-five for a mom, aunt, or sister)
- Cigarette smoking
- Hypertension (even if it's being treated)
- Low HDL (less than 35—the lower you are, the greater the risk)
- Diabetes (even if it's being treated)

Because higher HDL protects you from heart disease, if yours is over 60, you can cross one risk factor off your list.

The more risk factors you have in the picture already, the less you can tolerate the additional risk presented by high levels of LDL cholesterol—and the lower you'll want to get them. For some of us, changing our diets brings about major changes in our cholesterol counts. Try cutting back on the consumption of foods that are high in saturated fat (red meat, dairy products, certain oils). For others, diet simply isn't the answer—no matter how prudent, even austere they are, their cholesterol stays pretty much the same. In that case, medication is the only way to go.

The National Cholesterol Education Program offers the following guidelines for when to start managing cholesterol with medications.

Drug treatment should be prescribed for LDL cholesterol levels of:

- 100 or more if you have cardiovascular disease or have had a previous heart attack
- 130 or more if you have two or more risk factors for heart disease
- 160 or more if you have one risk factor
- 190 or more if you are a male under thirty-five or a woman under forty-five

29. Have Your Blood Sugar Checked to Detect Diabetes   Impact ★★★★

Diabetes, the non–insulin-dependent, adult-onset variety, results from our body's inability to take sugar absorbed from the food we eat and get it from our gut into the cells where it is needed. As a result, the sugar floats around in the bloodstream, damaging blood vessels. It's not difficult to tell that something's wrong once classic symptoms such as constant thirst, frequent urination, and unexplained weight loss appear. The trouble is that many people have this disease and are being harmed by it long before the signs are there. In fact, thirty-six million Americans have diabetes and *half of them don't know it.*

Diabetes is deadly in its own right. But its indirect effects, including two to four times the risk of developing heart disease, having strokes, or dying from a stroke, are just as devastating. Its potential to damage health and detract from longevity is so great that the National Institutes of Health have done away with the term *borderline diabetes.* That term implies that we are still safe, that we still have some wiggle room before we have to take the condition seriously and get our blood sugar levels under control. But if you are interested in a long, sweet life, you can't wait.

Get Tested and Take Control

Diabetes is detected by a fasting blood test. The blood sugar level that indicates the presence of a problem, which used to be 140 milligrams (mg) of glucose per deciliter (dl) of blood, has been lowered to 126 mg/dl. This is where diabetes' hidden but dangerous effects begin. I recommend that everyone over the age of forty have a fasting blood test at least once every three years, more often if:

- You have a number of relatives with diabetes
- You are Native American, Hispanic, or African-American
- Past tests showed you to be what used to be called borderline

All abnormal tests demand a further workup.

At least as important as screening for diabetes, timely treatment— including a concerted effort to control blood sugar levels through lifestyle changes and, if necessary, oral medications—can slow the progress of this progressive condition and help you avoid serious complications further down the line. Initial treatment is usually quite simple. It includes:

- *Dietary management.* The older, rigidly controlled diabetic exchange diets are rarely used today. A diet high in fiber and complex carbohydrates, with five or six small meals at regular intervals, is usually suggested now. You should keep the amount of sugar and simple carbohydrates to a minimum. Results from the Nurse's Health

Study show that the foods most likely to protect you from diabetes are unsweetened high-fiber breakfast cereal and whole grains, including whole-grain breads.

- *Exercise.* Any increase in physical activity will make a difference.
- *Weight loss if you are overweight.* Simply losing ten to twenty pounds can fully control diabetes in some patients.

If these measures don't get the job done, your doctor may prescribe oral medication to help you process glucose better. By controlling things now, you may avoid ever having to use insulin or at least postpone it for several decades.

30. Have Your Bone Density Tested for Signs of Osteoporosis   Impact ★★★

Our bones are not the hard, lifeless things you see on a skeleton in a museum of natural history. They are living tissue. Bones support our muscles, protect our vital organs, and serve as a storage depot for calcium, which is what gives our bones their density and strength. Bones are constantly changing, taking in calcium and releasing it to help our hearts beat and our muscles, nerves, and blood perform their essential functions. During childhood, adolescence, and young adulthood we build up our bone supply, always adding and storing a little more than we use or lose. By our thirties, however, our bones begin to break down faster than new bone can be formed. Then, at menopause, women, who have less bone mass than men to begin with, start losing bone even more rapidly. The dramatic drop in estrogen, which served to protect their bones when they were younger, now accelerates their deterioration.

The net result for millions is osteoporosis—a degenerative condition that culminates with bones becoming fragile and breaking easily. This can occur anywhere in the body, but causes the most concern when the hips or spine are involved.

There's absolutely no doubt that osteoporosis is a longevity buster. It causes more than three hundred thousand hip fractures annually, and 25 to 50 percent of people who suffer one die within a year, generally from complications such as pneumonia; 20 percent of those with hip fractures need long-term nursing home care. Spinal fractures also have serious consequences, including a decrease in height, severe back pain, and dowager's hump.

The givens that make you a prime candidate for osteoporosis are:

- Heredity
- Slight, thin body type
- Race (Caucasian and Asian-American women have the highest risk)

Risk factors we can do something about include:

- Estrogen levels
- Calcium intake
- Exercise
- Smoking
- Excessive alcohol consumption

If one or more of these apply to you, a bone density test along with a physical examination by your doctor can provide the impetus for lifestyle changes and medical treatment to slow bone loss and ward off this disease. I recommend this test for all women sixty-five or older who have one or more risk factors.

If a bone density test indicates that you are moving toward osteoporosis, there are a number of things you can do to change direction:

- *Increase your calcium intake.* Women between nineteen and fifty need approximately 1,000 mg daily. After that, and especially after menopause, this increases to 1,500 mg. Most can't get all they need from their diet, so a supplement is indicated (see page 252).
- *Get more exercise.* The weight-bearing kind—walking, biking, dancing, and so on—stimulates bone growth and increases density. Tai chi, yoga, stretch classes, and resistance training, which are geared toward building strength and flexibility, improve coordination, balance, and agility to prevent falls.
- *Take safety precautions, especially at home.* Potential hazards include throw rugs, extension cords, stairs without handrails, and poorly lit areas. Be careful when lifting or retrieving objects from high shelves.
- *Consider hormone replacement therapy* (see Booster 33, page 247). Highly effective during the period right after menopause, when bone loss is the most rapid, you will be able to see a noticeable

change in bone density within six months. You will need to take it indefinitely.

- *Talk to your doctor about bone-strengthening medications such as Fosamax and Calcitonin.* They work.

My best advice? Don't wait until you're fifty or sixty and osteoporosis is within striking distance. Start exercising and getting more calcium now. Encourage your daughters or other younger women to do the same.

VITAMINS AND SUPPLEMENTS

Do you: Have personal habits, a family history, or other characteristics that put you at risk for heart disease, stroke, colon cancer, or osteoporosis? Find it difficult to eat a well-balanced, varied diet? Follow a vegetarian diet? Have food allergies, sensitivities, or preferences that compel you to forgo certain food groups, especially fruits or grains? Feel less energetic than you'd like to? Consider your life to be excessively stressful? Are you: Over fifty? A postmenopausal woman? Heavy drinker? Smoker? Then the suggestions you find in the section that follows should help you add years to your life and sweetness to your years.

Like a finely tuned machine, the human body runs best when well fueled. It fairly hums when it gets just the right mixture of macronutrients (proteins, fats, and carbohydrates) and micronutrients (mainly vitamins and minerals). Under ideal conditions we would get all of these in the proper proportions from the foods we eat. Trouble is, few of us consume an ideal diet. Even when we stick pretty closely to the recommendations illustrated by the food pyramid, our individual food choices can leave us deficient in certain areas.

We've known for more than a hundred years that not getting sufficient amounts of certain vitamins or minerals promotes disease, from beri beri and pernicious anemia for those deficient in specific B vitamins to scurvy for folks lacking vitamin C. Fortifying foods, by iodizing salt, for example, or adding vitamin D to milk, helps prevent deficiencies and protect us from the diseases associated with them. So does taking vitamin and mineral supplements. But that's not the only longevity-boosting benefit of supplementing our daily diets.

Supplements also can help us avoid conditions that are not directly related to a particular micronutrient. Take heart disease. It is not the result of a vitamin deficiency, yet subjects of the Nurse's Health Study who started their days with vitamin- and mineral-fortified breakfast cereals were much less likely to develop it.

Supplements often produce positive health results in their own right as well. They strengthen bones and slow bone loss that could lead to osteoporosis (calcium and vitamin D), shore up the body's natural defenses (vitamin C and zinc), and possibly delay some of the effects of aging (vitamins A and E, beta-carotene, and other antioxidants).

And that's just the vitamins and minerals. There are several other substances that can be taken on a daily basis to promote wellness and/or prevent specific medical conditions. Aspirin (325 mg), wine (one glass for women, two for men), and estrogen for women after menopause (to replace what the body no longer makes), although not traditionally thought of as supplements, are administered in the same way and taken for the same purpose. They get an essential component of health into our systems every day. And their impact can be dramatic.

31. Add an Aspirin Every Day   Impact ★★★★

Undoubtedly one of the greatest compounds ever developed, aspirin relieves pain and reduces swelling. It is useful for lowering fevers, treating headaches, and preventing two of the top three causes of premature death—heart disease and stroke. Aspirin makes the platelets in our blood less sticky and therefore less likely to clump together and form clots that cut off blood flow in the arteries leading to our hearts and brains. Subjects of the Physicians Health Study who took an aspirin a day suffered 44 percent fewer heart attacks. In heart attack survivors, taking aspirin reduced the risk of having another attack by 30 percent. The FDA is even allowing aspirin makers to advertise these benefits and tell potential buyers to take an aspirin as soon as you think you might be having a heart attack.

Although the hows and whys are just now being uncovered, aspirin also appears to protect against colon cancer. In the Nurse's Health Study, women who took one full-strength aspirin at least five days per week (for headaches, fever, or cardiac protection) had as much as a 50 percent lower colon cancer rate. Lower doses did not have the same effect.

Aspirin is not without its drawbacks, of course. Many people who take it experience gastrointestinal distress. Its anticlotting effect can mean bleeding more or for longer if you cut yourself. This may also raise your risk of experiencing a hemorrhagic stroke, the kind caused by a leaky, bleeding blood vessel rather than a blocked one. If you've had such a stroke, this booster isn't for you. Others who should forgo it include anyone who:

- Has a bleeding ulcer
- Is taking drugs that leave you prone to bleeding, such as Coumadin
- Is prone to falls or injuries (if you hit your head, you could have a hemorrhagic stroke)
- Is allergic to aspirin

However, if you *are* going to take an aspirin a day, here's what I recommend. Although a low dose (half a regular tablet, or 162 mg) is enough to prevent heart attacks, I find the colon cancer data quite compelling. Consequently, I recommend the full 325 mg dosage per day for patients who can tolerate it. Coated tablets, also called enteric-coated, are easier on the stomach. And any aspirin should be taken with food or milk.

32. Drink a Little Wine   Impact ★★★★

It's known as the French paradox. Natives of France consume a relatively high-fat diet but suffer fewer premature heart attacks than Americans do. Their resistance appears to come from a bottle—a wine bottle. The French consume four times as much wine as we do. They drink it daily. They drink it modestly (without the goal of getting drunk). And more often than not, they choose red wines over white, possibly profiting from the vitamin-like substances known as flavonoids that are plentiful in red grapes.

Study after study has supported the notion that moderate daily alcohol intake can protect our hearts and prolong our lives. It may work by increasing "good" HDL cholesterol or in the same way aspirin does, by making platelets less sticky. And beer and spirits could be just as cardioprotective as wine. Overall, however, what we drink is not as important as not drinking too much. Moderation is crucial. Alcohol's adverse effects, from inebriation to liver damage, begin to kick in once women exceed one drink (1.5 ounces of hard liquor, 5 ounces of wine, or 12 ounces of beer) and men exceed two.

My recommendation? Skip this longevity booster if you:

- Are an alcoholic or problem drinker (see page 183)
- Have a liver disease such as cirrhosis
- Have ulcers or other gastrointestinal tract troubles
- Are a high-risk candidate for breast cancer, as alcohol consumption has been shown to slightly increase this risk

Otherwise, enjoy a drink once a day. Because its links to longevity are the most clearly established, select red wine if you like it and it is available. But never choose a fortified wine, such as cherry, as it's fortified with alcohol and *not* vitamins. If you're concerned about uncorking a bottle for just a few ounces, then purchase one of the nifty special bottle recorkers that will keep your wine fresh for a week or more. If a red doesn't fit your taste, then consider white wine as your next best choice, or a beer or a mixed drink.

If you don't want the side effects of the alcohol in wine but still want some of its benefits, then grape juice might be your choice. There is some provocative evidence that grape juice may confer some protection. Only time and more research will tell.

33. Take Estrogen   Impact ★★★★

The medical establishment's use of estrogen in postmenopausal women and the public's perception of it have fluctuated wildly over the past few decades. In the sixties it was prescribed and taken without a second thought for hot flashes or other signs of menopause. In the seventies its downside—an increased risk of blood clots and cancer—came to the forefront. Those factors seemed to overshadow estrogen's usefulness—until the nineties, when important new uses were found.

Estrogen is one of the most influential hormones in a woman's body. During her reproductive years, it plays a starring role in ovulation, conception, and pregnancy and a supporting one in maintaining bone strength and protecting the cardiovascular system. New research indicates that it may even slow the onset or progression of dementia. Unfortunately, as a woman's childbearing years wane and the amount of estrogen produced by her ovaries drops, or if her ovaries are removed along with her uterus during a hysterectomy, her protective shield is taken away. For some, menopause is a change with few symptoms. But many women have to cope with the hot flashes, mood swings, and often memory problems that accompany menopause or follow a hysterectomy. The longer a woman is without estrogen, the greater her risk for heart disease and osteoporosis. The solution seems simple: Replace the estrogen. But it's a lot more complicated than that. Recent studies have disputed estrogen's supposed cardio-protective role. And the risk of developing breast or uterine cancer must always be factored in.

During their lifetimes, one in eight women will develop breast cancer, while one in two will have heart disease. Osteoporosis, which strikes more women than men, causes incalculable pain. One of its common outcomes, a fractured hip, leads to a whopping sixty-five thousand deaths per year. When you come across something such as estrogen that can significantly lower women's odds of experiencing either of these conditions, you don't want to pass it up. Yet the cancer risks and other contraindications cannot be ignored.

Combining estrogen with another female reproductive hormone, progesterone, can greatly reduce the risk of uterine cancer. Unfortunately, it also increases the risk of breast cancer. Thus, a woman who has had this illness should not take any hormone replacement therapy. I would additionally advise against it for a woman whose mother and sister or mother and maternal aunt have had breast cancer as well; her risk, even without estrogen replacement, is very high. Additionally, estrogen may be a less-than-ideal option for women who have fibroids or endometriosis, gallbladder problems, or migraine headaches.

Although its protection against bone loss is not quite as strong, the newer "synthetic" estrogen, raloxifene, may be the answer for some. Whether it gives cardiac protection is unknown.

My recommendation? I feel strongly about estrogen's ability to ward off osteoporosis, but I am not sure that it shields you from heart disease. Whether it works in preventing memory loss remains to be seen. In the average woman, those benefits probably outweigh the cancer risk. But I wholeheartedly believe that the actual decision to accept estrogen replacement or not is one that each woman must make for herself. My best advice is to reexamine your personal longevity profile and thoroughly review the pros and cons of taking estrogen with your doctor. If you decide for or against it at menopause and change your mind later, that's okay. Recent studies show that women benefit even when they start it at an advanced age.

34. Take a Multivitamin	Impact ★★★

Proteins, fats, and carbohydrates keep our engines running. Vitamins and minerals do the fine-tuning. They play a crucial role in growth and digestion, healing wounds and fighting infection, as well as helping us avoid deadly or disabling conditions from heart disease to dementia.

With the exception of vitamin D, which we make when our skin is exposed to sunlight, our bodies don't produce these micronutrients. We obtain them from the food we eat. However, most of us don't have enough of them in our daily diets. Deficiencies in vitamin D, which builds bone strength, and in folic acid, which helps prevent heart disease and birth defects, are well documented. So is the difficulty we have absorbing vitamin B$_{12}$ as we get older, which can contribute to memory loss and dementia.

To fill in these or other nutritional gaps we could eat more fortified foods, such as the cereals that boosted longevity in subjects of the Nurse's Health Study. Better still, we could improve our overall eating habits, adding fruits, vegetables, grains, nuts, or foods high in specific nutrients (citrus fruits for vitamin C, dairy products for calcium, and so on). This allows us to take advantage of the fiber and other longevity boosters foods have to offer. Unfortunately, getting all of our nutrients this way is quite difficult for many of us. And that's where multivitamins come in. They are our nutritional insurance policies, providing reasonable compensation for the flaws in our daily diets. They are not a substitute for eating, however. You can't starve yourself and expect a multivitamin, or even a whole handful of them, to give you everything you could obtain from a day's worth of food.

I recommend a multivitamin with minerals that meets FDA standards (look for "USP" on the label). Make sure it contains B vitamins, (at least 100 percent of the recommended daily allowance) and a minimum of 0.4 mg (400 mcg) of folic acid.

Women with heavy menstrual bleeding should take iron. If you are a man or a postmenopausal woman, select a multivitamin that does not contain iron. If you're eating right, your body does not require the extra iron, and the common side effects of iron supplementation, constipation and bloating, are simply not worth it. Some theorize that taking iron when you don't need it actually increases the risk of heart disease and hinders the discovery of colon cancer, because it can mask the anemia that is often associated with it. Therefore I do not recommend it for men or for women after menopause.

35. Take Advantage of Antioxidants: Vitamins C and E, Beta-carotene, Selenium   Impact ★★★

Every day unstable molecules known as free radicals bombard our bodies. These natural by-products of our own metabolism try to stabilize themselves by grabbing electrons from our cells. Those cells are damaged in the process, and over time that damage adds up, leading to much of the physical deterioration and many of the health problems we associate with aging. Higher levels of free radicals, generated by cigarette smoke, ultraviolet rays, and pesticides, have been linked to heart disease, cancer, cataracts, macular degeneration, and signs of premature aging.

Antioxidants are the vitamins, minerals, and other substances that chemically neutralize free radicals and keep them from overrunning our systems. They also seem to lessen the effect of "bad" LDL cholesterol, which can translate into less plaque buildup and fewer heart attack– or stroke-precipitating blockages in our arteries. We would be in big, big trouble without these defenders, and we can help ourselves by making sure there are enough of them available to get the job done.

Our bodies produce some antioxidants. Others are found in the food we eat. They are plentiful in whole grains, fruit, and veggies—things we should be consuming anyway. Study after study has shown that when we eat foods loaded with antioxidants, we seem to have less heart disease, cancer, and stroke. Supplement capsules do not appear to have the same protective shield as mother nature; they are supplementary to good eating. However, since the downside is minimal, I recommend considering these two:

- *Vitamin E.* Found in green leafy vegetables, shrimp, eggs, wheat germ, whole-grain cereal, nuts, and vegetable oils, vitamin E protects against heart disease, cutting premature heart attack rates by one-third. It may also prove valuable for shoring up our immune systems and combating Alzheimer's, Parkinson's disease, or breast cancer. I recommend 400 IU (international units) daily.

- *Vitamin C.* As a cure for the common cold, vitamin C has been a bust. But this micronutrient, found in citrus fruit, papaya, strawberries, kiwi, cantaloupe, tomatoes, broccoli, Brussels sprouts, and peppers, does seem to play a role in preventing cataracts, cancer, and coronary artery disease. It may prevent inflammations in our arteries, stopping the formation of artery-blocking clots that cause strokes and heart attacks. Extra-low levels are associated with memory loss. My recommendation? Take 500 mg twice a day. A double dose is needed because water-soluble vitamin C leaves our systems quite quickly.

Now, here are two the jury is still out on:

- *Beta-carotene* is the best-known member of a class of vitamin-like substances known as carotenoids. They promote good vision and help maintain healthy skin, teeth, bones, and muscle. Beta-carotene, which the body converts to vitamin A as needed, is believed to go several steps further. A diet that contains lots of beta-carotene-rich foods such as carrots, spinach, broccoli, cantaloupe, winter squash, mango, papaya, and apricot has been linked to lower cancer rates, less coronary artery disease, and fewer age-related problems such as macular degeneration. However, no such correlation has yet been made for beta-carotene supplements. In fact, one study showed *higher* lung cancer rates for smokers who took beta-carotene than for smokers who did not. A sensible dosage would be 6 to 15 mg a day. But at this point your best bet may be to stick with dietary sources.

- *Selenium.* Selenium, found in meat, poultry, fish, and vegetables grown in soil that contains large concentrations of this mineral, fires up our immune system and may protect against lung, colorectal, and prostate cancers. When taken with vitamin E, selenium enhances the antioxidant effects of that vitamin. However, dosage can be a problem. We need only a little bit, and too much can be toxic, causing hair and nail loss. Between 200 and 400 mcg should be enough.

36. Make Room for Calcium and Vitamin D   Impact ★★★

Calcium is a mineral with many functions. Ninety-nine percent of it goes toward building and maintaining strong, healthy bones and teeth —an absolute necessity if you hope to avoid the pain, fractures, and premature death associated with osteoporosis. The other 1 percent helps your heart beat, your muscles contract and relax, your nerves send and receive messages, and your blood clot. No wonder you hear so much about this micronutrient!

Throughout our lives, we must take in enough calcium daily to replace the calcium our bodies are using. If we don't, we begin depleting the calcium in our bones, leaving them weak, porous, brittle—and fracture-prone. This devastating end result is most often seen in older women. Female skeletons have less calcium than males' from the start. So when they lose calcium they have less reserve. But men are not immune—their hips fracture, too.

The solution is simple, and hardly news. If you aren't consuming 1,000–1,500 mg of calcium daily, increase your intake. Start immediately. It is never too early—or too late—to benefit from calcium. Your best source, as always, is dietary. Calcium is most plentiful in dairy products, tofu, sardines and salmon, spinach, and other dark green vegetables. If you find that you are unable to meet your daily requirement even after you change your diet—a common occurrence—then turn to a supplement.

I recommend 1,500 mg a day of calcium from all sources—food or supplements. Most of us do not get enough calcium from our diets. If you eat dairy products such as milk, yogurt, and cheese every day, one 750 mg tablet with vitamin D would suffice. If you consume little or no dairy, I recommend two 750 mg tablets. That breaks down to roughly 1,000 mg a day from all sources for men twenty-five through sixty-five, and women twenty-five through fifty. Women over fifty who are postmenopausal, and men over sixty-five, need a total of 1,500 mg a day.

When choosing a calcium supplement, consider calcium carbonate first. It is the most readily available and the least expensive option. If you develop gas or constipation, you can switch to calcium gluconate, calcium citrate, or calcium lactate.

Vitamin D is calcium's ally in the fight against osteoporosis. Our bodies use it for bone growth during childhood and adolescence, for bone maintenance in adulthood, and for help absorbing calcium at any age. We obtain vitamin D from milk fortified with it, other dairy products, fish, eggs, fortified breakfast cereals, or sunlight. Many of us fall short of optimal intake, especially in the winter, when we spend more time indoors. I recommend 600 IU a day for adult men and women, increasing to 800 IU a day after women hit menopause and men turn sixty. Take it as a separate vitamin tablet or combined with calcium.

REGULAR MEDICAL VISITS

37. Get Periodic Tune-ups   Impact ★★★★

We all have heard stories about someone going to a doctor's office for an annual checkup and dying in the parking lot on the way out. That's because there really is no assurance that a physical exam and blood tests will pick up everything that may cause you harm. It would be wonderful if an annual EKG would detect heart disease or an annual chest X-ray would pick up the beginnings of lung cancer. But both of these tests have been proven to be relatively worthless as screening exams to pick up any disease before it's significant.

But I am not a naysayer. I do believe, based on standards developed by the U.S. Task Force on the Preventive Medical Examination and the Canadian equivalent, that there are certain tests and exams that should be performed routinely to help you stay well. The following chart is a guideline of major recommendations:

TUNE-UP GUIDELINES

PREVENTION/SCREENING TEST	AGE					
	30	40	50	60	70	80
Blood pressure every 1–3 years	X	X	X	X	X	X
Cholesterol testing every 1–3 years	X	X	X	X	X	X
Pap test every 1–3 years	X	X	X	X	X	X
Mammogram						
Every 1–2 years		X				
Yearly			X	X	X	X
Stool for occult blood yearly		X	X	X	X	X
Flexible sigmoidoscopy every 5 years			X	X	X	X
Osteoporosis screening every 5 years			X	X	X	X

38. Have a Good Relationship with Your Doctor   Impact ★★★

More than just an examination goes on when you visit a doctor. It's a time of consideration, a time to:

- Think about getting immunized
- Reflect on your diet and exercise regime
- Decide whether or not you should take supplements such as aspirin, wine, or estrogen
- Examine your mental sphere—are you happy or depressed?
- Look at your kinship sphere—what about those relationships?

But to do this well you need to have a good relationship with your doctor. It's crucial. Your doctor should be your advocate, not your adversary. Times have changed, thank goodness, since a passive patient sat with a physician and the physician told him or her what was wrong and what needed to be done. If we trust the person who gives us advice and believe that the information is good and his or her intent honest, if we analyze and dialogue about what we are being told, then everyone feels something positive has taken place from both sides. But in today's world of HMOs this scenario is not always the first one you enter into. So you have to be an advocate for yourself and remember at all times that you are a consumer. Choosing and staying with a physician should at least be as important and take as much work as investigating and buying a car.

You want a doctor who is compassionate and knowledgeable, who takes the time to know who you are. But how do you choose a doctor you can have confidence in? That may take a little hunting.

Set Up a Short Interview

A get-acquainted interview is a common medical practice. Plan an initial short period for this. Take notes if you feel more comfortable. The responsiveness to this first request will tell you something about them immediately. Here's how I suggest you script it: When you walk in the door, is the receptionist friendly? Is he or she too rushed to answer your questions? Ask one crucial question: "If I am sick, can I usually see the doctor that day?" If the answer is no, then I would suggest shopping around. You want a physician who is available, or has someone else who might be, when you're ill, not a week later.

When you are brought into the office or examining room, is the nurse courteous and friendly or hassled? Does he or she seem professional? Trust your judgment and intuition—they're probably right.

When you meet the physician face-to-face, your goal is to observe his or her attitude. Is he or she open to your queries? Concerned with you? Do you feel comfortable? Then go right ahead and ask questions that might be important to you. You initiated the interview, so you should direct the conversation. Ask pointed, short questions on any of these topics, or others that might interest you:

- What are the doctor's views on medicines? Does he or she give medications out fairly freely?
- Does the doctor believe medications are usually the way to go when lifestyle changes might work just as well?
- What are the doctor's views of complementary and alternative medicine, such as chiropractic, megadoses of vitamins, and other supplements?
- What does the doctor think about personal issues of importance to you, such as breast-feeding, jogging, yoga, estrogen replacement therapy, mammograms, and so on? Many people—including doctors—have strong opinions on these topics.

Do the answers fit into your worldview? If you believe that alternative and complementary medicine or natural health modalities are good for you, ask about them and listen to the response. You certainly want a doctor who's not hostile to a view that you hold; at the very least you want a reasonable explanation as to why the physician doesn't share that view, since you're gathering information to review and reflect upon later. Also, rapport is extremely important in an initial interview. Remember at all times that you are asking legitimate questions, just as you would do for any other important issue. Is the physician antagonistic? Are you? Then, as they say in the game shows, it's not a match.

When you're finished, you should ask yourself:
- Did the doctor have an interest in you?
- Was the doctor courteous and compassionate?
- Did you trust that the doctor knew what he or she was talking about?
- Does the doctor have time to be a partner in your care?
- Does the doctor simply wish to give you advice, and you must take it or leave it?

If not, look elsewhere.

Sometimes you may need to set up an interview in the same office with a colleague of the doctor you just rejected because that's the way your insurance works out. Just do it. It may feel awkward, but in reality you do yourself and the doctor a favor if you choose someone who fits your tastes and needs.

Here are two stories that illustrate how much this relationship means. A woman patient, who just moved from a different town, came to my office to establish her care. She was a runner. When we had our first regular visit she asked about blood pressure medication because her previous doctor had put both her and her husband on a hypertensive agent called a beta-blocker. This is a very good pill to control hypertension, but not for runners. Beta-blockers slow down your heart and retard the pulse, so that you would not be able to run a marathon in the time you'd want. She asked her last doctor to switch drugs. He replied that he thought the beta-blocker was the best one for her and refused to listen to her reasoning. In fact, she said, he seemed upset that she even asked. In reality, she was right and he was wrong.

In another case, a friend's son saw a specialist for a significant neurological injury. Although the family was comfortable and confident with the specialist, when the issue of surgery came up they asked the specialist if they should seek a second opinion. Without missing a beat, the doc said, "Absolutely. You should talk with anyone else you feel might help you to decide the best course of medicine." That's the kind of answer you want. A good doctor is one who's personally secure in his or her opinion but not defensive.

The Informed Consumer

If you're unhappy, switch. I am continually amazed at people who are unhappy with their doctor but are afraid to switch. Maybe they think that they have no rights in their HMO, or the doctor will think less of them, or the next doctor will look askance because they switched. The first thing to realize is that you're in charge. It's your life, and the doctor is simply a resource for your care. We switch cars, houses, and restaurants over the course of years. It's at least as important as that to get the best match we can with our physicians.

My mentor, Bob Mendelsohn, always said that the best patient is an informed consumer. Even today some physicians complain that patients always come in with questions about new drugs, new procedures, or cures that they've discovered on the Internet or in a magazine. In fact, it is good to bring in that information, because it will help you decide if your doctor is well informed, and it provides a perspective on their advice. I think any reliable information that you can have assures you of a better result. A good doctor-patient relationship is ongoing and needs periodic fine-tuning to keep you satisfied and happy.

39. Get Immunized   Impact ★★★★

Shots aren't fun for kids *or* adults. Pain is the most common reason given for not taking advantage of flu shots or getting tetanus boosters or being immunized against hepatitis B. Other obstacles include the time it takes to go to a doctor and get a shot, the cost of the shot, and simply not knowing that immunization is important.

In addition, some folks just don't believe in immunization. They feel there's something inappropriate about having shots when they aren't sick, or they fear that the shot, which is intended to keep them well in the future, will make them ill now.

Vaccines work by stimulating your body to produce antibodies to a virus or bacterium without having to actually suffer through the disease caused by that particular bug. People are often afraid that they will develop diseases from immunizations. They've heard that certain vaccinations trigger seizures, give you Alzheimer's disease, or cause autism in children. The best scientific evidence we have today is that immunizations' side effects are usually limited to pain at the site of the injection, fever, and sometimes mild symptoms of the illness you're being immunized against.

Immunization is available for a wide range of diseases, although many you'll need to have only if you're traveling to places where sanitation is questionable or where a disease that is virtually unheard of in the United States remains active. The ones you should get are:

Influenza	Get it yearly.	75 percent effective. It's only good for a single season.
Pneumonia	Especially if you are sixty-five or older.	80 percent effective. Protects against some common forms of pneumonia.
Tetanus Booster	Every ten years.	100 percent effective.
Hepatitis B	A three-shot primary series protects you for life.	98 percent effective. If your job puts you in contact with blood or bodily fluids or if your personal behavior puts you at risk for sexually transmitted diseases, it's worth getting.

40. Use Medications Effectively   Impact ★★★★

From penicillin, first used in the 1920s, to Prozac today, every era has its so-called miracle medications. These breakthrough drugs and others like them capture our attention and often earn tidy profits for the companies that manufacture them. But do they work? Perhaps not as miraculously as their advance publicity suggests, but yes.

You might think that because of the rigorous approval process they must go through, all medications on the market today do what they're supposed to. But that's not the case. All drugs that are purported to fight the same disease are not equivalent. Some are more effective than others. Some need be taken only once a day, making it easier to take the drug as prescribed. Others have side effects, making us drowsy or irritable, nauseated, "hyper," or depressed. Some of us even have life-threatening allergic reactions to them. Certain medications can interact dangerously with each other or with food or beverages or herbal remedies. Very few, if any, are right for everyone all the time.

That's why longevity-minded medication takers will want to become familiar with any drugs they are now or soon could be taking. Always, the goal for you and your doctor to shoot for is the most effective medication with the fewest side effects at the lowest dosage necessary to get the job done.

As a physician, there are a number of drugs that I'd hate to have to work without. Simple analgesics such as acetaminophen (Tylenol) and ibuprofen come to mind, as well as antihistamines for allergies. And of course antacids and acid blockers (Zantac and Prilosec) have made great strides in making our lives more comfortable and easy. Let's not forget hypertensives, cholesterol-lowering agents, and antibiotics, to name a few. But using pharmaceuticals correctly means knowing their effects and side effects.

Prevent Adverse Reactions

Even the best of medications administered with the best of intentions by the most conscientious medical professionals sometimes create unforeseen and potentially fatal complications. It's estimated that seventy-six thousand deaths and more than two million serious but non-lethal incidents involving adverse drug reactions occur annually.

- Make sure that your doctor and pharmacist are aware of your past experiences with various medications.
- If you're asked to fill out a questionnaire prior to an outpatient procedure or hospital admission, complete it as thoroughly and accurately as possible.
- Because you sometimes may be too sick or too anxious to fill out forms completely, jot down important information ahead of time and bring it with you.
- Avert potentially harmful reactions among various medications and treatments. If you're taking drugs prescribed for you by another

doctor, over-the-counter medication, pills left over from a prescription written for your sister, even herbal preparations such as Saint-John's-wort or ginkgo biloba, be sure to share this information with the physician who's treating you.

- Consider medical-alert jewelry if you are allergic to certain classes of medicine—sulfa or penicillin-type drugs.
- Educate yourself, especially if you will be using a relatively new product. Find out what side effects to look for. Utilize the drug-information sheets every pharmacy should give. Similar information can be found in books on prescription medications such as *The Pill Book* or the *PDR (Physician's Desk Reference)*. The Web is also an excellent source of medical information.
- Try not to be "pill happy." The law of averages dictates that the more medications you take, the greater your chances of being harmed by one of them.

41. Consider Complementary and Alternative Medicine   Impact ★★

Complementary or alternative medicine (I prefer the term *complementary,* because conceptually it fits my view) is often used in addition to standard medical care. For the most part, complementary medicine can be useful when regular medical care doesn't meet your needs. Examples of conditions for which it may be suited include sore throats, backaches, insomnia, fibromyalgia, and chronic fatigue syndrome—Western medicine does not offer a superlative treatment for any of these. Many physicians are broadening their practices to integrate traditional and complementary health care despite the fact that it doesn't stand the tests of scientific rigor. Why? Because people want it: Studies show that nearly one out of three Americans uses complementary medicine.

When we look at alternative therapies, we might find:
- Chiropractic
- Acupuncture
- Mind-Body skills (guided imagery, yoga, self-healing techniques)
- Dance therapy and tai chi
- Relaxation and stress reduction
- Hypnosis
- Biofeedback

- Craniosacral body work, reflexology, and massage
- Homeopathy
- Herbal medicines
- Rolfing
- Aromatherapy
- Natural hormone balancing

The field is diverse, and some approaches are worthy while some are less so. My feeling has always been that if you benefit from something and it doesn't harm you in any way, you may want to continue with it. But some things bleed your pocketbook while providing no real benefit, such as chelation therapy.

If you choose a manipulative technique, such as chiropracty, massage, acupuncture, or reflexology, make sure that your healer is certified, licensed, and recommended. If there is no licensing for a particular technique, such as craniosacral therapy, then choose a healer who's recommended by someone you trust.

If you choose an herb or botanical treatment, be sure that the remedies are manufactured by a reliable source. The FDA does not regulate supplements as it does drugs. That means that even though the label may *say* that a particular supplement contains a certain ingredient, there is no guarantee that it actually will. I find this lack of government regulation repulsive. I think that if the label says feverfew, ginkgo, or milk thistle, it should have that in it. If it says 10 mg, it should have 10 mg. Sadly, that is not the case. Know thy supplier.

Read about the treatment you're considering adopting. Study after study shows that those who use complementary medicine are usually more knowledgeable about all forms of healing.

I believe more research is definitely needed on alternative cures. Western medicine clearly does not have all the answers; some issues are not dealt with satisfactorily and are answered better by alternative views. A good example is vitamins used for heart disease prevention. For years I thought taking a multivitamin, vitamin C, and vitamin E was baloney—not as useful as eating foods that contained these vitamins. Alternative healers were touting it, and they were right. It took Western medicine more than twenty years to discover what health food devotees have known for years. Now I recommend eating the foods themselves *and* taking reasonable doses of certain ones.

And let's not forget that vegetarianism, which we now consider a healthful diet, was always—and still is—an alternative lifestyle. In fact, we appreciate and acknowledge the superiority of veggies and fruits. So I find it disingenuous that mainstream medicine pooh-poohs vegetarianism when balanced vegetarian diets are sensible and healthier.

The problem with alternative medicine is that it is hard for doctors and laypeople to evaluate. Commonly, the way we weigh such information or treatments is anecdotally. A friend says, "It worked for me, maybe it'll work for you." So we try it. And it might be great. The danger is that alternative medicine, just by being called a form of medicine, cloaks itself in the trappings of science. It uses scientific terms to gain credibility without adhering to the rigors that science demands. I take umbrage with this. My opinion is if you're going to use science to show the credibility of your treatment or therapy, you have to apply the rules of science. That means not just the words but the research. If you don't apply scientific rules, then don't use scientific terms. Some approaches, such as the vitamins I mentioned above, have been scientifically proven to work. Unfortunately, some remedies are bogus and some are merely unproven, and at present there's just no way to know which is which.

42. Drink Plenty of Water   Impact ★★

Like the air we breathe, water is absolutely essential. It helps cool our bodies, convert food into energy, burn fat, and carry away waste. It keeps our body chemistry balanced, our brains (which are 75 percent water) sharp, and our kidneys healthy.

Our bodies easily go through sixty-four ounces of fluid a day—more if we exercise or are ill and running a fever. So we need to take in at least that much daily. All fluids count toward that goal, including water, coffee, juice, soda, even beer—and food (there's some water in practically everything we eat or drink). The Harvard School of Public Health recently reported that men in their Health Professionals Follow-up Study who drank six or more cups of water a day were 50 percent less likely to develop bladder cancer than men who drank less than one cup. Drinking lots of water may reduce your risk of prostate cancer as well.

You don't have to get fancy about this. Buying bottled springwater isn't necessary. Although you can drink it if you prefer that taste and have money to burn, it is really no purer than the tap water in most communities. You can purify water by running it through a filter before drinking it—an especially good idea if you use well water that has not been tested or your home has lead pipes.

43. Get Enough Sleep   Impact ★★★

There are few things in life more pleasurable and refreshing than a good night's sleep. So when was the last time *you* got one? If you're like most of us, you'll have to rack your brain to remember. Most of us are chronically sleep deprived.

Two out of three people surveyed by the National Sleep Foundation did not get the recommended eight hours of sleep nightly. One-third got less than six. This deficit has an adverse effect on hormones, brain cells, and our immune systems. It prevents us from combating fatigue or replenishing our energy stores, which in turn wreaks havoc with our waking hours. Sleep deprivation can be deadly. It dulls our minds, increases irritability and depression, and makes us more accident prone. Driving while drowsy causes an estimated hundred thousand car crashes annually and more than fifteen hundred fatalities. Cheating ourselves of sleep may make us age faster and expire prematurely. Human Population Lab researchers tracking sleep patterns in men thirty or older found that those who slept just four hours a night were nearly three times as likely to die within six years as those who slept seven or eight.

We all function best with around eight hours of shut-eye. If you have trouble getting yours, try to:

- *Keep a regular bedtime hour.* Make it a little earlier each week until you're getting enough sleep time.
- *Make your bedroom as conducive to sleep as possible.* For many of us this means keeping the TV and anything related to work outside our bedroom walls.
- *Avoid caffeine, alcohol, and heavy meals* for three hours before going to bed.
- *Get more exercise during the day.* It helps tire you out and bring stress levels down. But avoid it at night, when vigorous activity may pump you up instead of wind you down.

Nap Your Way to Health

If a good night's sleep continues to elude you and daytime drowsiness threatens to overpower you, a nap may help. Nappers report feeling rejuvenated, less stressed, and better prepared to handle problems after catching a mere fifteen to twenty minutes of sleep at some point during the day. Buoyed by recent studies linking naps to increased alertness, accuracy, and productivity, some companies are even making "nap stations" available to their employees.

---

44. Take Care of Your Teeth and Gums   Impact ★★★★

Few of us actually *like* going to the dentist. And flossing? Well, it's exceptionally easy to skip when we're busy or tired. But taking care of our teeth and gums has more than cosmetic value. It also:

- *Helps us keep our own teeth longer.* When I arrived in Nova Scotia, Canada, to complete my medical training, I encountered what seemed like an inordinate number of adolescents and young adults with some or all of their teeth missing. It didn't take me long to figure out why. I could see that they consumed lots of candy. I knew that their water supply was not fluoridated. And I learned that they rarely went to the region's few dentists. These deficits in dental care were directly responsible for the sorry state of their teeth.

Nobody wants a bridge or dentures. To avoid having them, setting up a program of good dental hygiene can:

- *Contribute to better nutrition as we get older.* The pleasure goes out of eating when we experience discomfort with every bite. Sadly, that's the case for many seniors who let their teeth and gums go.
- *Prevent gum disease.* Periodontal disease has recently been linked to serious health problems elsewhere in our bodies. Research shows that gum disease may be a major risk factor for premature heart attacks and stroke. It works like this: The bacteria present in our gums enter our bloodstream, ultimately getting stuck in the cholesterol plaques that line our arteries. They produce a chronic inflammation that eventually swells and leads to a blockage that can cause death. What's more, if you have an artificial joint or valve, these same bacteria can easily infect them. A dangerous situation indeed.

So do what you've been told since Mr. Tooth first visited your preschool classroom. Brush well, preferably after every meal. Floss daily. Have your teeth cleaned by a professional once or twice yearly. Get regular checkups.

Mental Sphere

DETRIMENTAL CONDITIONS

45. Treat Depression	Impact ★★★★

Depressive illness is extremely common in this country and all too often overlooked, minimized, or misunderstood. It can be divided into two categories: exogenous or endogenous. Exogenous depression is situational, often precipitated by the death of a spouse, dissatisfaction with a career change, financial worry, or other stress. It tends to be limited by the circumstances that caused it. Endogenous depression is a different character. It comes from the inside, from you. It's often called chemical depression. Most researchers in the field believe that this is due to a neurotransmitter imbalance.

Depression's effect on longevity, though rarely talked about, is well documented. A recent article looking at depression in a sample of seventy-five hundred women sixty-five or older found that 24 percent of the women who had six or more symptoms of depression died during the next decade compared to 7 percent of the women who had no symptoms at all.

There is overwhelming evidence that major depression is a risk factor for heart attacks and stroke, one commensurate with cholesterol. It seems to predict your chances of having both a first heart attack and subsequent heart attacks. For both heart attacks and bypass surgery, recovery is better and the risk of dying less if you are not significantly depressed. In both the young and the old, depression also has been linked to an increase in cardiac arrhythmias, those extra heartbeats that can kill you.

Depression also predicts physical decline. Anyone with a physical illness or disability who suffers from major depression as well will be less likely to function well. It's hard to get on top of things when you're depressed.

Finally, the pain of depression is sometimes so relentless or becomes so unbearable that people end their own lives to escape it. There are more than sixteen thousand suicide deaths in this country each year; many of those are because a patient has been seriously depressed.

Are *You* Depressed?

Signs that this illness has crept up on you include:

- A sad or "empty" feeling that persists despite your efforts or desire to relieve it
- Feeling hopeless, helpless, worthless, pessimistic, or apathetic
- Increased use of alcohol, prescribed medications, or illicit drugs, often with the goal of numbing or blocking out painful thoughts and feelings
- Fatigue that no amount of sleep seems to overcome
- Losing interest in ordinary activities, including sex, and also finding it difficult to feel pleasure or enjoy any activity for more than a fleeting moment
- Disturbed eating and sleeping patterns—you may have no appetite or want to eat constantly, sleep more than usual or less, have trouble falling asleep at bedtime, or wake early in the morning and be unable to get back to sleep
- Irritability, crying jags, general anxiety, panic attacks, or believing that something bad is about to happen to you
- Difficulty concentrating, remembering, or making decisions
- Thoughts of suicide, or suicide plans or attempts
- Aches, pains, or other physical symptoms that do not respond to medical treatment, including headaches, stomach problems, or neck, back, joint, or mouth pain

When several or many of these symptoms last for most of the day nearly every day for at least two weeks, you could be suffering from a major depressive illness. You can overcome it. Plenty of people have. But it won't go away on its own.

If You Have It, Treat It

If you suspect that depression is dragging you down, get help. With help, four out of five people with this illness get better. So why do only

30 percent of those who suffer the kinds of problems I just listed actually seek professional assistance? Because we feel guilty about having it. It has a social stigma. We think that we should be strong enough to pull ourselves out of it. If we take medication for it, we feel guilty about that, too.

In a small number of cases, perhaps 10 or 15 percent, depression is a symptom of another disorder or the side effect of prescription medications. Under these circumstances, treating the underlying illness, changing prescriptions, or taking a more active role in managing your chronic conditions may relieve depression's symptoms.

More often—and always when no other medical condition is behind it—the depressive illness itself must be treated. Antidepressant drugs are designed specifically for this purpose. They effectively relieve depression in 60 to 80 percent of the people who take them. They aren't habit-forming and usually won't interfere with your ability to carry out your normal activities.

Prozac, Zoloft, and Paxil, the next generation of antidepressant drugs, generally are the best ones to use. They do not control depression any better than the older medicines, but they have fewer unpleasant side effects. As a result, patients stay on them. All antidepressants take at least six weeks before they really take effect.

And don't forget counseling. For many, this alone may be all that's needed to get people back on their feet and stay there.

A HOLISTIC VIEW OF DEPRESSION AND STRESS MANAGEMENT

For centuries, healers made few distinctions among illnesses coming from your body, mind, or environment. They believed everything was integrated, interdependent. The five-sphere concept updates this ancient paradigm.

You know yourself better than anyone. Trust your own intuition and insight when solving health problems. Muscular problems, headaches, weight issues, job or family conflicts can produce stress, agitation, sadness, and pain. Try looking inside for answers before you try to fix problems from the outside. Then be your own best advocate in finding the help you need. A strictly rational, logical approach to any medical condition can provide some answers, but usually not all of them.

DEPRESSIVE ILLNESS IN A NUTSHELL

Major Depression

People with major depression get hit with symptoms that can last months or years and significantly impair their ability to function on all fronts. With effective treatment, patients return to feeling normal and resume their normal lives.

Bipolar Illness or Manic-Depression

Sufferers swing back and forth between emptiness and euphoria, lethargy and excess energy, depression and mania.

SAD (Seasonal Affective Disorder)

Symptoms of depression, including low energy, fatigue, overeating, and irritability, appear in the fall, when days begin to get shorter, and last through the winter months. Often treated by having the SAD sufferer sit in front of a bank of lights for thirty minutes each day.

Dysthymia

Analogous to walking through life surrounded by a gray cloud, dysthymia appears to be more of a predepressed state than a full-blown depression. It is chronic in nature, and some folks suffer from it for decades. Because of its low-grade blueness, it often goes unrecognized and untreated.

Help Yourself, Too

In conjunction with counseling, medication, or a combination of the two, the following lifestyle changes and mood-lifting measures also can help you with depressive illness.

- *Curtail alcohol and drug use.* Because they create a comfortable numbness or offer a brief euphoric respite from the dreariness that engulfs you, many mistakenly self-medicate with alcohol, marijuana, cocaine, or other illicit substances. Unfortunately, they are not good antidepressants. When the initial effect wears off, the depression is often worse. What's more, the impaired judgment and tendency to act on impulse that accompany alcohol and drug highs are behind many suicide tries.

- *Seek emotional support* from friends, self-help groups, or professional counselors when making life changes. Change is often scary, even if it is positive.

- *Get more exercise.* Inactivity prevents you from reaping the biochemical and psychological benefits that getting up, getting involved, and moving around can bring. The endorphins released during aerobic exercise are natural antidepressants. Any time you fill with productive action is time not spent ruminating about your unhappiness.
- *Develop more and better skills for coping with stress.* Try out the tools on pages 272–276. They're all designed to help you look at the world from a more optimistic point of view.

46. Manage Anger   Impact ★★★★★

Anger kills. If it turns into aggression and there's a weapon handy, anger may end in homicide, suicide, domestic violence, child abuse, or fatal accidents. But anger also kills slowly and cumulatively, its ill effects on our heart, arteries, blood pressure, and relationships adding up over time.

The evidence is mounting. In a University of Michigan ten-year study of two thousand men in their fifties, the men who got angry most often were twice as likely to have strokes. If they also had atherosclerosis (hardening of the arteries), their odds were six times higher. Of particular interest was the finding that suppressed anger (the kind we keep a lid on) and controlled anger (the kind we channel into problem solving or constructive action) did not have the above effect. Only expressed anger—screaming, stomping, hitting, ranting, and so on—increased stroke risk.

These results certainly make you think twice about the advice we were given a few years back to get anger off our chests by "telling it like it is" and "letting it all hang out." But they make perfect sense physiologically. Each time we become angry, we experience a fast, intense burst of adrenaline and cortisol, which overstimulate our nervous system and wreak havoc on our heart and arteries. Our blood pressure rises. Our heart beats erratically, and blood flows in and out of it improperly. Our bodies, anticipating the physical attack the primitive part of our brains believes is coming, try to prevent us from bleeding out profusely by preparing our blood to clot quickly. So with each angry episode, there's a chance that a clot will form in and block an artery. No wonder research keeps linking this emotion to heart attacks

---

PRACTICE PATIENCE

Take a deep breath to calm your mind. Try square breathing: four breaths in, four breaths out, four times. What if you can't calm down, if you just can't stop being angry? What if you're angry at so much more than the present interaction? Can it ever get better? Well, it's hard to be compassionate to someone who is annoying you—but are they really your mortal enemy? Do you truly wish them unimaginable, unending suffering? Or do you just wish that they would give you some space? Who better to teach you compassion and patience than your enemy? You act warmer toward the people you care the most about. The more you practice compassion for the one set of folks, the more you may recognize the negative emotions that are causing you to be unhappy with the other set of folks. That's when I suggest you exchange them. *Replace the negative with the positive.*

---

and life-threatening arrhythmias. In the United States, angry outbursts precipitate thirty-six thousand heart attacks a year.

After we've pitched a fit or burned rubber passing the Sunday driver we were stuck behind for ten miles, our bodies return to normal —slowly. At least physiologically, we stay angry for a long time. And we don't help matters by a "venting" to uninvolved parties after the fact. When we relive anger-provoking incidents with anyone who makes the mistake of asking how we're doing, our bodies reexperience the anger, too.

Because the damage to our hearts and arteries is cumulative, hostile individuals—folks who grumble and growl and react furiously to the slightest provocation—fare worse than those of us who occasionally lose our tempers. High levels of hostility lead to a death rate from all causes that is 68 percent higher than the general population's. In one study, men with the highest hostility scores had a 50 percent higher death rate than that of the men with the lowest.

Signs of excess anger and hostility include:
- Frequently feeling angry (although not always knowing why)
- Usually expressing your anger by yelling, shouting, striking, or verbally abusing the person who angered you
- Putting up with what you believe are slights, injustices, and good causes for anger until you "can't take it anymore" and explode

- Having little or no tolerance for delays or frustration
- Getting into a lot of physical confrontations
- On a fairly regular basis, confronting people or creating scenes that you later feel guilty about or ashamed of
- Believing that, given the opportunity, most people would betray or mistreat you
- Constantly being on the lookout for people who could be taking advantage of you

If more than one or two of these beliefs and behaviors apply to you, anger is probably undermining your efforts to live a longer, sweeter life. You need to defuse this ticking time bomb and find more constructive ways to deal with frustrating events and infuriating individuals.

Clearly, "letting it all hang out" when we're angry isn't good for us. And it's no picnic for the target of our fury, either. No one likes being on the receiving end of someone's anger. Having someone shout at you is frightening and often demeaning or humiliating. Tantrum-throwing bosses don't boost their employees' productivity. Parents who angrily smack or verbally abuse their children and call it discipline don't teach them to be well behaved and respectful. Instead, they learn that it's okay to hit or say horrible, hurtful things when they're angry.

Yet some anger isn't all bad if you consider it in a larger context. It can stir us to change jobs, get out of unhealthy relationships, start petition drives, campaign for political candidates who share our view of a particular problem, plant a community garden on an unsightly city lot, and much more. *This is the key to managing your anger. Instead of allowing it to compel you to do something destructive, channel it into something constructive.* Taking positive action puts you back in control of your anger rather than having it control you. Look at your anger as a motivator to teach you patience.

Of course, you may have to take a few interim steps before you reach that point. Some of those steps follow.

- *Know what triggers your anger.* Most of us have pet peeves or people in our lives who "push our buttons," situations we just hate to be in and behaviors we just can't tolerate. We can predict how we'll react. And we can plan to react differently. The more triggers we are aware of, the more prepared we can be to keep our anger to a minimum.

- *Count to ten.* Yes, this old chestnut really works. It's distracting enough to flip off your anger switch or at least give you a few seconds to cool down.
- *Put things in perspective.* How important is the situation that's provoking you? Is it absolutely necessary to react to it vehemently? Is it worth giving your nervous and cardiovascular systems another pounding? As Dr. Redford Williams asks in his book *Anger Kills,* if you only had twenty-four hours left to live, would you really want to spend any of that time fighting this battle, reaming out this person, or getting this point across? If not, then don't.
- *Step away.* If things get too hot, excuse yourself for a moment.
- *Set anger aside for the moment.* Think of anger as an insistent child clamoring for attention. Mentally acknowledge it, then send it away for a while.
- *If you seem particularly short-tempered or overly sensitive on a particular day or in response to certain situations, look for reasons in the past or present.* Perhaps you're working too hard or getting too little sleep. Maybe you're misdirecting your frustration over a job you hate or a situation at home.
- *When you identify an anger-provoking problem, get help solving it.*
- *Look into anger-management courses or counseling.*
- *Consider antidepressant medications.* They appear to keep chronically angry people on a more even keel, perhaps by slowing the time it takes for them to react to precipitating events.

47. Develop More and Better Skills for Coping with Stress   Impact ★★★★★

Jean Cassidy had done everything she was supposed to in life. She married a kind, hardworking man and had three kids, gave up her teaching job to raise them when they were young, and then went back to work part-time to help out with expenses as they got older. She attended church every Sunday. She helped raise funds for local charities. And in doing all this, Jean had effectively erased every trace of her past—except the bitter taste thinking about it brought to her mouth. It wasn't easy growing up with an alcoholic mother, and even though her mother had been sober for a while, Jean still harbored resentments. Yet she couldn't refuse her mom's request to come live with her after Jean's father died.

It was a tense situation from the start, and only got worse as Jean's kids complained about the space they'd lost to accommodate Grandma. Jean's husband groused about giving up their yearly vacation because Jean's mom couldn't be left alone. Feeling obligated to her mother and sorry for everybody else, Jean struggled to get life back to normal again. But then Jean learned she had breast cancer, which in her mind was one more thing her mother could be blamed for.

"It's the stress," she said by way of explanation as soon as the diagnosis sank in. "Running here, going there, making sure everything's right for her—not that she ever went to such lengths for me. I know I volunteered to take her in, but I didn't know then how hard it would be for everyone to adjust." Jean's roles as a caretaker, peacekeeper, mother, wife, and that year's chairperson for her church's winter ball had pushed her to her limits. Sleepless much of the night, she would be irritable most of the day. She yelled at her kids and everyone else and was generally unhappy.

All things considered, it was a miracle she made it in for her mammogram, and a good thing, too, since her cancer was still in the very early stages and her breast could be spared. But did stress cause that cancer? I told her that from a purely scientific point of view, I didn't think so, that there were many studies that showed stress does not cause cancer. Looking at all the demands in her life, the more important question seemed to be what role stress would play in her recovery. There was evidence that women with breast cancer live longer when they have less stress. If she wanted to improve her odds of survival for five years or more, she would need to start changing things now. Jean agreed and went into counseling with her mother to work on their relationship. She got involved with Al-Anon and started taking time for herself, which she used to go to movies and take up sailing. As a result, five years after her surgery, Jean is not only cancer-free but calm, content, and hopeful as well.

Stress comes in many flavors. The exhilaration of starting a challenging new project is stress. So is the trepidation that comes along for the ride when you bring your first bundle of joy home to the nursery. Being roused from a deep sleep by your alarm clock creates stress, even when you're getting up to do something you love. From the smallest to the largest, the long-dreaded to the totally unexpected, when circumstances require us to change or adjust in any way, we experience stress.

Back in prehistoric times, most stress was triggered by physical stressors—a raging forest fire, neighboring tribespeople coming to invade us, or a saber-toothed tiger blocking our escape route. Our primitive brains, with our survival in mind, released a chemical known as cortisol, which put every inch of our bodies on red alert. Our hearts beat faster, our breathing became shallow and rapid, and our extremities got icy cold as blood rushed to our torso to protect our vital organs. Eyes wide, jaws clenched, muscles tensed, we were ready for a fight or to flee for our lives. Today, even though most of the stressors in our lives are psychological, our physiological response is almost identical. Our bodies react to the threat of missing a deadline or overdrawing our checking account or having a parent start drinking again in the same way they used to when a saber-toothed tiger came around the bend. This isn't always harmful.

Indeed, *some* stress is inevitable. A reasonable amount—enough to snap us to attention and make us aware of something in our lives that needs changing—may motivate us to take action. If we respond appropriately and succeed at solving a problem, accomplishing a task, or meeting a demand, a stressful situation may even increase our confidence and effectiveness. But too much stress for too long with too little we can actually do to change or resolve matters spells trouble. It means that we are spending too many hours of every day with stress hormones racing through our veins, raising our blood pressure, blood sugar, and serum cholesterol levels. The eventual result is a host of physical, psychological, and relationship problems that can add up to an increased risk of premature death. Science has linked acute or chronic stress to heart attacks and stroke; depression, anxiety, and suicide; gastrointestinal problems, including ulcers and colitis. We may smoke, drink, or eat more than usual, and we're more likely to have household or motor vehicle accidents. Even our immune system stumbles.

I probably don't need to tell you how stress messes with our minds, stirring up feelings of anxiety, hostility, frustration, and hopelessness. We tend to get trapped in details. We worry excessively and criticize ourselves endlessly. Our memory for daily details takes a holiday. Yet we can't seem to get distressing thoughts out of our minds.

Excessive stress spares no sphere of wellness. Our work lives suffer as absenteeism, chronic lateness, lost productivity, and more on-the-job injuries take their toll. Our relationships suffer. We can be abrupt, short-tempered, impatient, and argumentative. Kids and colleagues start to avoid us. People may tire of listening to us. And the strain on our relationships adds to our stress, especially if those relationships were tense and on shaky ground to begin with.

Finally, spiritual pursuits seem pointless to us when we're stressed out. But that's exactly when we need them. Walks in the woods, meditation, church attendance, and artistic endeavors all feel frivolous and needlessly time-consuming, when in fact they are feeding our souls.

This widespread impact is probably one of the reasons stress is such a killer. It barrels through our lives like a runaway train—but it doesn't have to. There are numerous actions you can take to lower your stress level and cope more successfully with stress you can't alter or avoid.

- *Know your stressors.* Which daily demands really get to you? What external circumstances can bring on your physical, emotional, or mental stress symptoms? How many do you create or magnify by trying to do the impossible or to do things perfectly at all times? And which are truly threatening to your health, happiness, and peace of mind?

- *Put them in perspective.* All demands are not created equal. A last-minute report or an overflowing toilet is not equivalent to hearing that your child has been in an accident or that floodwaters from a hurricane are on their way up the street. If you reacted to the former with the same intensity warranted by the latter, you'd reach stress overload by lunchtime every day of the week.

- *Try rating demands on a scale of 1 to 10 before responding to them.* If you're facing anything less than a 5, roll with it. Leave your teen's socks instead of fighting with him about it. Pull over and let the tailgating semi pass you.

- *Concentrate your efforts on the things you can change.* Identify stressors that could be eliminated or rolled with if you made a few attitude adjustments.

- *Exercise.* Taking time out to tune your body often alleviates stress. Physical activity has been shown to speed the exit of cortisol from your body. What's more, the healthier your mind and body are, the greater your resilience when plagued by excess stress.

- *Do some deep breathing or practice meditation, deep muscle relaxation, and/or creative visualization.* These are all excellent methods to reverse the effects of raging cortisol and to find some serenity.
- *Beef up your social and spiritual spheres.* Spend more time with supportive friends and family members. Try prayer or singing in the gospel choir, yoga, volunteering, or other spiritual pursuits.
- *Time management is crucial.* Most highly stressed men and women are also pressed for time. So make room for stress-relieving activities and other longevity boosters. Learn to delegate.
- *Get your head out of the sand.* We create our own stress when we identify a problem but do nothing about it, the way Jean did with her hard feelings toward her mother. If much of your stress comes from a major life issue such as job satisfaction or marital problems, look for viable ways to change things. This may mean getting some counseling or consulting a job recruiter or moving to another part of the country. It's up to you to find out.
- *Keep reading.* Many of the longevity boosters that follow this one are tailor-made for stress reduction.

48. Stop Worrying Yourself to Death   Impact ★★★★

At 2 A.M. on Friday, Lori Anderson lay awake worrying about all the things she needed to do before her brother and his wife arrived for Sunday dinner. She was determined to impress them but knew that wouldn't be easy to do. After all, her brother owned several L.A. eateries and his wife was an interior decorator to the stars. She wished they had not suggested "real family time" in her modest home.

She wanted the house to be spotless and the meal perfect. Had she ordered the right cut of meat? She would call the butcher again. Would her sister remember to bring back the roasting pan she'd borrowed? Would Jake like the wine? Would her children behave? What if it rained? There was no way everyone could mingle inside while she was cooking. She'd have a nervous breakdown—that is, if she didn't have a heart attack first, Lori thought as she felt a twinge in her chest. Every muscle in her body felt tense enough to snap.

Now, that's anxiety—a compendium of stresslike symptoms, only more narrowly focused and more likely to be generated by threats that exist primarily in our own minds. Indeed, you might think of anxiety as stress of your own making or as a negative form of anticipation, one that doesn't involve looking forward optimistically but rather bracing ourselves for the future warily. Even when there really is a potential calamity waiting in the wings—a ruined dinner, a flubbed speech, or the possibility that a lump will be discovered in your breast at your next checkup—it is our thoughts and beliefs that trigger our anxious feelings. We tell ourselves that we can't cope, that we aren't good enough, that people will laugh at us or find out the truth about us and reject us, but most of all that something horrible is going to happen. Just like threats to our physical survival or the demands on our time and energy that create stress, these threats to our self-esteem and self-confidence also trigger a fight-or-flight reaction, and often a very intense one.

During a bout of anxiety, our body goes through many of the same changes I described in the sections on stress and anger. It is not uncommon to also experience tension headaches, racing heart rate, dizzy spells, trembling and sweating, nausea and diarrhea, and hyperventilation. When symptoms like these strike occasionally (such as before a big test, first date, or important audition), or situationally (whenever we have to fly or visit a doctor or socialize with people we barely know), anxiety is unpleasant, uncomfortable, and maybe even a bit frightening. But for many of us anxiety is so severe and so unremitting that it becomes almost completely debilitating and may develop into distinct anxiety disorders.

Both occasional or situational anxiety and anxiety disorders take their toll on our bodies, increasing our risk of heart attack, stroke, cardiac arrhythmia, hypertension, suicide, and accidents. They frequently go hand in hand with self-sedating behaviors such as prescription drug abuse, heavy drinking, and compulsive eating. But anxiety's greatest impact, beyond the immediate discomfort it causes, is on the quality of our lives.

We limit life's sweetness by limiting our activities, movements, relationships, careers, and more. Anything that makes us anxious is cut from our life. We don't make presentations—and miss out on promotions. We stay out of social situations—and become lonelier and lonelier. We put off doctor's visits—and wind up with an illness that could have been cured if it had been detected earlier. People with obsessive-compulsive disorder can become paralyzed by their self-imposed rules and rituals. And panic disorder sufferers as well as people with agoraphobia, who are terrified to go anywhere or do anything that might trigger a panic attack, can turn themselves into virtual prisoners in their own homes.

With all of this in mind, I recommend the following action steps:

- *Consider getting professional help.* This is really a must-do if you have an actual anxiety disorder that is limiting where you travel or what activities you participate in. There are a number of very effective cognitive and behavioral therapies available. They can also help those of you who simply worry way too much or suffer from diffuse panic attacks.

- *Take an antidepressant.* Low doses of Paxil, Zoloft, Wellbutrin, or any of the others do a good job of controlling symptoms on a daily basis. Your doctor or therapist may suggest an antianxiety drug, such as Xanax or Ativan, to take when you actually feel anxious or panicky. Antianxiety medications can be habit-forming, however, and shouldn't be relied upon long-term.

- *Pinpoint anxiety-provoking thoughts and beliefs.* An old rational-emotive therapy tool works well for this. Start at point C—your anxious feelings. Look back until you find the event that triggered them. That's point A. Then try to uncover the thoughts that came to mind right after you encountered point A. Did you anticipate failure or remind yourself that you had messed up situations like this before? Did you make negative predictions or jump to extreme conclusions? If you run through this exercise often enough, perhaps keeping a daily anxiety diary, you'll start seeing irrational beliefs and anxiety-provoking thought patterns that need to be changed.

- *Talk about your feelings and the events that led up to them.* Share these with your friends, spouse, family members, or other supportive people. They may shed new light on how you may be contributing to your own anxiety.

- *Learn to relax.* There are any number of audiotapes that can walk you through relaxation exercises, and one in particular—deep muscle relaxation—that has been included in many books on stress management. It's filled with breathing exercises, stretches, and visualizations that can soothe your mood.

- *Create a calm scene.* This is a detailed image of a real or imaginary location that you associate with relaxation and serenity. Write it out ahead of time and conjure it up after you have relaxed your body. Also try shutting your eyes and recalling it for a minute or two when you feel yourself getting anxious.
- *Change what you can.* Sometimes you have good reason to be anxious—living in a dangerous neighborhood or with an abusive or explosive spouse, working for a supervisor who sexually harasses you or around occupational hazards that should be corrected. The cure for your anxiety may not be easy to execute, but it is straightforward: Change the situation as soon as possible.
- *Try helping someone else.* Kindness is always in order, and it will help you as well as someone else. Put your personal concerns on the back burner for an hour or a day, and do something for someone else that nourishes your heart.
- *Broaden your perspective.* We can get caught up in details and fail to see the big picture. Happiness comes from a calm mind, not from clinging to rigid expectations.
- *Bring laughter into your life.* Surprise yourself by doing something outrageous or spontaneous. Let down your guard and be silly (even for a short time). Allow others in on the fun.

49. Address Alzheimer's, Senility, and Dementia   Impact ★★★

Senility, or dementia, is a permanent, progressive decline in intellectual function—the ability to process facts, memorize information, and act on it. Over time it interferes substantially with a person's normal social and economic activity. Alzheimer's disease is the example we hear about most these days.

My mom died of it back in the 1970s before *Time* magazine announced that it existed. From the onset of this devastating disease until her death eight years later, the quality of my mother's life declined steadily. It was painful to watch. There was little anyone could do. Now the situation has changed some, although not much. The average life expectancy for an Alzheimer's patient is still about eight years from when the condition is identified. (It can't be conclusively diagnosed except through a brain autopsy following death.) And most Alzheimer's sufferers still tend to die from aspiration pneumonia (from food going down the wrong way, irritating the lungs, and causing infections), accidents, and a host of other problems.

We still don't know the reason people get Alzheimer's. Loss of cells in the cerebral cortex, a marked disorganization of the brain connections, and an increase in the protein amyloid have all been suspected at one time or another.

But we finally do know a few things that might help prevent it or slow its progress. Several longitudinal studies, including the Baltimore Longitudinal Study on Aging (BLSA), note that long-term use of NSAIDs, anti-inflammatory drugs such as naproxen or ibuprofen, appears to reduce the incidence of Alzheimer's. Men and women who took five to seven NSAIDs a week displayed a significantly lower risk for Alzheimer's. It's too soon to tell if this is a cause-and-effect relationship or merely a coincidence. The people taking these anti-inflammatory drugs just might have had more brain function to begin with, or a better genetic makeup. No one knows.

We can also draw some encouragement from the results of the nun study, a famous longitudinal study of 678 Catholic nuns between the ages of 75 and 102. The study, which is profiled in more detail on page 282, indicated that education (especially higher education) and mental exercise through crossword puzzles and word games may keep Alzheimer's symptoms at bay. It appeared that the nuns who continued to learn throughout their lives were shielded against the ravages of Alzheimer's.

Alzheimer's is only one form of dementia. Some of the other forms are treatable, or preventable, or both.

- *Multi-infarct dementia* is caused by small strokes to the brain. Hypertension is the chief contributor, but other risk factors include excessive alcohol consumption and arteriosclerosis.
- *Alcoholic dementia*, as you might expect, is the result of drinking too much for too long.
- *Injury dementia* is brought on by head injuries sustained in accidents, in sports such as boxing, or from other severe trauma.
- *B_{12} deficiency dementia,* actually a disease caused by the body's inability to absorb B_{12} from the intestine.
- *Thyroid deficiency dementia* is reversible with proper medication if caught early enough.

Given this, I suggest the following dementia busters:

- *Take an aspirin a day to lower your likelihood of having a stroke.*
- *If you have a family history of Alzheimer's and you can tolerate anti-inflammatories, then take one.* Naproxen and ibuprofen are inexpensive and available over the counter. One a day of either is probably enough. Several long-term studies looking at these and the newer anti-inflammatories called COX-2 inhibitors may have the answer soon. You may take one aspirin in addition to the anti-inflammatory, provided that the aspirin is coated or low-dose.
- *Take a multivitamin with minerals and vitamin B$_{12}$.* This is important for anyone with a dementia amplifier. A simple blood test at your doctor's office can determine if you're deficient.
- *If you have high blood pressure, treat it.*
- *If your cholesterol is sky high, treat it.*
- *If you drink too much alcohol, cut back.*
- *Protect yourself from injuries.* Kickboxing with contact does put you at risk, for instance. So do headers in soccer. Wearing a helmet when in-line skating, skiing, or riding a bike or motorcycle is wise. And please, make sure you know how deep a body of water is before you dive into it! If you've had a concussion, all of these tips are doubly important for preventing future concussions.
- *If you start to notice memory changes, have your thyroid checked.*
- *And absolutely most important: keep learning.* The nun study showed that lifelong learning may be the best protection we have against Alzheimer's.

INTELLECTUAL ACTIVITIES

50. Commit to Lifelong Learning   Impact ★★★★★

When it comes to factors that predict longevity, education goes to the head of the class. Simply put, the better educated we are, the longer we live. For instance, researchers at Johns Hopkins University found that middle-aged men who had dropped out of high school were more than twice as likely to die before their sixty-fifth birthday as men who had attended college. Numerous other longitudinal studies have uncovered similar connections. And the benefits of education are even more pronounced when learning continues throughout our lives.

Education and lifelong learning keep us healthy in body and mind. Some think they allow us to build up a reserve of brainpower that we can draw upon when Alzheimer's disease or other forms of dementia strike. Their impact on thinking and memory as we get older was most dramatically demonstrated by a study of 678 nuns whose ages ranged from 75 to 102. The nuns provided writing samples (drawn from autobiographies they wrote when they first entered the convent), completed questionnaires and mental status examinations, and underwent brain autopsies upon their death. These autopsies helped researchers identify nuns who had Alzheimer's disease or other forms of dementia.

The results held a surprise or two. The nuns who learned throughout their lives, as evidenced by their jobs, their habits (such as reading, writing, doing crossword puzzles), or how many college courses they took, did not show signs of Alzheimer's disease even though some on autopsy actually had Alzheimer's. And the same was true for other forms of senility such as the dementia caused by stroke. Researchers were amazed. One explanation may be that the nuns who exercised their brains had more reserve when their brains were ravaged.

While evidence abounds that people with more education stay healthier and live longer, we have not yet pinpointed the reasons why. We do know that people with more education tend not to smoke cigarettes. They're less likely to drive recklessly and more likely to wear bike helmets or follow lower-fat diets. And these are the kinds of health habits that lead to a longer, sweeter life.

Likewise, better-educated men and women generally make more money in jobs that provide them more satisfaction, not to mention health care coverage. They have easy access to medical care, less stress because their higher-level positions give them a greater sense of control, the wherewithal to take vacations, and fewer opportunities to be injured or exposed to toxins on the job. Add it all up and it is easy to see how these consequences of higher education boost longevity.

People who learn all the time are more likely to learn about what they can do to prevent disease. No surprise there. What's interesting is that they're also more likely to put what they learn into action. Perhaps a better understanding of the importance of change accompanies the facts they pick up, or maybe, because they are continuously expanding their horizons, change comes naturally to them.

Finally, lifelong learning may simply leave us better equipped for getting through life's ups and downs. When Darwin came up with the concept of "survival of the fittest," he was not just referring to the physically strongest or fastest or least sickly. The most likely to survive were also the best able to adapt, switch gears, plan for contingencies, and at times blend in. Learning is a big part of this kind of adaptation. It gives you more options, more escape routes, more coping skills—and more longevity.

So go for it. Let lifelong learning keep you young. We all have different learning styles. Learn yours! If you're concerned about a subject, get the facts. If you're curious about a topic, look into it. If you're worried about something, investigate it. For the longevity boosting power of it:

- *Read to stay informed about the medical problems you have or are predisposed to.* There's tremendous power in knowing everything you reasonably can about a disease or condition that is likely to directly affect you.
- *Read how-to and self-help books.* Whether you want to build a birdhouse or conquer an eating disorder, manage your money or manage your time, there's a book to tell you how to do it.
- *Read for pleasure.* It's a real treat right before bed and a great temporary escape from your worries. Make it a mainstay of your stress-reduction efforts.
- *Read for your job.* Increasing knowledge and skills can make a significant difference in your pay, status, and job satisfaction. Increasing your knowledge and skill in a new area can be the first step to a much-needed career change.
- *Listen to public radio shows.* Public radio is undoubtedly the best broadcast medium around.
- *Watch less television.*
- *Learn a foreign language.*
- *Take a course in medieval art or bicycle repair, bird watching or Web page design, or anything else that interests you.* When you sign up for a course, you get the added benefit of socializing with people who like the same things you do.
- *Visit a museum or other education site.* Tour museums, aquariums, historic battlefields, or any environment where you can learn something new.

- *Travel.* Learn as much as possible about the history and culture of your destination both before and during your visit.

51. Cultivate a Resilient, Optimistic, Can-do Attitude   Impact ★★★★★

Does our attitude truly have an impact on the length and sweetness of our lives? You bet it does. A negative, self-blaming, fatalistic attitude can end our lives prematurely. It did for those men and women in the Terman Life Cycle Study who displayed catastrophic thinking that convinces you that bad things happen to you all of the time, that this will go on forever, and that each time these bad things happen they'll reverberate through your life, ruining everything. More men than women in this study felt that way, and the men who did died in greater numbers at all ages than their noncatastrophizing counterparts.

How about the flip side of the coin? A recent study published in the *Journal of the Royal Society of Health* looked at middle-aged men and women to see what affected their longevity. They found, as you might expect, that genetics, economics, diet, smoking, alcohol, and physical activity played a role. But they also found that attitude mattered. That those who cultivated a positive outlook and looked at challenges optimistically were often longer-lived than those who did not.

The idea that a positive outlook would be preferable to a negative worldview isn't tough to swallow. But what about the notion that people who believe they will live longer or recover from an illness are actually more likely to? In another study involving two hundred patients with physical complaints but no identifiable disease, half were told that what they had wasn't serious and that they soon would be well again. The other half simply were told that the cause of their illness was unclear. Two weeks later 64 percent of the first group had recovered, compared to 39 percent of the other group.

Our thoughts are powerful—perhaps not powerful enough to replace surgery for appendicitis, but certainly influential enough to lift some depression, stabilize blood pressure levels, and even bring cholesterol levels down. Conversely, they can also trigger anxiety, exacerbate depression, precipitate anger, and increase the stress of an already stressful situation. Their positive power lies primarily in their ability to get us to do what's best for us. If nothing else, we pick healthier behaviors for ourselves when we look at the future with optimism and prepare rather than view it through a veil of pessimism and brace ourselves to fail.

Here's an action plan for revitalizing your attitude:

- *Learn coping skills.* There's more than one way to solve a problem.
- *Stop when you hear yourself dwelling on how awful things are.* Visualize a big stop sign. It really works.
- *Use visualization in other ways.* Picture your troubles and negative thoughts being crammed into a trash can, mentally attaching the trash can to a hot-air balloon, and watching it float away.
- *Plant positive thoughts.* Like seeds in your garden, they will grow into new attitudes. Find or compose some positive, life-affirming, confidence-boosting statements and repeat them to yourself every day. Books by Louise Hay are a good source, especially for affirmations geared toward healing illness and pain.
- *Identify people you know who are happy and funny and make a point to see them.* Make them dinner, invite them to a show, and just be with them. Humor and a positive mental attitude are infectious.
- *Check out the humor sphere.* Laughter is an antidote for negativity.
- *Look at the spiritual sphere—it's important when it comes to a positive attitude.* Volunteering, spending time with nature, and seeking a spiritual path can all help your attitude.
- *Read different viewpoints.* Sometimes you may have a bad attitude because you've never researched the other side.
- *If you have chronic pain, consider a different way to treat it.* Chronic pain often causes unhappiness.

52. Hang on to Your Sense of Humor Impact ★★★★

Go ahead. Giggle. Guffaw. Chuckle. Snort. Or let out a great big belly laugh. It may not cure any deadly diseases, but laughter does disarm several killers, including worry, stress, and attacks on our immune systems. In 1964. Norman Cousins, author of *Anatomy of an Illness,* used it to help him over the effects of an autoimmune disease (where your body literally makes antibodies against itself). Following prescriptions that could have read "Take one Laurel and Hardy tape with breakfast" or "Watch the Marx Brothers before bed," he found that fifteen minutes of hearty laughter brought him two hours of pain-free sleep. His daily blood samples even showed a difference.

In the years since Dr. Cousins's one-man experiment succeeded (he walked out of the hospital healthy several weeks later), researchers from Loma Linda University in California have shown that laughter increases immune system activity and decreases the production of stress hormones. Other studies have chronicled our physical response to humor, which includes an improvement in respiration, circulation, digestion, and blood pressure. Exuberant laughter works like aerobic exercise, conditioning our hearts and bringing oxygen to our lungs. The word from one Stanford University psychiatrist is that a hundred ha-has can be as beneficial as ten minutes on a rowing machine or fifteen on a stationary bike. And at the University of Akron, a study of elderly siblings found that the brother or sister with the better sense of humor lived longer than the more serious or subdued sib.

Getting more humor into your life may just be one of the easiest— and certainly most amusing—of all longevity boosters.

- *Pinpoint the things that make you laugh out loud and bring more of them into your life.* Some of us are punsters, others slapstick lovers. We may adore stand-up comics or Second City skits or watching Saturday cartoons with our kids. If it tickles you, take in more of it.
- *Think like a comedian.* Find the humor in everyday life or stressful situations by trying to imagine how your favorite comic might react to it. What would Jay Leno do in a traffic jam? How would Jerry Seinfeld cope with his in-laws?
- *Watch comedy films or go to comedy clubs.*
- *Maintain a laughter library of books, videos, and audiotapes.*
- *Have daily jokes e-mailed to you.*
- *Spend time with people who share your sense of humor.*
- *Go get three scarves and try to juggle them.* Or watch someone else try it.

---

53. Fight Forgetfulness   **Impact ★★**

Memory lapses happen to all of us throughout our lifetimes. We only need to think back to our teens or to observe today's adolescents to see memory gaps galore. Between raging hormones and "more important stuff" on their minds, teens are too distracted to remember everything.

Distraction plays a role in our mental fumbles regardless of our age. We may simply have too many concerns occupying our minds. Or we are so thoroughly focused on one subject that we inadvertently shut out stimuli from all other fronts. It happens. There's no need to panic or worry that we're developing Alzheimer's disease just because we have to write down locker combinations or computer passwords.

Depression, sleep deprivation, or the side effects of a medication we're taking can trigger memory difficulties. Overscheduling and multitasking may leave us grasping for day planners or handheld computers with scheduling software. There is no pathology behind this.

Having a harder time retrieving certain information from our memories as we get older does not mean that senility is setting in. It's normal for the memory of names and phone numbers to decline a bit. Although our long-term memories are not affected, as we get older it usually becomes a little harder to learn a foreign language or calculate complicated sums quickly.

Fortunately, it's fairly easy for most of us to learn to cope with, compensate for, and maintain a sense of humor about these gaps. Almost anything works, because often the major reason for memory failure is our failure to pay attention.

When it comes to remembering things, ego—or vanity—will be your downfall. There is no shame in Post-it notes or grocery lists or voice-mail messages to yourself. My other recommendations:

- *Get organized.* Have designated places for your keys, wallet, or sunglasses, and use them. Mark dates on a calendar as soon as you learn about them. Make to-do lists.
- *Remain intellectually challenged.* If you use your memory for lifelong learning, you're less likely to lose it (see page 281).
- *Get regular physical exercise.* It helps to keep the arteries that feed the brain clear. Studies show that aerobic exercise increases mental ability by 20 to 30 percent.
- *Practice.* Memory-training books and courses do a pretty good job in whatever they specialize in. But they specialize in different things. Before signing on for anything, make sure that the course's objectives match your own.

- *Try the tricks.* Use rhyming words to remember names, or acronyms to remember instructions. If a technique works for you, keep at it.
- *Take care of yourself.* Get enough sleep, eat well, and keep stress and anxiety to a minimum.
- *Keep Alzheimer's, senility, and dementia away* (see page 279).
- *If it's really significant, seek help from a memory disorder clinic.*
- *If you're on any medications check the side effects* and see if memory or concentration are affected. Antihistamines, antidepressants, the smoke-ending pill Zyban, and many hypertensive medications can cause forgetfulness.
- *Are you depressed or stressed-out? Any form of mood disturbance can cause forgetfulness.*
- *Learn a new subject that requires you use your memory.* Studies have shown that the brain is like a muscle—the more you use it, the stronger it becomes.

Kinship Sphere

54. Extract Yourself from Abusive Relationships   Impact ★★★★★

Victims of battery vary—there's no stereotype, save high percentages of women. Abuse crisscrosses society, ignoring economic lines, employment status, education, class, religion, ethnicity, race, age, and national origin. It sabotages heterosexual as well as gay and lesbian couples. It hurts our elders and may permanently damage our children. Sadly, the majority of future perpetrators witnessed abuse as children—and 3.3 million children are exposed to physical or emotional torment each year.

Because it carries a stigma, domestic violence is rarely talked about. Yet its occurrence is easy to determine. We know that between 2,500 and 11,000 cases of abuse occur nationally every single day. That means some of you have been, or are about to be, a victim of violence.

Take Mary, a patient of mine for more than twenty years, with three good-natured, healthy children who played all the sports in which small towns take pride. She and her husband, Bob, appeared to be soul mates. One day Mary came into the office because she had slipped on the sidewalk. In fact, when I thought about it, could Mary really be such a clumsy person—tripping in her garden, falling down the stairs when carrying laundry, and on and on? Turns out Mary came to see me for only some of her falls; for others she went to the ER in the next town. (In this Mary is typical. Most battered women are likely to see a physician frequently, although the rate of detection by emergency-room doctors remains low.) She was embarrassed and didn't want anyone asking her questions. Perhaps that is why it took so many years to admit the truth. This time was different. This time Mary was scared. This time Bob had hit her with a bat.

Mary is fine now. She sought help through counseling, ultimately divorced Bob, and, after a five-year time-out for healing and growth, has remarried. For Mary the violence is gone. But the violence could have been—and should have been—eradicated sooner.

Studies show that abused women consider themselves worth far less than they ought. This fact is not surprising, since intimate partners torment their victims in many ways: broken arms and spirits, coercion, intimidation, isolation, calls at work, death threats, suicide threats, stalking, sexual, emotional, and economic abuse.

Verbal deprecation, however, challenges evaluation. It can be subtle or severe; it can be rare or ongoing. The person being abused may or may not know what is happening. Nevertheless, the syndrome is the same: The ridiculed person feels worthless. Those being battered or verbally assaulted believe—wrongly—that they deserve what they get.

Studies show that acrimonious and abusive relationships can definitively affect the well-being of children, too. In such situations, researchers have found that adolescents who live in violent homes have a higher incidence of anxiety, depression, and violence. Boys who witness violence tend to fight more, hurt pets, and destroy personal property. When they grow up, they not only tend to continue being depressed, they are more likely to abuse their spouses. They frequently do not have a high quality of life. It's the same for girls, except instead of being violent they tend to withdraw.

What to Do If You Suspect Someone You Know Is Being Abused

- *Speak to them.* Offer your support.
- *Ask.* "Did someone hit you?"
- *Call the police* if you hear violent arguments in your neighborhood.

- *And most important, risk involvement.* It is so terribly difficult for some of us to step in and help. But that's the only way to combat abuse.

What to Do If You're Being Abused

- *Seek help.* This is clearly your most pressing need. Help may come from a doctor, friend, parent, sibling, or clergy member. A hotline counselor or a hospital ER nurse may help you get started.
- *Plan an escape route to safety.* Start by knowing different exits from your home. Decide how to get out if you leave at night.
- *Know what public places are always open.* Know the routes to the police station, hospital, fire station, or twenty-four-hour convenience store.
- *If you leave by car, lock the car doors immediately.* If you have no car, know the bus routes, train stations, or subways. Call a cab. Or find a safe place close to home where a friend can pick you (and your children) up.
- *Take your essentials.* Make sure you have money, checkbook, credit card, and other essential ID.
- *Consider an order of protection.*
- *Don't be discouraged.* Many women try many times before they finally leave. You deserve more.
- Contact the National Domestic Violence Hotline: 800-799-SAFE, (TTY 800-787-3224). Every city and county has abuse specialists who can help.

55. Have a Satisfying, Long-term, Committed Marriage or Its Equivalent	Impact ★★★★★

Think of it this way: Marriage is a clear-cut way to craft a positive social environment, right in the comfort of your home. The "marriage effect" boasts consistent results from study to study—married men and women live longer than those who have divorced. Incidentally, those who never married are situated right in between.

An imposing collection of evidence shows that marriage benefits both men and women. The classic default belief is that with marriage men enjoy better health habits and women gain economically. Ultimately, however, the greatest advantages occur in the social realm. We're social creatures. We have fun going out together for walks or to plays, baseball games, or the opera. We want a long, sweet life; we want fun. And our spouses often encourage us to diversify our interests. Marriage ultimately increases our outlook and our hopefulness. In addition, stress is reduced, because having a partner to talk to makes challenges easier to take. You know that if you have a medical problem, it's harder to make decisions alone. Indeed, social connections are important all your life, and marriage is an incomparable form of social connectedness.

The Terman Life Cycle Study, begun in 1921 in Stanford, California, took a sample of fifteen hundred children, born around 1910, who had been labeled bright, and followed them for decades. First the researchers observed their progress through school, then evaluated how they made out in life. In 1950 these students—now middle-aged—were asked a series of personal questions about social relationships, economic life, and marriage. In 1991, when this now elderly sample was revisited, the striking finding was happily married people lived longer than those who suffered a marital breakup.

Undeniably, something happens in marriage that seems to be protective. Why is this? When people marry, they agree, tacitly or explicitly, to share many things: finances, homes, friends, extended family, and habits. Married couples often eat more nutritiously. They tend to engage in more constructive hobbies and live a healthier lifestyle. If one spouse doesn't drink to excess, the other is less likely to get sloshed. Their mental health improves. And with children at home, parental health habits are often better than when no children are present. Smoking, again, provides a great example. I have lots of patients who smoke, then quit smoking as soon as they have kids. Even those who don't quit usually go outside so that their progeny won't be affected by their smoking.

Married couples are more likely to follow a doctor's advice or even see a doctor if sick. How many of us have had a loved one tell us to go to a doctor when we thought our malady would go away. Now, even though most maladies do go away, for some that is not the case. In my family, for example, we share a predisposition to malignant melanoma, the type of black mole you don't ever want to see. When my dad was fifty he had a bump that my mom did not like. He refused to see our doctor, saying the mole was nothing. She refused to cook him supper—or at least that was the story that I was told. Within short order, Dad's mole and melanoma were removed, and he was cured. Two of his older sisters were not so lucky, because they simply waited too long. Within a marriage, health becomes a shared relationship.

Women are more likely to engage in healthier habits, eat well, exercise, and take fewer risks. Women are also more likely to seek help for symptoms and diseases. When a man is married, he is more likely to be affected by his wife's behavior. And, in fact, he may be a healthier person because of it. Nevertheless, because of companionship, the marriage effect is vitally important for both men and women.

If your marriage is not ideal, and you want it to be, look at some of the following problems:

- Use of alcohol and/or illicit drugs
- Sex outside of marriage
- Financial problems
- The question of having children or not having children
- Lack of honest communication
- Unwillingness to be flexible

What do you do to turn it around? Seek help. Listen more. Talk to a marital counselor, friends, relatives, clergy; then implement their suggestions.

Divorce

Divorce affects health and happiness. When divorce happens, several things occur. Poverty increases, especially for women—in one study five years after divorce a woman's income was only 70 percent of her marital income, while a man's was 114 percent of his marital income. Social support suffers.

Divorce affects children. Looking again to the Terman Life Cycle Study, we find that children in divorced families have a higher incidence of premature mortality themselves. They are more likely to have their own marriages end in divorce, and often obtain less education. On the other hand, research has shown that children reared in a conflict-filled home have similar outcomes. Clearly, children are affected by what they see in the home. I counsel people to take the most appropriate action to reduce a continuously negative environment.

Marriage can be protective if it's productive. Implications for marriage satisfaction, however, may lead those involved in struggling marriages to work on the friendship—or the exchange of ideas—as a first step toward improving the situation.

56. Build a Strong Social Network   Impact ★★★★

Our society intuitively understands that social supports benefit the vulnerable—our children and the elderly, the sick, and those with mental or physical disabilities. At the same time, we tend to admire people for being independent rather than interdependent. Consequently, when we conjure up the image of the independent, successful executive, thoughts of ulcers and stress readily come to mind. The good news is that philosophies are changing. More people collaborate at work. Social supports are intangible, but they create a pathway to success and good health.

Social networks prevent disease. Research supports the theory overwhelmingly, although no one understands exactly why. Does the neighbor who carpools to soccer help reduce your level of stress? Does your mother-in-law who shares her famous minestrone recipe increase your joy? Does your coworker's recommendation of a perfect preschool promote your well-being? Whatever the connection is, studies show that social supports protect health, enrich life, prevent disease, and promote longevity. The haunting truth is confirmed by health statistics of the French, Japanese, and Italians. All three cultures experience significantly less heart disease than Americans, although they smoke considerably. So what's the scoop? All three cultures are vastly different in lifestyle. Their foods vary significantly—they do eat fewer calories than we do, and much of their fat is healthier fats from olive oil or fish, but that doesn't explain it all. And although they walk more than we do, none of them can boast an exemplary exercise regimen. The answer may be that the three societies enjoy a level of social connectedness that protects them from the ravages of disease. Why social supports and not, say, red wine? Because when Italians, French, and Japanese emigrate to America, they lose their cultural armor and begin to log the same rates of disease as Americans do. Genetics do not account for their cultural shield, otherwise residency would not factor into the equation so resoundingly.

In a way, the phenomenon of social networks is difficult to grasp because it's harder to measure than cholesterol and hypertension. Keep in mind that a century ago, in the 1890s, we couldn't measure cholesterol. Still, cholesterol factored prominently in heart attacks. In the same fashion, we can't quantify social connectedness at present, but we see from literature and social trends that social relationships play an important role in health and disease.

Take an easy example, the common cold. One study, which actually infected healthy people with cold viruses, found that the more social ties you had, the less susceptible you were to developing a cold. In addition, those with the strongest networks produced less mucus. But fighting colds are a mere minor advantage of a healthy social engine. A study from Kaiser Permanente showed that patients with strong social networks were less likely to die from cardiovascular disease.

In the final analysis, ties binding you to a variety of community groups add to longevity. How this works within the body takes a little explaining. People under stress tend to be hyperalert, with more adrenaline and cortisol in their system and consequently a greater chance of sudden death from stroke. The opposite is also true: With little stress present, there's less adrenaline and cortisol. A study from Rockefeller University shows that social networks and the environment may affect neuroendocrine regulation by reducing production of hormones such as adrenaline; perhaps the social supports provide a buffer against stress. Consequently, over time social relationships may reduce death.

The Alameda County Study from the Human Population Lab looked at nearly seven thousand adults around San Francisco over a nine-year period. They found the most isolated individuals were more likely to die—at rates 2.3 times higher for men and 2.8 times higher for women. Social ties were independent of self-reported health status and other health habits such as smoking, alcohol, obesity, and physical activity.

In Baltimore, researchers found that extreme social isolation was a major predictor of increased mortality among African-American women. Extremely isolated women were three times more likely to die prematurely. Researchers from the University of Utah compiled eighty-one peer-reviewed studies examining the relationship between social supports and physiological processes. Findings indicate that social supports are beneficial in reducing cardiovascular disease, making the body's

immune system more effective, and positively affecting endocrine function. They postulate the following reasons this occurs:
- Social relationships buffer life's stressors and emotions.
- Familial support may be important in nurturing health.
- Emotional support helps relieve stress.
- A relationship with one close friend adds longevity to life.

If you lack social supports, make an action plan for yourself:
- Consider joining a group that explores an interest of yours.
- Share your knowledge and skill with people less fortunate.
- Share your energies. Consider helping on a community project, such as Habitat for Humanity.
- Take an adult education class.
- Go out of your way to befriend someone at work.
- Volunteer. Tutor at local schools. Mentor a student.
- Join a health club or music ensemble. Take a class on computers, parenting, language, or art.
- Reconsider religion. Investigate different spiritual pursuits.

57. Build Good Relationships with Your Family   Impact ★★★★

Family relationships usually enrich life. Calling up Mom, Dad, and your brothers or sisters can rekindle warmth and remind you of the happiness you had years ago. Those memories can give you joy and happiness. But for some of us families are a prominent source of stress. Sometimes the leftover frustration of childhood manifests itself in relationships today.

We're all someone's child. Your immediate family is like a school for many of the behaviors and values you take to the larger world. How fortunate are those of us who had good teachers. So if you have children, you know a good relationship with them is paramount. They are a mirror of your innermost spirit and a window to your immortality. If you do not have solid, healthy, and comfortable communication with your child, now is the time to mend that fence. Just work on making interactions a level or two friendlier every couple of months. Keep the old stuff out of the new stuff. Use an eraser and start making some quiet contracts where you divide up the responsibility for the relation-

---

IF CHILDHOOD ABUSE IS AN ISSUE

Consider counseling. The stress of childhood abuse is constant and enduring. Individual and, if appropriate, family therapy can help free you from the horrible memories that abuse evokes. Whether these nightmares were physical, emotional, or sexual, you may find support from others who shared similar experiences. But nobody's experience was exactly like yours. Be compassionate toward yourself first, and then try to connect with someone you can trust.

---

ship. And stay out of each other's way politely by showing each other an uncommon amount of respect.

As an adult, you can always investigate a relationship without the mental and physical restraints you had when you were a child. Do you want to visit a grandparent whom your parents say wronged them? Or see the uncle who swindled his brother, your father? Every person has stories, and they are all powerful. It's always a good decision to find the ones that shaped your family, just as you are doing with your children. Many people find that studying their personal genealogy opens up a world of family hitherto undiscovered.

In some religions there is a time each year set aside for forgiveness. These times open the opportunity to purge the resentments of an exceptionally foolish past and start anew. Each of us does thoughtless things. Forgiveness is a blessing that can relieve stress and open links with someone you love.

Stepparents and stepchildren in blended families present unique opportunities to practice patience, suspend judgments, and to develop a great sense of humor. Possibly the best way to relate to someone who at one time was not part of your family and now is, is to get to know them personally, as a separate individual.

Sibling to Sibling

Another source of cheer and stress is the sibling link. Many people agree that our strongest bonds in life, just as influental as marriage, are with our siblings. Many of us share wonderful memories with our siblings and continue today to thoroughly enjoy each other's company. Our siblings remain some of the dearest people in our lives.

Sometimes old patterns of childhood rivalry surface and interactions replay themselves. But hopefully you've grown up and have learned to resolve conflicts. Talking with your brother or sister is worthwhile, because you shared some of the same experiences as children, and mending relationships with them can be powerful. Often obstacles you perceive as standing in the way of relating are the same obstacles that exist for them. Make the first move. If you can simply move an acrimonious relationship from the negative to a neutral sphere you will have improved your situation.

Perhaps we should think of our children as a reason to repair the relationship with our siblings. We are role models for our children, and when children see their parents enjoy a healthy friendship with their siblings, it invites them to do the same.

A story from one of my patients illustrates how powerful and meaningful bonds of the immediate family can be. I have an older gentleman in my practice who is, well, highly opinionated. He was suffering from diabetes, lung disease, and heart disease when he came into my office complaining of a chest cold. Knowing how sick he was, I put him in the hospital. That turned out to be a good move, because six hours later he was intubated and placed in intensive care. Now, this man had a large blended family, three kids from one side and three from the other, and the two groups did not get along. None lived in town, but because he was now in the process of dying, about half the kids from both sides showed up. The mix included a nurse, a doctor, a malpractice lawyer, and two who had struck it rich. Everyone had an opinion. He was aware of the kids being there and knew they wanted to be with him. At the point the medical staff thought about shutting off the ventilator, he rallied and started breathing. Afterward he told us that he had been ready to let go of life—but, as he said, "I just couldn't leave the kids. They'd be so disappointed. Especially after traveling all that way to see me." So he stayed around. In fact, he's still around today. And a little mellower, I might add.

Redefining Your Relationship with a Relative

If a relationship with a particular relative just seems so frustrating, I have a suggestion for the long run: Change your perspective. Visualize this person as someone who lives down the block from you. They're full of opinions (usually the opposite of yours) and tons of advice. How would *you* most likely respond?

I recommend that you hear them out and thank them for the advice. Then say, "Maybe I will." *Maybe* is a big word with lots of wiggle room. That's it. Now it's time to plead an excuse and hang up the phone or tell them that you're going to do some volunteer work. And you know what? Go do it and forget about them. No negative reaction. No mental engagement. Just a neutral reaction.

What you may need to do is form an action plan.

- *Make peace.* Start by talking. A phone call or note may be the best way to begin.
- *Invite your would-be loved one to lunch.*
- *Talk about neutral topics.* Pretend your relative is someone you've just met and have no opinion about. Then you would have a very different mental image to react to.
- *Either bury the hatchet or agree to discuss the problem.* If you agree to bury the hatchet, don't discuss the incident. If you agree to discuss the problem, set up ground rules. Pick a stress-free time and a tranquil place. Remember that hearing takes more attention than listening, and you have to do both. If you believe the two of you can't discuss the issue rationally, invite someone along to mediate.
- *Plan to see your relative again, soon.*
- *Leave your ego at home.*

Remember, it may not be necessary to become best friends with your relative, but it is important for your well-being to have cordial or at least neutral ties. Together you can work on moving the relationship from anger and resentment to neutrality and perhaps someday to peace.

58. Build Good Relationships with Friends   Impact ★★★★

Friends reduce social isolation. The stronger your social supports, the longer, sweeter, and happier your life. Real friendships are precious and deserve loving attention. The world is open for us to choose friends from every sphere we encounter: at work, at worship, at school, in the neighborhood, walking our dog, or buying plant food.

We intuitively know the benefits of friendship with someone who has common values, who is warm, with whom we laugh and reinvent ourselves. We are by nature social creatures. Doing activities with other people strengthens our self-esteem, our sense of well-being, our playfulness, and our sense of fun.

If we don't have friends and have only a significant other, our lifestyle is not as healthy. After all, we need other relationships to bounce ideas off. And if you have marital conflicts, your friends are often the first ones you turn to. Friends become people who help you decide your path in life, who give you perspective, congratulations, advice you can't use, and advice you need. Friends help our social and psychological well-being. Friends are the bonus of life. We may call our good friends "unrelated relatives," because our families are in other geographical areas and for many kinds of support in our lives our friends have taken their place.

Some men often excuse their lack of friendship by claiming they are too busy. But this is quite the contrary for most of the men I know. We place great value on friends—both male and female—and fondly know that they add a rich dimension of shared interests to our lives. I cook with some women friends and am a proud member of the Bad Movie Club with my male peers. Different activities attract people who become your friends, and as the warmth in your relationship grows so do the number of pursuits you may share. Women's schedules are often overloaded, stretching their time between home, work, family commitments, and extended family. Leaving time for friends adds to the tenuous balancing act, but the benefits are enormous in enhancing the quality of our lives. Women value and help each other in countless situations, extending a sisterhood of spirit outward to others. Historically, women formed strong matriarchal societies where feminine wisdom and intuitions were passed from generation to generation. Today the descendants of those wise women continue these traditions in friendship.

As Ralph Waldo Emerson wrote, "The only way to have a friend, is to be one."

What to Do If You Want to Expand Your Circle of Friends
- *Start a book group.* Oprah did; you can, too.
- *Start a movie group.* Same idea.
- Other thoughts:

- Poker night, bowling night, gourmet cooking night
- A "wise woman" group to discuss mythology, past or present
- A church group that meets to read, give service, or debate
- Membership in a gym
- Share or trade kids so you can have times out with other friends, with and without your kids

What to Do to Expand a Friendship with One Friend
- Meet for Sunday brunch, or lunch, or coffee.
- Suggest going to a lecture, or just a walk.
- Suggest going for a bike ride, or cross-country skiing. Plan any activity together that makes you both happy. Be honest.
- Try something new. Visit somewhere you've always wanted to see.

---

59. Savor Sex and Intimacy   **Impact ★★★**

In a way, sex and intimacy are just two points on a spectrum of contact. Intimacy welcomes us as infants; it warms us and teaches us and nurtures us. Touch plays a central role in our physical and mental fitness. We yearn for this kind of nurturing all our lives.

Young children are exceptionally physical. In middle school and junior high the priorities reorder themselves. Conflicting emotions—especially for girls—over the pressure to have sex at a young age may lead to lifelong esteem issues. But as kids move on toward high school they change once again and exhibit lots of overt friendly contact. Teenagers hug all the time; they enjoy a natural intimacy that tends to disappear as we get older.

As we mature, intimacy and touch evolve to an act of passion. Sex nourishes both physical and emotional longing; thus, lovemaking is key to a good long-term relationship. There is intimacy in sex; they commingle, but they are not the same. Even with a healthy sexual relationship, we continue our need for simple intimacy and touch.

We know that strong social supports improve longevity, but whether sex itself will lengthen your life is still debated. Certainly sex is not vigorous exercise, as the average energy expenditure in sex is 20–30 calories per orgasm. At present, the scientific data are too sketchy to make a firm statement on longevity. Still, the need for sexual and physical intimacy persists throughout our lives, although as we age sexual encounters tend to decline in number. In our society more than 50 percent of married men and women in their seventies are sexually active. More vacations, earlier retirement, and the continuing dedication to action-oriented lifestyles can play a positive role in sex and intimacy.

Should You Have Sex When Your Relationship Is in Trouble?

Actually, the answer must be a function of the relationship. In some instances, engaging in lovemaking is refreshing and beneficial; other times it is not. For example, if the union is stressed because of money, sex may represent a positive encounter. If, however, the relationship is stressed because of power issues, such as dominance or abuse, the answer is totally different. In such cases, using sex to solve relationship problems is similar to getting pregnant to solve a failing marriage. Also, victims of sexual abuse and rape often have great difficulty coming back to the point of trust. Deal with the main issue first before you try to fix it with sex.

Sex Addiction

Can there be too much of a good thing where sex is concerned? Unfortunately, yes. Sex addiction does occur, and people obsessed with sex should seek counseling. However, a healthy interest in sex can easily accommodate occasional use of sex aids. Addiction concerns itself with larger issues such as control, little regard for your partner, and lack of safety concerns such as those involving condoms and drugs.

Intimacy and Touching

Human intimacy is an issue from babyhood on. Studies show that people of all ages want to be touched, and in some cultures people touch nonsexually all the time. European women walk everywhere hand in hand. In Mexico, for example, where I've visited very often, people hug you as they greet you. Traveling there, you notice that friends are as warm and outgoing as close relatives. In Asia I observed that men are very often physical in gentle gestures toward each other.

What to Do If You Have Lost Your Libido

Sexual problems may be best addressed by consulting with a physician, counselor, clergy, family member, or friend. But quite often a loss of desire may be more easily fixable than you think.

- *Check with your doctor to see if your medications are the issue.* Blood pressure and cardiac medications are notorious in this regard.
- *Are you a postmenopausal woman and not on estrogen?* Consider it.
- *Are you a man with erectile dysfunction?* Viagra and other newer medications may just change your life.
- *Are you worried about your performance?* Sometimes sexual counseling or reading one of the excellent books on the subject with your life-long companion can help.
- *Do you drink too much?* Alcohol clearly is an obstacle to sex, especially when you're older.
- *Are you depressed or angry about something?* Psychotherapy and antidepressants can play a significant role in the short run. Examining what is happening to you now is crucial.
- *Just too busy?* Make time for sensuality. Relationships prosper when there is an effort to be tender and not always sexual.

60. Own a Pet	Impact ★★

The effect that pets have on senior citizens is well documented. In the *Journal of Personality and Social Psychology* a study reported that senior citizens who were pet owners didn't frequent the doctor as often. Another study showed that seniors with pets were happier and healthier. Pets can even help those suffering from dementia. Researchers from the University of Nebraska showed that people with Alzheimer's who were visited by a dog were less agitated and more social.

For many of us a pet can provide a fellowship that buffers us from the outside world in a positive, fun way. And animals don't talk back.

Spiritual Sphere

61. Explore the Spiritual Within You	Impact ★★★★★

The search to find happiness and inspiration can be an eternal quest or a clear road map. Everyone is different, so the spiritual journey for each of us is unique.

Are you attending a Sunday service or fasting on the high holy days? Do you pray at a certain time of the day or meditate? Some find comfort in a mainstream religion; some prefer a nontraditional path. For many the search lies within themselves. It is difficult to put into words what is really not definable. For me, silence and art are spiritual. Hiking in the mountains with my family can be spiritual. Each of us pursues the spiritual when we rummage for meaning in our lives.

Each millennium has borne myths and mystics, traditions and wisdom. We've watched science and technology pass from taboo to become a form of theology. We are a global family with different cultures living side by side. Sometimes we don't have far to go. In my rural Wisconsin town, we can journey down the road to the east to a Tibetan Buddhist temple or to the west to a local Bible study group. The new millennium brings us an opportunity to redefine and broaden our concepts of religion. Personal investigations become a kind of spiritual yellow brick road, which allows us to explore ourselves, our own backyards, and the world at large.

A spiritual sphere awaits us, ready to add a dimension to our lives that material success and good health alone may not provide. Like breathing, thinking, interacting, and working, your actions as a spiritual human being can be automatic. Daily. There's no need to meditate in a cave for years or leave the world around you. In fact, finding some personal peace while engaging in the world around you is the essence of a spiritual path. Just try to be a better person. Follow the Golden Rule and any version of the Ten Commandments that suits your lifestyle. Think about the people you are living with and dealing with day in and day out with compassion. Be a generous person, materially if possible. But it's far more important to be generous in spirit. Take care of yourself in a loving manner so you know the boundaries of your physical and mental needs. And when you need spiritual replenishing, find it in your own way. Deal with people ethically. Respect the basic integrity that each of us has and be a little more flexible, a little less judgmental. If you treat others with love and respect, ultimately those good feelings will be reciprocated. When you are kind you feel better about yourself and develop a more positive outlook on life. Why? Because what goes around comes around.

Can you simply decide one day to incorporate more spirituality into your life? Of course you can. The Dalai Lama wrote in *The Path to*

Bliss, "What is very obvious to us is that a positive state of mind and positive action lead to more happiness and peace, whereas their negative counterparts result in undesirable consequences. Therefore, if as a result of our practice we are able to alleviate our sufferings and experience more happiness, that would in itself be a sufficient fruit to encourage us further in our spiritual pursuits."

What Can We Do to Cultivate a Spiritual Path?

Start out by believing in yourself and what you are capable of doing. See yourself as a good person who is trying to take care of yourself and not harm anyone. Then start thinking of compassion toward others— first the people you know, and then the people you don't. Try to be a little kinder. It almost seems too simple. But a simple formula toward spiritual practice starts with maximizing the good things you do for yourself and others and minimizing the bad things you do to yourself and others.

This advice is thousands of years old, but we can adapt it for today. Let's take one principle: *If you show compassion, you'll be happier. If you want to be happy, cultivate compassion.* For example, say you have teenager trouble. Think back to something outrageous *you* did when you were that age. Did it ruin your life? Were you eventually able to recoup? Share the unembellished story with your teen, lace it with a little humor, and confess you learned one of life's lessons. By exchanging places with your teen, or any person you're angry with, you show your humanity. Instead of judging, you share how you're more alike than different. And remember this: If you don't feel strong enough to help someone in a critical moment, never harm them. Sometimes verbal outbursts are very negative, very harmful. And we all feel terrible after they happen. So think of your child first, not how this affects you. That's practicing compassion.

Two more illustrations: (1) *Money equals generosity.* We all need money to survive, but when we can support our favorite causes, we find pleasure in something that doesn't represent the usual material symbol. (2) *Time equals contemplation and study.* We all know people who fill their extra time with more and more projects, spreading themselves too thin. If we take the time to read, study, contemplate, analyze, we find a calmness within ourselves. We feel less scattered, more centered, more able to say yes to those things that matter most. A spiritual path helps you examine life. It's a different focus.

Recall or imagine a time when you were rushed, irritated, and had a bad day. What happened? The wrong tone or look suddenly transformed a simple interaction into a contest. Now replay the same set of circumstances, but replace your irritation with kindness. Where you felt your ego attacked, replace it with a smile of forgiveness.

If you think about it, under a different set of circumstances or on a different day, we might not have reacted the same way. Some people with a problem get stuck—they see only one way to solve it. Others analyze a problem and creatively consider all the angles in solving it. They may even distance themselves as they search for a solution. You might try to stop focusing on yourself as you step back and consider any problem. A problem doesn't have to drive you crazy. What are you doing that someone else in the same situation might not be doing?

My friend Stephanie developed fibromyalgia at fifty-six. She tried conventional therapy and responded well to anti-inflammatory medications, but not entirely. For a number of years she came into my office complaining, but refused to try different approaches. After an especially bad flare-up she phoned and said, "Tell me everything I can do." Stephanie tried meditation, began to swim daily, and returned to her first childhood love, the violin. Her joy about her return to music filtered into other areas, producing positive effects. Things slowly improved, and now she manages her disease with diverse treatments. She still meditates daily. Stephanie showed great kindness to herself, which made her happier.

Spiritual insight encourages you to deal with other people who may have suffered from the same thing and distracts you from dwelling on yourself. We need lots of practice to cultivate these attitudes and not get stuck in the small stuff. Instead, work toward finding a consistent calmness and sense of humor—every day.

If you feel the need for some spiritual solace, consider these:
- Going back to your spiritual or religious roots
- Taking up tai chi or yoga
- Joining a meditation class
- Finding a local Bible, Torah, Koran, or Dharma study group

- Reading one of the excellent books on religion and spirit available at most bookstores
- Finding some beauty in nature to replenish your spirit
- Volunteering service for others

A More Detailed Action List

- *Wake up every morning, look in the mirror, and think positively.* Affirmations are self-nourishing and self-fulfilling.
- *Share your story of illness or sadness.* Stories give us healing power when we can verbalize grief, feelings of loss, and traumatic events. Stories connect us to one another because we find a kindred spirit.
- *Think about what inspires you.* Could you bring a symbol of it to a group meeting, or to your desk or your kitchen shelf? Inspiration doesn't have to be a big formal thing. It might be a symbol or picture that comforts your mind.
- *Form your own circle of spiritual friends.* Create your own rituals. Circles are sacred ancient symbols, and the people within them are all equals. Everyone is encouraged to speak at least once, from their own experience and from the heart. Listeners are encouraged to be nonjudgmental and to listen from the heart. Insight often comes from silence, so a silent period is suggested.

---

62. Get Involved in a Spiritual Community   Impact★★★★

There are numerous opportunities to practice a life infused with spirit by yourself, but you also can be part of a community that shares your vision. People believing in the same traditions often find comfort and support being together. Have you found a group of people who share some common spiritual values with you? It's a prime motivator to extend your longevity on a few different levels. Social interactions stimulate active involvement in life. People sharing a vision demonstrate hopefulness as they move through life's challenges and obstacles together. And when multiple generations interact in the same environment, lifelong learning takes place between the young and the old.

Your mind-set in a spiritual gathering is different than the office. You're more likely to observe participants demonstrating love over hate, kindness over violence, and patience instead of anger. Sometimes it's like coming out of the rain and under an umbrella of tranquillity, if only for a short respite.

The kinship and social spheres are in full play here as we reach out to others and receive nourishment from them in return. Opportunities abound in sharing time with old friends and actually meeting new people who might be interested in something very important to you. Family members often commit a special time in the week and prioritize their other activities to spend this period together. Sociologists contend that these types of positive rituals create continuity and positive memories in a child's life.

Research again and again confirms that people who go to church and synagogue regularly live longer. Any place of worship offers us a time to reflect with others and to nourish our souls. When we stop thinking about ourselves, we really do become happier. This impacts longevity. In fact, whenever we practice kindness, it's a spiritual act. You may have volunteered for the library fund-raiser, picked up some food for a neighbor who's sick, tutored someone, fixed the leaky sink at pre-school, or donated money for an animal shelter.

63. Take Time with Mother Nature   Impact ★★★

Nature is always rejuvenating itself. And its predictable rebirth every spring is another of life's lessons. We are physical beings and the children of Mother Nature. Nature gives her beauty to us with unconditional benefits. All we have to do is honor and protect these sacred spaces.

What happens to us when we take a walk in the woods? Simply put, the distractions are different. They invite us into the philosophical. We are distracted by a sunset, a tree we can't identify, where a path will take us and who took the path before. In nature, we share a joyous curiosity.

The path outdoors leads us to an internal spiritual path. We tend to look broadly at our environment and realize we're not the only ones around. We share the planet with other living organisms. Most everyone finds pleasure experiencing nature, whether seeing a flower garden, the rain forest, or going white-water rafting. Our world's beauty touches our inner souls, and we gain joy every day we take time for nature. How many times have you looked out of the window on a beautiful day and wished you could be outside? Simply doing something outside for fifteen minutes instead of wishing will make a difference in your calmness, your energy.

If you are the sort who needs a scientific explanation for why a walk in the woods makes you feel good, here's my best shot: Beyond being innately enjoyable, walking in a relaxed manner, on a hiking trail, for instance, probably reduces adrenaline in the body. That makes you feel calmer. When we're calm, we gain perspective. Perspective increases hopefulness.

Try these action plans for connecting with nature:

- *Plant something and nurture it.* You can do this indoors or outdoors.
- *Join a group that enjoys nature.*
- *Join a group that protects the environment.* It will nourish your spiritual sphere by volunteering, while their outings will connect you directly with Mother Nature.
- *Hike today.* Visit your community park or perhaps a nature preserve that you've never been to. Take a friend, and your kinship sphere will be enhanced.
- *Volunteer to help at any outdoor activity, such as a marathon.*
- *Take up a hobby such as fishing, orienteering, bird watching, skiing, walking.*
- *And think about sleeping outside.* Find somewhere away from city lights and noise if possible. Listen, watch, smell, feel.
- *Find nature in art and use it for solace.*

64. Don't Avoid Thinking About Death   Impact ★★★★

Planning for death would be a lot easier if we knew a few of the specifics. At the very least, a rough idea of the date would be helpful. With moving, graduation, marriage, a new baby, there are proper announcement cards, and we can do a little preparation. But death doesn't announce itself, does it?

So it's a paradox. We know that death is inevitable and unpredictable. In many religious traditions and cultures it is not a taboo or a scary topic. It's part of life and worth thinking about because it brings more balance and thoughtfulness to your daily decisions. Just ask anyone who's survived a major health, social, or financial crisis. They're apt to tell you how much more they appreciate each new day. They value having a new opportunity to do things again, maybe even better. Sometimes I think of life as a giant chess game: Your next move is always exciting. But what if we never value the time we have together and never prepare for death?

First of all, avoiding thinking about death produces a lot of stress, and that's one additional thing we don't need when we're dying. Being unprepared for death also produces another source of mental anguish: regret. "I should have done this. I could have done that. I would have changed those." Shoulda, coulda, woulda. It's time to finally give up all of those self-recriminations.

What to do? I asked a friend of mine (who is also my patient) how he felt after surviving some rather traumatic heart problems. "Well," he said, "I think before the episode I had sort of a casual denial of what I was afraid of. The sense wasn't a fear of dying. It was more like a fear of missing the point of why I'm here. Kind of a sublevel panic. Then something happens to you, like immediate surgery, and you lose all of your control. Picture taking your dog for a ride in the car and you're in the driver's seat and he's next to you. And he is incapable of knowing who's driving the car; that's how I felt. I had no idea who was driving the car. But my diagnosis and subsequent treatment created space in my head. Things like money, schedules, problems, interpersonal relationships lost their weight. Before the episode, I wasn't able to tell you what I wanted to do. Now, I simplify." For perennial deniers, having a healthy fear of death is good; it produces positive action during your life.

Think about all of the things that make you who you are: your physical body, your mental agility, your accomplishments (splendid and not so splendid), your friends, your loved ones, your material possessions, your spiritual practice. Our preoccupation with the business of living often consumes all of our time and energy. Even those of us who have had experience with someone dying whom we cared about do not believe that we could die today. And we can.

It's scary to think about death. It starts you thinking about how impermanent everything is. And then you wonder, "What's important in life, anyway? Am I satisfied with my life if I were really to die today? Did I do enough? Did I contribute anything at all? How will I be remembered? Why should I bother thinking about death if I can't do anything about it anyway?" And bingo! You've got it.

The reason to think about death is that it forces you to think about your life and your future. And at that very moment you can begin to make preparations for it. You can make longevity choices that enhance your life. You can make spiritual choices to be ethical, show equanimity, and bring compassion to your everyday actions.

You can live your life in such a way, every day, that if you were going to die tomorrow, you would have no regrets.

Here's an action plan.

- *Consider your personal views of what happens after your physical body dies.* Does it make sense to you?
- *Consider your spiritual outlook.* Does it correspond with your view of death? Or do you wish to look in another direction?
- *Talk to your minister, rabbi, spiritual friend, or close friend.*
- *If you are grieving, give yourself some time to grieve.* Slowly, when you are ready, try writing about it.
- *Think about forgiveness.* Don't forget about forgiving yourself. Is there anyone you would like to write some thank-you notes to?
- *Think about your gratitude to others.* Share these words and experiences, if it seems right, with others.
- *When you write your will, think about your legacy.* Consider not only the money you may leave behind but the memories.

Birth is a beginning
And death is a destination,
But life is a journey.
A going—a growing
From stage to stage,
From childhood to maturity
And youth to age.
From innocence to awareness
And ignorance to knowing
From foolishness to discretion
And then perhaps to wisdom.
From weakness to strength
Or strength to weakness—
And, often, back again.
From health to sickness

And back, we pray, to health again.
From offence to forgiveness,
From loneliness to love,
From joy to gratitude,
From pain to compassion,
And grief to understanding—
    From fear to faith.
From defeat to defeat to defeat—
Until, looking backward or ahead,
We see that victory lies
Not at some high place along the way,
But in having made the journey, stage
    by stage,
A sacred pilgrimage.
Birth is a beginning
And death is a destination
But life is a journey,
A sacred pilgrimage—
Made stage by stage—
    To life everlasting.

              —ALVIN I. FINE
           from *Gates of Repentance,* 1973

65. Prepare Your Living Will and Advance Directives   Impact ★★★

It's not a fun job, but somebody has to do it and you're the somebody. Technically called advance directives, commonly called a living will, this document allows you to specify what you want done to keep you alive if you are too sick to express those wishes yourself.

Eleanor was a patient of mine since the first week I went into practice. She was a wonderful, award-winning teacher who always had time for a needy child. Never quite having time to get married or have children, Eleanor called our rural community her family. She was the peripatetic volunteer whom everybody loved. Her one living relative, her sister, Denise, lived five hundred miles away in Cleveland. They cared for each other enough, but their worldviews were different. Eleanor was eclectic, Denise rigid and narrow.

Then came Eleanor's first stroke. She survived and prospered as I knew she would, throwing herself full force into physical rehab and speech therapy. One year later the only sign of what she had gone through was a slight facial droop.

Several years ago Medicare mandated that all seniors must be offered a living will when hospitalized. Before that, doctors rarely discussed it. When I spoke with Eleanor she really wasn't interested. She wanted to get well and not think about death. I disagreed and tried to gently cajole her into thinking about signing the document to specify her wishes. She said, "Doc, you know what I want. No tubes, no IVs, no life support if you think that I won't return to my old self."

After her second stroke two years later she developed "locked-in syndrome," where you can hear and see but cannot respond. Patients are clearly aware but have totally lost the ability to communicate by words or nodding.

Eleanor thoughtfully stared at me every day I made my rounds. She refused totally to eat and drink. It was obvious that she wanted out. But we kept her on IVs until her sister arrived.

That's when things happened. Denise insisted on putting in a feeding tube. When I demurred, Denise went to the courts to establish that, as the closest relative, she was in charge and would take it from there. I was temporarily removed from the case. Eleanor had a feeding tube placed in her, after which she was transferred back to our local nursing home, where I was asked once again to take over as her family doc.

It took Eleanor three years to die. Every time I stopped by to see her, I could easily see in her thoughtful face this message: "Remove the danged tube and let me go." I felt wretched, and still do. Had she signed a living will, I could have abided by her wishes. Perhaps you should consider drawing up this document now.

Here are four ways to draft a living will:

- Go to your community hospital. Every hospital in the country *must*, under federal mandate, have an easy-to-fill-out living will form. You do not need a lawyer, just a witness or two.
- Buy one of several excellent self-help books with detachable forms.
- Get computer software that has a living will form.
- Go to your lawyer and have him or her draft a document.

Here are the most important things you should specify:

- When to keep you alive with IVs, feeding tubes, breathing tubes, and the like.
- Whether you want CPR.
- How much pain medication you wish. Massive amounts of morphine may keep you pain-free but retard your breathing, thereby hastening your demise. Be specific.

66. Volunteer Service to Others   Impact ★★★★

Volunteering is a small act of giving that often brings a big difference to someone else's life. It strengthens and gives us a sense of purpose and a connection to other people.

A close friend of mine epitomizes the spirit of volunteering. Along with other compassionate people and mentors, she works tirelessly teaching a support group called "Renewing Life," for people with life-threatening illnesses One day a few years ago the teacher became a student. She had a heart attack. After bypass surgery, she went through cardiac rehab, made dietary changes, faithfully took her cholesterol medication, and continued her lifelong habit of meditation. In short, she practiced what she had been teaching and felt safe in the knowledge that she was doing everything right.

Then she had her second heart attack. This time the road to recuperation was much more devastating emotionally, and she came to understand what a "non-death experience" was. It was a grieving for what she had lost, the person she had been before the heart attacks. It was coming to grips with the fear of dying, all the imagined and all the real fears. But she no longer feared death itself, because she knew it was inevitable. What she feared was not living, not being able to live life every day with the same sensitivity and altruism she always had. Her volunteer work proved to be the key for overcoming that fear. As she became stronger and stronger day by day, she began to ask herself, "Right now, at this very moment, have I done all that I can?" And the answer was a resounding *"Yes."*

We live in the human community in order to share our lives with others. No one person can do everything. No matter how self-sufficient we wish we could be, we all rely on one another for some things. When we volunteer goods or services or time, we always get *something*. Sometimes voluntarily helping others through a painful tragedy allows us to get a better sense of our own mortality. Sometimes we chaperone the high school band and learn more than their musical selections.

Helping one another, reaching out to the larger community, is a dance of changing partners. One week a family with youngsters may need clothing. At a future time the senior who spearheaded a clothes drive may need some extra meals.

Whether we give directly to people we know or do our part to advance the efforts of a larger network, it feels good to help people. The lines blur between the giver and the receiver, because both benefit. Time is not an issue in volunteering once we learn to say "yes" to those things we can handle and "no" to those things we cannot. "If you can't give a beggar a dollar, give him a dime," my grandmother used to say. To put an updated spin on that teaching, if you can't be the chairman of the AIDS walk, just walk. Kids can spearhead recycling drives in their neighborhoods. Teens can organize fund-raising dances. Often the simplest offer of aid becomes all the more valuable because of its timeliness.

Volunteering is an act of kindness—and awareness. It makes you more conscious of the world you inhabit, close to home or far away. There is some project, some cause, some need that stirs your passion. Go look for it. You'll meet some great, like-minded people along the way.

Material Sphere

EXERCISE 12–WORK LIFE

You spend thousands of hours in a work environment. Do you believe that:

- ❑ What you do in your occupation each day usually gives you pleasure?
- ❑ You are safe from avoidable accidents?
- ❑ You will be doing the same thing in five years?
- ❑ You will be at the same physical workplace in five years?
- ❑ The benefits outweigh the specific work that you do?
- ❑ You are making enough money?

❑ You are sharing the responsibility with the primary people you see every day?

❑ Your creativity is undervalued and underused?

❑ There are simple ways to improve your work situation in terms of physical risk?

❑ You are willing to stay where you are so that you can do what you want when you retire?

❑ The people you work with are important to you and support you?

❑ You are contributing some good?

67. Pursue Job Satisfaction — Impact ★★★★★

It's obvious that job satisfaction or lack of it influences your health. Certainly your mental sphere is intimately tied up in your job. Studies show that five fundamental criteria affect job selection: working with people, money, social status and prestige, and having the opportunity to use your talents and be creative.

All of the spheres of your life are affected by the work you choose. A job you don't like is stressful mentally or physically, while a job you feel is worthwhile is not. Sometimes there's a conflict with the material sphere: You like the job you have but simply cannot manage to live on the money you are making, or you like the salary you're making but feel very dissatisfied with the work you are doing. Let's face it—you spend too much of your life connected with the work you do to live with perpetual dissatisfaction.

If you knew you were going to live a shorter life than you hoped for, would you stay in the position you're currently in?

Do you hate your job?

Would you rather be in a different occupation?

Would you rather work in a different city?

Would you rather move to another country?

Does your job impact your family far more than you'd like?

Are you underpaid?

Does your job simply stress you out?

Job satisfaction is also affected by your home life. Do you have children who are seeing you as often as you wish? Can you give the needed attention to nurturing your own relationship and creating a loving household? Do you balance the demanding schedules and household work, or is one partner doing an unequal share? Frustration over inequity, in anything, is a big piece of job satisfaction, especially if your household has two wage earners.

If these questions bring up some discussion, you can figure out why you're dissatisfied at work. Are you showing up at work so preoccupied with the issues in your personal life that you're not functioning? Time to do some homework. Or are you receiving much more personal satisfaction from your time at work than from your home? Evaluate this very closely when you think about the profound relationship of the five spheres.

Work in the home has its own criteria of job satisfaction. Certainly (and hopefully) we all equally value the work that's done in raising a family and managing a household. The trouble is that there is still no outside wage paid for staying at home. There are also no delineated shifts, scheduled breaks, worker's compensation, and often no intellectual stimulation from other adults for long periods of time.

Job satisfaction has a plus or minus rating when people participate in work that makes them feel that they are contributing something worthy to someone else. A taxi driver who prevents drunk people from getting behind the wheel of their car may have more personal job satisfaction than a corporate executive who knows the pitiful conditions of the company's overseas labor force.

Your job influences a lot of life's choices, especially in the social sphere. We often share common interests with our friends from work. As such, job satisfaction can rise or fall with these social bonds.

Too much commuting time ranks high on the list of factors that affect job satisfaction. A commute of under thirty minutes still represents 250 hours a year. Here's a startling statistic: If you commute two hours a day, at the end of twenty years you'll have spent the equivalent of five working years in your car. Besides, commuting causes a profusion of negative emotions, including stress, anger, and irritability.

Are You Doing What You Wish, or Do You Wish to Do What You Love?

When our oldest son was starting college, he received the best advice from a dear family friend: "If you do the work you love, it's never a job." Ask yourself: "What do my job and my leisure time mean to me?" If you're not doing the job you want or you're not satisfied, you may be at risk for a heart attack because you're stressed out. We've all heard someone say, "This job is going to kill me." Well, sometimes it does.

Obviously, quality of life and the quality of our work life are significant. But do we see direct evidence that job satisfaction translates into longevity? For that we will go back to the Terman Life Cycle Study, which found that men and women who changed careers frequently were more likely to die prematurely. The most common explanation of this is that moving frequently between jobs is a stressful activity and translates into poor health for the primary person making the move. Just think what it must do for the rest of the family.

David's story helps us see how the various spheres interrelate. David embodied the American dream. A prosperous, award-winning architect, he and his wife had five children and sent three to expensive private colleges. Contracts kept coming until his partner, whose life had just fallen apart, embezzled the firm's capital. At fifty, David was out of work in the only town he had ever lived in.

Needing cash quickly, and unable to find acceptable work, David headed to Chicago and a prestigious firm. The money was excellent but the hours were not. The grind of sixty-plus hours a week suited the younger competition, who were intent on moving up the ladder. That's when David started to drink. Soon he developed high blood pressure, got an ulcer, and became morbidly depressed. His wife wanted a divorce. His life was in shambles.

His crises all seemed to stem from his job, and my suggestion was terse: Quit the job and come home. Tell the kids you'll help pay tuition at a state college, and they can foot the rest with loans and grants. Go into marital counseling and alcohol recovery. In the short run, start taking an antidepressant such as Prozac to give you some breathing space. In fact, investigate some quiet ways to calm yourself—maybe biofeedback or deep breathing meditation. You need some time to *be*; don't work for a month. Think. Use your savings. That's what savings are for—emergencies and illness.

This was not easy advice to follow, but after counseling they accepted most of it. The result? Their marriage survived. The kids graduated from college—though not the ones they started in. David now teaches at a local technical school and loves it. They sold their house, and their vacations are not as exotic (the north woods of Wisconsin rather than the sumptuous beaches of Hawaii). But he's happier and will undoubtedly live longer. These changes did not go unnoticed by their children, who shared in this happy ending. A spiritual decision is making those choices in life that bring you and your loved ones the greatest amount of happiness.

Many people today are downsizing their lives. They are selecting less stressful jobs because they want to *enjoy* life. People are looking for more integrity and simplicity in the way they spend each day. Many volunteer and give back to the community some of the wonderful life skills they have mastered. Although you may earn less money, living where you want to and doing what you want clearly benefit your longevity.

Action Plan

If talk of job satisfaction makes you sneer, you're probably stressed at work. You may want to change your life, but a good place to start may be changing your job. This is a five-star arena of life, and that means your longevity depends on it. If you've been told your cholesterol is high, your first step may be not to take a cholesterol-lowering drug, stop smoking, or start a low-fat diet, but rather to quit your job.

- First get a résumé together and start listing your skills.
- Read about redirecting your career.
- For some, an interest inventory—a test that tells what careers people with your interests and personality might enjoy—can help.
- A key step in career revamping is the informational interview. Find someone working in the career you fancy and ask questions about it.
- If necessary, retrain. You may or may not be at the job you had ten, twenty, or thirty years ago. You changed then; you can change again.
- Volunteer or apprentice to gain experience in your desired job market.

68. Ensure Job Safety

Impact ★★★★

The latest federal statistics show that the most dangerous occupation in America today is driving a truck. Almost one quarter of deaths occurring at work transpired because of highway crashes. By far the road remains the most dangerous place to be, with the farm a steady second-place finisher. If you work in sales, homicides and highway accidents serve equally as causes of death. For construction employees, mortal danger lurks from falls and things falling on workers.

As you can see, this list is no David Letterman matter. The list describes on-the-job death, and it might include you. Making your job safer is a joint responsibility. Some of the issues are obvious: Fire and police departments have obvious dangers. But only recently have we recognized that the main danger to people who work in a bar is smoking rather than violence.

My recommendation is to take a good objective look at your job. Lots of hazards are in plain view but others are not as obvious. My mother-in-law was a hospital social worker for twenty years in a neighborhood that continued to deteriorate. She was finally forced to quit the job she dearly loved because of the physical threat of violence as she left work late at night.

Not all workplace environmental problems are covered by the Occupational Safety and Health Administration (OSHA). However, most companies have safety programs. If you have questions about your job safety, call the OSHA hotline: 800-321-OSHA.

Consider the following in your action plan:
- What's the air like? Is it smoky or not? Are there fumes? Chemicals?
- What are the transportation problems?
- Is work located in a dangerous neighborhood?
- Does your job involve excessive or dangerous driving or equipment?
- Is your employer following the common safety rules it should?

69. Procure Adequate Job Benefits   Impact ★★★★

Not having adequate benefits adds stress to your life. Should you become sick, you want to be optimally cared for. Should you become disabled, you and your family are at risk for financial disaster. In fact, the risk of disability is far greater than the risk of death for anyone raising a family. Yet too few of us have a plan should this occur.

Health Insurance
The perfect health insurance package would offer a choice of any doctor, any hospital, and any dentist anywhere in the world. It would include all drugs with no copay. It would cover any surgery with no

preexisting-condition limitation. Unfortunately, it's not a perfect world, so benefit packages vary.

Optimally you should have your benefits package reviewed by someone who knows—a friend or relative who's a bit further down the path than you are. Or perhaps consult a financial planner, who can take your whole situation into consideration.

Disability Insurance

Disability insurance protects you if you become too ill or injured to work. Disability insurance pays you a percentage of your former earnings in the event of a serious accident or sickness. Proof of prior earnings and proof of disability are usually mandatory. In some states, certain professions are excluded, such as interstate truck drivers.

Life Insurance

Many states require employers to provide minimal coverage, so that in the event of a worker's death there's enough money to cover funeral expenses. Most people elect to purchase their own life insurance to provide further for their family. This topic is replete with information on the benefits and disadvantages of different kinds of policies. Remember to compare.

Vacation

Here in America, two weeks of vacation time is standard, while European workers enjoy three to four weeks of vacation. Occupations such as teaching tie vacation to the school academic calendar. Lifestyle choices may prioritize time over money, or money over time. Some people change job descriptions and go from corporate work to independent consulting in order to have more flexible personal schedules. Increases in salary reflect additional vacation time in many professions.

70. Make Your Workplace Fun   Impact ★★★

In this workaholic world, we might spend more time with our fellow workers than we do with friends and relatives. A suitable or constructive environment allows us to work productively, efficiently, comfortably, and creatively. But we also need respect, joy, and compassion.

- *Respect.* Do you respect your coworkers? And are you respected by them for the work that you do? If not, maybe it's time to take action. Sometimes just a conversation at the right time can make a substantial difference. Mutual respect is imperative. Without it, issues will surface that make your career much more difficult. In the workplace, think "we," not "I." Respect does breed respect.
- *Joy.* Are you happy at what you do? Do you show it? We all have off days, but the humor and happiness we enjoy in life can easily translate into your job. If your coworkers are constantly unhappy, inevitably you will be, too. Talk to them; befriend them. Try to put humor to work at work—it can make a difference. Joy does breed joy.
- *Compassion.* Whether you're the top banana at the office or the lowest apple on the tree, the key is to try to look at your coworkers with a compassionate eye. How would you treat them if they were your favorite relative or neighbor? If they were your children? If they were yourself? Developing a compassionate attitude can indeed take a work situation that is arduous and make it less so.

But what if all this fails? What if you're not happy? First you want to do everything possible to fix your job. But if that fails, leave. Take time to plan. When aiming for a long, sweet life, look at the horizon. Where do you want to be five years from now?

EXERCISE 13—FINANCIAL LIFE

The monetary decisions you make in life impact on your health and happiness. Have you decided to:

- ❑ Work in a job that pays you enough for your current material needs?
- ❑ Continue your education in order to have more options in work?
- ❑ Spend money now on setting up a place to live and buying a car?
- ❑ Take advantage of company retirement plans.?
- ❑ Spend more than you make?
- ❑ Live with people who can't control their spending?
- ❑ Look toward changing your job location so your life becomes less stressful?
- ❑ Take a brutal look at your debt and start paying it off?
- ❑ Retire and simplify your life?
- ❑ Work so that the money is enough to make you happy?

For hundreds of years we have observed an association between money and longevity. Traditionally, people who have more money live longer because they enjoy more nutritious food, superior health care and better living conditions. People with lower socioeconomic status tend to smoke more, live in more crowded and polluted environments, suffer financial stressors, and be more physically inactive, among other things. But researchers also found two significant issues. One, the poorer you are, the less likely you are to have social support and social relationships; two, poverty makes the stress of racism, classism, and the like weigh heavily on you.

We worry about money for our needs and wants, about being in debt and getting out of debt, about buying a home, about college costs, about vacations, about saving for retirement. Money is clearly a major preoccupation with many of us.

Money greatly affects the social and mental spheres. Questions about where you live, who your friends are, what you do, and how you feel about yourself are often tied up with money and money concerns. All these questions and issues can affect how sweet your life is and how long it is.

71. Calculate How Much Is Enough   Impact ★★★★

Talk about money, and one thing is clear: If we don't have enough, we're stressed. But what's enough? Basically, if we have job benefits and spend within our means, save some for a house, retirement, and college education, plus a little reserve to go to a movie or restaurant and take a vacation, then things are off to a good start. We call that middle-class.

The Whitehall Study from Britain looked at civil servants in London, all middle-class workers making middle-class salaries and all with equal access to medical care, for thirty years beginning in the 1960s. They found that money predicts longevity. Those who made more lived longer, regardless of their health habits. Lower-middle-class workers were more likely to have monotonous work, less job satisfaction, less control, and less longevity.

In summary, three main points can be gained from these British studies:

1. How much you make is a marker for education. Education predicts

job status; the better-educated had higher-level jobs. Education also predicts income; people with college degrees make two to three times more money than high-school graduates. All this means that education predicts social status, too. In addition, the more educated you are, generally the better your health habits.

2. How much you make affects how long you live, even with equal access to medical care. Education not only predicts income, it also predicts longevity, regardless of health habits. If you are a rich smoker, you will generally live longer than a poor smoker. Shocking, isn't it?

3. How much money you make is a marker for control in your life, control on the job, vacation opportunity, and job satisfaction. People in the upper strata of government work—again, these were middle-class civil servants, not CEOs of corporations—had more control over their lives. If you're the bureau head, you can take off for your daughter's preschool play. The bureau supervisor can often take vacation time more liberally, too. Moreover, those in the upper tier of income had more control over the job and surroundings, which translates to more praise and esteem at work. Granted, with more responsibility comes stress. But when you control the project and use your creativity, you get credit for the results.

But the critical factor to remember is perspective. How much is enough? Money doesn't buy longevity per se. Once you reach the threshold of the middle class—you have a little in the bank and spend within your means, with some extra for dinners out, entertainment, and vacations—ultimately your life is less stressful, and you have bought the basic longevity pie. For example, the difference between having a reliable car and no car or a car that barely works is a major difference. Having a reliable car gives you ease of life and mobility. But the difference between having a reliable car and an expensive reliable car is minimal.

Scientifically, we believe that when you relieve stress, you reduce the cortisol and adrenaline levels in your body. These chemicals are implicated in sudden cardiovascular death, heart attack, and stroke. So you take away the major causes of early death, and you'll live longer—it's as simple as that.

Determining how much is enough requires that you evaluate your needs and expectations. Because money is a key driving force in most of our lives, calculating what we need allows us to plan how hard we wish to work, and, conversely, how soon we wish to retire. I recommend that you:

- Evaluate how much money you need now and when you retire.
- Determine what you wish to do when you have met your goals.
- Go to a financial planner.
- Conclude what you would do if you met your financial goals prematurely.

If you meet your goals early, then you might spend more money earlier, as did a successful lawyer patient of mine in her forties. She discovered to her dismay that she was saving more than she needed to meet her children's educational goals. She did not plan on retiring early, since she loved what she did. So instead she took her family to Europe for a prolonged vacation and tripled her donations to the local homeless shelter. When she had more than she needed, she made an active choice on how to utilize it. But you cannot do that until you know how much is enough.

72. Minimize Your Debt	Impact ★★★

Okay, you're thirty and don't have a shekel in the bank. You're young enough to get on top of things, so you'll just keep buying on plastic and maybe go to one of those Web sites that promise to consolidate all your debts into one loan payment that's supposedly lower. Is that stressful? Yes. Can it make a difference in your health choices? Most assuredly.

I have a lot of patients who come into my office complaining that they'd like to exercise but can't join a health club because they have too much debt already. We talk about the possibility of taking a walk in one of our beautiful state parks instead, but it's not the answer they wanted to hear. They'd like to go on a nice vacation but have no money. I again suggest some of the fabulous wooded or lake retreats we have in our state, but again we're not on the same page. Usually these patients fail to take their whole financial picture into consideration. You have a set amount of money; it all depends on where you decide to spend it.

For instance, if you smoke cigarettes, you have to generate roughly $1,200–$2,000 per year in cash—or, for most taxpayers, possibly $2,500 per year in pretax salary—to pay for a pack-a-day habit. If you took that money and invested it, you'd have a nest egg, or at least a pot you could grab for that vacation you crave.

If you spend lots of mental time puzzling about how you're going to pay things off, then it's time to take action in this sphere. Financial issues are rarely thought of as health issues. But they are. The issue here is to reduce your debt so you can reduce your stress.

Here's what you should do if you have too much debt:
- *Take a course on financial planning and budgeting.*
- *Cut your credit cards up and pay them off.*
- *Stop spending.* Look at every purchase.
- *Start putting all loose change in a big container.* Sounds hokey, but it provides Christmas presents without using credit.
- *My mother-in-law used to say, "Those who understand interest earn it. Those who don't, don't."*
- *See a financial counselor, because that spurs you to action.*

On the other hand, if you really want to work something out on your own, first assess all your income, then list all your expenses in a year. Look at your canceled checks, your credit card statements, and your receipts, and try to think of all the incidentals, like music lessons, compact discs, and library fines, for which you think you might have paid cash. Itemize and regroup. Figure out what you spend on which items each year for each person in the house, then figure out how much you can afford to spend. If your income doesn't stretch that far, figure out where you can reasonably cut back. Start budgeting.

73. Maximize Your Savings and Retirement Income — Impact ★★★

We know that debt is onerous; too much debt is debilitating. The stress it causes destroys feelings of wellness. Once you've conquered your debt, you're at a neutral spot. Savings should be your next goal. Looking at the plethora of books on the subject in any bookstore, you can see that debt reduction and savings are important issues. But is your health actually affected? And how?

Take Frank. He worked for the state for more than twenty years as a guard at our local prison. By carefully saving something from his paycheck every week, by putting the maximum amount he could into the state retirement plan, Frank was able to quit his job at fifty. He was free to do what he really wanted to do—build houses and design perennial gardens. Was Frank happier? Of course he was. His job had not been his passion; it was simply a way for him to support his family. And because his wife, Kate, still worked for a large banking firm, health insurance continued; so Frank was able to work as he wished, knowing that they would be able to retire comfortably in the future. Some of you may ask, "What about those twenty years Frank worked at a job he didn't like?" His decision may have been different from what yours would be, because he had different goals and circumstances.

Then there's Alice. A farm wife with six kids, she saved some of the milk money every week and stuffed it into an IRA. She and George planned on selling the herd when he was sixty-five. But arthritis took over, and they could no longer farm. George sold the herd when he was fifty-five with one big question: How were they going to survive? Alice's planning paid off. With an IRA, they could both get some part-time jobs in town with health care benefits, and still retire. Had she not saved, there would be money problems.

I could go on and on. But the issue is that the money you save today will bring you opportunities tomorrow. I don't pretend to be a financial counselor, but from the family doctor's perspective, many a family's stressors are related to what's stashed away. It determines the success of future financial commitments: Whether or not you can leave your job to retire, whether or not you can switch occupations, whether or not your kids go to summer camp—all that is a function of what you save.

Right before your death, with fifteen seconds left in your life, will you think about the money you have in the bank? Probably not. And that means it's not your first priority. So prioritize. Money may be up there, but if it's not number one, spend time and energy on the things that *are* number one.

Here's an action plan to maximize your savings:
- *Create a five-year plan.* Articulate your goals and dreams; start saving.
- *Fund your company's 401(k) to the maximum.*
- *If you're eligible for an IRA, set it up now.*

- *If you have kids, start a savings plan now,* at the earliest age possible.
- *Use direct deposit* to put retirement money and savings directly in an account before you cash your paycheck.
- *Quit smoking* and save up to $2,500 per year in pretax salary toward retirement or a vacation.
- *Shop wisely and pay with cash.* People who purchase with plastic usually buy more than they need.
- *Live within your means.* Pay off all debt, bit by bit by bit.

EXERCISE 14—YOUR SURROUNDINGS

There's no place like home—especially yours. Do you come home to:
- ❏ A friendly neighborhood?
- ❏ People who respect your space?
- ❏ An outside environment that's safe?
- ❏ A house that you find relaxing because of its colors, furniture, location?
- ❏ A quiet, peaceful environment?
- ❏ Little touches of nature that nourish your soul?
- ❏ Somewhere you want your family and friends to join you?
- ❏ A space that is comfortable, where you put your feet up and relax?

74. Don't Live in a Violent Environment	Impact ★★★★★

I remember riding my bicycle to medical school in the Windy City. It was usually a delightful respite from hard days of studying and long hours at Cook County Hospital's emergency room, waiting for the next gunshot victim to arrive. What I hadn't bargained for was that I could be the next casualty. I was riding my bike past Cabrini Green, a notorious housing project, but the couple of blocks distance set it mentally far away. Suddenly five boys standing on the corner bolted after me, perhaps coveting my bike.

I pedaled and pedaled; they raced on, hurling stones at me. In the nick of time I crossed into a very busy street, stopping my bike in the middle of traffic. I stayed put, the cars whizzing by on both sides, until they finally left. I could have easily suffered a serious injury or perhaps been killed. Who knows? Of course, at the time, like many twenty-one-year-old males, I thought I was invincible.

The issue is that danger I never thought about existed in a place

I passed every day. The same may be true of you. How do you determine your risk? Any urban or rural community with an established record of gang activity, drug trafficking and use, or high larceny or burglary rates will provide general indications of an unhealthy living environment. Moreover, streetfights, barroom brawls, domestic squabbles, and just the absence of kids playing on the streets can give one pause.

Take Clare. I remember her well because she was a mother of three who nearly died on her way home from working at the hospital. She was in housekeeping, working 3 to 11 P.M., while her husband, Rick, worked the day shift at the local Schwinn bicycle plant. By working different shifts, they saved on child care expenses. Every day she took the bus, then walked four blocks to her house. She never really noticed the two bars at the corner bus stop—until one night when she stepped off the bus and two fighting men tumbled out of one of the bars right in front of her. She was knocked to the ground, and though several bystanders pulled her to safety, she nonetheless ended up with twenty stitches in her head and a concussion to boot. In Clare's case, economics prevailed, and she continued to walk home, though she got off at a different bus stop.

Urban centers are not the only dangerous areas. Where I live now, in the country, we take care on the third week in November because that's deer hunting season. A walk in the woods that weekend may be your last.

The point is that with just a little forethought, you can avoid violence. For example, take the two anecdotes above. In both the bicycling and bus incidents, taking sensible action prevented further trauma. I never biked down that road again, and Clare chose a different bus stop.

Whatever your situation, consider the following self-preservation tips:

- *Walk defensively.* Be prepared.
- *Look objectively at your destination* and determine if the possibility of confrontation exists.
- *Carry a whistle* with you in case a problem occurs.
- *Tell people where you're going* and when to expect you.
- *If possible, have someone meet you* at the bus stop or train and walk you home.

- *Don't be afraid to yell* if you find yourself threatened. Yelling may save you.
- *Check out public service rides,* offered in many communities for those with late-night schedules.
- *Consider taking a taxi* if you are worried that danger is imminent.
- *Get to know your neighbors.* Violence decreases in neighborhoods where residents know and trust one another.
- *If possible, move.* But if that's not possible now, then at least consider it and plan for it. It should be part of your future.

75. Nurture Your Home	Impact ★★

Our personalities, our tastes, and even our ethics are reflected in the rooms and spaces we live in. Some are personal efforts to bring artistic beauty into our lives. Others create peaceful, personal signature spaces that nurture and relax us. Surroundings can spur you to cowboy dreams or Hollywood visions of grandeur. Some people design their living space to reflect a minimalist view of harmony and focus, while others use secondhand and recycled materials to produce creative new combinations.

It is the small pleasures that distinguish one home from another. Many homes are a personal expression of love. They may include a child's drawing or an original work of art. If you bring in some beauty, some creativity, some joyfulness to show who you are and what you enjoy having around you, you have created a home. Whether you live in a college dorm room or a sumptuous mansion, an oceanfront cottage or a New York apartment, a heartland farm or western ranch or northwestern houseboat, it says something to you and about you.

Feng shui, an Asian art of arranging space, teaches us that the intermingling of heavenly influences and earthly influences affects our surroundings. Some say unseen elements such as magnetic fields and celestial influences comprise the heavenly: color, shapes, furniture arrangement, location, decor, and layout are the earthly elements we can see. Indeed, color research shows that we can be influenced toward hunger, anger, calmness, irritability, physical activity, and even bodily temperature changes depending on the interplay of shades around us. The important reason for considering feng shui is to have a beautiful, harmonious environment inside and outside. The goal of creating a specific environment in the place you live is to produce a peaceful respite for your heart and soul.

So do your thing. Invite your friends and loved ones to share your space. Make your home beckoning, and fill it with joy and gladness.

Here's an action plan for creating a sweet place to live:

- *Be sensitive to the likes and dislikes of the people you live with.*
- *Buy yourself or someone else you live with an unexpected small pleasure gift*—flowers, linen napkins, something that says, "I thought of you."
- *Use different paint colors to express a room's personality.*
- *Create small, personal spaces for reading, working, being.*
- *Share the physical work* of maintaining a household with everyone.
- *Use fabric creatively.* Build small projects.
- *Let kids decorate their own space* and be responsible for it. Then let them redecorate it.
- *Change your rooms and bedding to reflect the seasons.*
- *Bring the outside indoors* with objects and live plants from nature. Notice and interpret the world around you and let your home reflect that diversity. Start collections.

---

76. Reduce Air Pollution, Radon, and Indoor Toxins   Impact ★★

Air Pollution

In nearly every urban environment, our air is cleaner than it was twenty years ago. Still, it's not as clean as the Environmental Protection Agency would like. Though it is difficult to quantify the risks air and water pollution pose, many prominent cancer researchers believe that it contributes significantly to the number-one cancer killer, lung cancer.

We know that air pollution aggravates asthma, chronic bronchitis, and emphysema. Some researchers have shown that air pollutants can aggravate sinusitis and allergies. Its effect on heart disease and stroke has yet to be determined, but we know that severe pollution makes exercise difficult.

Asthma is one of the chronic diseases where modern medicine has failed to cut the death rate. In fact, more asthma deaths occur today than one and two decades ago. This is puzzling, since pollution has abated over the past twenty years. Some theorize that the over-prescribing of asthma inhalers is at fault; others believe that pollution, although decreased, is still the cause. Asthma disproportionately strikes people who are poor and live in inner cities or industrial neighborhoods. Simply put, the closer you live or work to a source of pollution, the more your asthma is likely to bother you.

But not all air pollution is outside. The chemicals that abound within can make your indoor air more toxic than the air outside. The list includes the chemicals you clean and paint with, pesticides, and cleaning solutions.

Passive Smoke

Actually, the worst air pollutant that exists is tobacco smoke. Twenty thousand people die from passive smoking every year. If you or your spouse smokes, then take it outside. Making a smoking parlor outdoors will enable you to live smoke-free. When you spring this decision on your spouse, relatives, and friends who smoke, you may have to tolerate some grumbling for a while. But you only need to make this decision once to live in your home smoke-free.

Asbestos

Used in buildings until the late 1960s, it was thought of as a wonder fiber. Cheap and easy to use in insulation and in flooring, asbestos was ubiquitous. But then researchers discovered that asbestos fibers that float in the air you breathe are a significant risk for lung cancer, especially for smokers. Whether in your house, at work, or at school, asbestos is not toxic until it's tampered with or someone tries to remove it. If you're unsure if you have asbestos in your home, call your county hazardous waste management office and ask. They can show you how to test for it and get it safely removed.

Lead Poisoning

Lead paint, commonly used until the 1970s, is still a problem in many older homes. Lead is toxic, and we know that children who breathe in lead dust or eat lead paint chips can suffer brain damage and score lower on IQ tests. If you strip existing lead paint to refinish an area, take precautions. Breathing in lead dust is a serious hazard. Every state operates a lead control office that can guide you on the right way to remove lead paint.

Radon

How much lung cancer is caused by radon is debatable. For several years the EPA thought that radon was a serious threat to our lungs, but later data question that assumption. I think the radon issue has been blown out of proportion. If you are in a radon-prone area and you're concerned, I suggest you get a home radon tester. If you find your house shows high quantities, then contact your county inspector. But my read is that radon is not nearly as lethal a pollutant as compared to tobacco smoke.

Here is your action list for achieving a healthful environment:
- *Consider moving to a community with clean air.*
- *Search for toxic chemicals* and dispose of them properly.
- *If your house is old, check pipe insulation for asbestos, and check for lead paint.*
- *Make sure that you do not have indoor tobacco pollution.* Remove all ashtrays, and divert smoking friends or relatives outside.

Epilogue

TO HAVE A LONG, SWEET LIFE is an ancient desire. Within the last century we've made great strides toward achieving that goal. Yet, as you have just read, there is even more to be had. Each of us is handed a different set of genes, the initial cards in the card game one might call life. How we play our hand determines, to a great extent, the outcome.

In Part I, I showed you how a long, sweet life is much broader than diet, exercise, and quitting smoking. The five spheres of wellness are a shorthand method to help you identify and master the longevity boosters and busters that impact so much in your life. Understanding their underpinnings—lifelong learning, active involvement, and hopefulness—undoubtedly aided you in putting the spheres into perspective. In the Introduction I promised to show you a life that was not just long but also filled with optimism and hope. I trust that I have done so.

In Part II, I explained how to crack your longevity code—as easy as 1-2-3: identifying what is unique in your life, completing your longevity questionnaire, and pulling the longevity cards that fit your needs. These are all vital steps in developing your particular plan.

In Part III, you found the set of longevity boosters you need to put your plan into action. The suggestions and tips were not meant to be an exhaustive list of what you may do, but rather guideposts. So when should you begin? In fact, you already have by reading this book. Congratulations!

References

General

Anda, Robert, et al. Depressed affect, hopelessness and the risk of ischemic heart disease in a cohort of U.S. adults. *Epidemiology* (1993): 285–94.

Anstad, S.N. *Why We Age*. New York: Wiley, 1977.

Battista, R.N. Practice guidelines for preventive care: the Canadian experience. Canadian Task Force on the Periodic Health Examination. *British Journal of General Practice*, 43, 372 (July 1993): 301–304.

Bernarducci, Marc, and Norma Owens. Is there a fountain of youth? A review of current life extension strategies. *Pharmacotherapy*, 16, 2 (1996): 183–200.

Butler, Robert N., and Jacob A. Brody. *Delaying the Onset of Late-Life Dysfunction*. Springer Pub. Co., 1995.

Cousins, Norman. *Anatomy of an Illness as Perceived by the Patient: Reflections on Healing and Regeneration*. New York: Bantam Books, 1979.

Evans, Robert G.; Morris L. Barer; and Theodore R. Marmor. *Why Are Some People Healthy and Others Not?* New York: Aldine De Gruyter, 1994.

Ferguson, Tom. *Health Online*. New York: Addison-Wesley, 1996.

Futterman, L.G., and L. Lemberg. The Framingham Heart Study: a pivotal legacy of the lost millennium. *American Journal of Critical Care* 9, 2 (March 2000): 147–51.

Glass, Thomas; C. F. Mendes de Leon; and A. Marottoli. Population-based study of social and productive activities as predictors of survival among elderly Americans. *British Medical Journal* 319 (1999): 478–83.

Healthy People 2000. U.S. Department of Health and Social Services, Public Health Services, Washington, D.C.: July 1990.

Idler, Ellen L., and Ronald Angel. Self-rated health and mortality in the NHANES epidemiologic follow-up study. *American Journal of Public Health* 80 (1990): 446–52.

McGinnis, Michael, and William H. Foege. Actual causes of death in the United States. *Journal of the American Medical Association* 170, 8 (1993): 2207–12.

Olshansky, S. Jay, and A. Brian Ault. The fourth stage of epidemiologic transition: the age of delayed degenerative diseases. *The Milbank Quarterly* 64, 3 (1986): 355–91.

Preventive Guidelines: Their Role in Clinical Prevention and Health Promotion. Preventive Health Services, Health Canada, Ottawa: 1996.

Vaupel, J. W. The remarkable improvements in survival at older ages. *Philosophical Transactions of the Royal Society of London—Series B: Biological Sciences* 352, 1363 (December 29, 1997): 1799–1804.

Vital Statistics of the United States, 1994—Life Table; U.S. Department of Health and Human Services, Washington, D.C.

Physical Sphere

Adams, Alexandra, et al. Antioxidant vitamins and the prevention of coronary artery disease. *American Family Physician* 60, 3 (1999): 895–902.

Ainsworth, Barbara E., et al. Compendium of physical activities: classification of energy costs of human physical activities. *Medicine and Science in Sports and Exercise* 25, 1 (1993): 71–80.

Alessio, Helaine, and Eileen Blasi. Physical activity as a natural antioxidant booster and its effect on a healthy life span. *Research Quarterly for Exercise and Sport* 68, 4 (1997): 292–302.

Allaire, S. H.; M. P LaValley; S. R. Evans; G. T. O'Connor; M. Kelly-Hayes; R. F. Meenan; D. Levy; and D. T. Felson. Evidence for decline in disability and improved health among persons aged 55 to 70 years: the Framingham Heart Study. *American Journal of Public Health* 89, 11 (1999): 1678–1738.

Ascherio, A.; E. B. Rimm; M. A. Hernan; E. L. Giovannucci; I. Kawachi; M. J. Stampfer; and W. C. Willett. Intake of potassium, magnesium, calcium, and fiber and risk of stroke among U.S. men. *Circulation* 98, 12 (1998): 1198–204.

Astin, John A. Why patients use alternative medicine. *Journal of the American Medical Association* 279, 19 (1998): 1548–53.

Blair, S. N., et al. Physical fitness and all-cause mortality. *Journal of the American Medical Association* 262, 17 (1989): 2395–400.

Brown, L.; E. B. Rimm; J. M. Seddon; E. L. Giovannucci; L. Chasan-Taber; D. Spiegelman; W. C. Willett; and S. E. Hankinson. A prospective study of carotenoid intake and risk of cataract extraction in U.S. men. *American Journal of Clinical Nutrition* 70, 4 (1999): 517–24.

Calle, Eugenia, et al. Body-mass index and mortality in a prospective cohort of U.S. adults. *New England Journal of Medicine* 341, 15 (1999): 1097–106.

D'Agostino, R. B.; M. W. Russell; D. M. Huse; R. C. Ellison; H. Silbershatz; P. W. Wilson; and S. C. Hartz. Primary and subsequent coronary risk appraisal: new results from the Framingham study. *American Heart Journal* 139, 2 Pt. 1 (2000): 272–81.

Dunn, Andrea, et al. Comparison of lifestyle and structured interventions to increase physical activity and cardiorespiratory fitness. *Journal of the American Medical Association* 281, 4 (1999): 327–34.

Gaartside, Peter S. Prospective assessment of coronary heart disease risk factors: the

NHANES I epidemiologic follow-up study (NHEFS). *Journal of the American College of Nutrition* 17, 3 (1998): 263–69.

Golier, Julia A., et al. Low serum cholesterol level and attempted suicide. *American Journal of Psychiatry* 152, 3 (March 1995): 419–23.

Gueguen, Reginald. The French paradox and wine drinking. *Novartis Foundation Symposium* 216 (1998): 208–22.

Hu, F. B.; M. J. Stampfer; J. E. Manson; E. B. Rimm; G. A. Colditz; B. A. Rosner; F. E. Speizer; C. H. Hennekens; and W. C. Willett. Frequent nut consumption and risk of coronary heart disease in women: prospective cohort study. *British Medical Journal* 317, 7169 (1998): 1341–45.

Int Veld, B. A.; L. J. Launder; A. W. Hoes; A. Ott; A. Hofman; M. M. Breteler; and B. H. Stricker. NSAIDs and incident Alzheimer's disease: the Rotterdam study. *Neurobiology of Aging* 19, 6 (1998): 607–11.

Iribarren, Carlos, et al. Effect of cigar smoking on the risk of cardiovascular disease, chronic obstructive pulmonary disease, and cancer in men. *New England Journal of Medicine* 340, 23 (1999): 1773–80.

Jacques, Paul F. The effect of folic acid fortification on plasma folate and total homocysteine concentrations. *New England Journal of Medicine* 340, 19 (1999): 1449–54.

Jiang, He, et al. Passive smoking and the risk of coronary heart disease—a meta analysis of epidemiologic studies. *New England Journal of Medicine* 340, 12 (1999): 920–26.

Joshipura, K. J.; A. Ascherio; J. E. Manson; M. J. Stampfer; E. B. Rimm; F. E. Speizer; C. H. Hennekens; D. Spiegelman; and W. C. Willett. Fruit and vegetable intake in relation to risk of ischemic stroke. *Journal of the American Medical Association* 282, 13 (1999): 1233–39.

Joshipura, K. J.; E. B. Rimm; C. W. Douglass; D. Trichopoulos; A. Ascherio; and W. C. Willett. Poor oral health and coronary heart disease. *Journal of Dental Research* 75, 9 (1996): 1631–36.

Keys, Ancel. Coronary heart disease in seven countries. *Nutrition* 12 (1997): 249–53.

Krinsky, Norman. Overview of lycopene, carotenoids, and disease prevention. *The American Journal of Clinical Nutrition,* 62(6) (supplement).

Lamberg, Lynne. Diet may affect skin cancer prevention. *Journal of the American Medical Association* 279, 18 (1998): 1427.

Lauer, Michael S. Association of cigarette smoking with chronotopic incompetence and prognosis in the Framingham heart study. *Circulation* 96, 3 (1997): 897–903.

LeBopff, Meryl S., et al. Occult vitamin D deficiency in postmenopausal women with acute hip fracture. *Journal of the American Medical Association* 281, 16 (1999): 1505–11.

Lefevre, Michael. Prostate cancer screening: more harm than good? *American Family Physician,* August 1998: 112–19.

Leitzmann, M. F.; E. B. Rimm; W. C. Willett; D. Spiegelman; F. Grodstein; M. J.

Stampfer; G. A. Colditz; and E. Giovannucci. Recreational physical activity and the risk of cholecystectomy in women. *New England Journal of Medicine* 341, 11 (1999): 777–84.

Levy, D.; C. N. Merz; R. J. Cody; F. M. Fouad-Tarazi; C. K. Francis; M. A. Pfeffer; N. A. Scott; H. J. Swan; M. P. Taylor; and M. H. Weinberger. Hypertension detection, treatment, and control: a call to action for cardiovascular specialists. *Journal of the American College of Cardiology* 34, 4 (1999): 1360–62.

Lloyd-Jones, D. M.; M. G. Larson; A. Beiser; and D. Levy. Lifetime risk of developing coronary heart disease [see comments]. *Lancet* 353, 9147 (1999): 89–92.

Manson, JoAnne, et al. A prospective study of walking as compared with vigorous exercises in the prevention of coronary heart disease in women. *New England Journal of Medicine* 341 (1999): 650–58.

Manton, Kenneth, et al. The dynamics of dimensions of age-related disability in 1982–1994 in the U.S. elderly population. *Journal of Gerontology: Biological Sciences,* 53a, 1 (1998): B59–B70.

Marshall, Kenneth G. Prevention. How much harm? How much benefit? *Canadian Medical Association Journal* 155, 2 (1996): 169–76.

McGeer, P. L.; M. Schulzer; and E. G. McGeer. Arthritis and anti-inflammatory agents as possible protective factors for Alzheimer's disease: A review of 17 epidemiologic studies. *Neurology* 47, 2 (1996): 425–32.

Michaud, C. Food habits, consumption, and knowledge of low-income French population. *Santé Publique* 10, 3 (1998): 333–47.

Mueller, O. Smoking in women. *Journal of the American Osteopathic Association* 982, 12 (1998): S7–S10.

Muldoon, Mathew F.; Stephen B. Manuck; and Karen Matthews. Lowering cholesterol concentrations and mortality: a quantitative review of primary prevention trials. *British Medical Journal* 301 (1990): 309–14.

Overview of Lycopene, Carotenoids and Disease Prevention. Proceedings of a symposium held in Berlin, Germany, October 10–12, 1994, by guest scientific editors Norman I. Krinsky and Helmut Sies. Bethesda, Md.: American Society for Clinical Nutrition, Inc., 1995, 12995–15405.

Paffenbarger, Ralph, Jr. Life is sweet: candy consumption and longevity. *British Medical Journal* 317 (1998): 1683–84.

Rantanen, T.; J. M. Guralnik; R. Sakari-Rantala; S. Leveille; E. M. Simonsick; S. Ling; and L. P. Fried. Disability, physical activity, and muscle strength in older women: the women's health and aging study. *Archives of Physical Medicine and Rehabilitation* 80, 2 (1999): 130–35.

Rowe, John W., and Robert L. Kahn. *Successful Aging.* New York: Pantheon, 1998.

Ruxton, C. H. S., and T. R. Kirk. Breakfast: a review of associations with measures of dietary intake, physiology, and biochemistry. *British Journal of Nutrition* 78 (1997): 199–213.

Ryff, Carol D., and Burgton Singer. The contours of positive human health. *Psychological Inquiry* 9, 1 (1998): 1–28.

Sano, M.; C. Ernesto; R. G. Thomas; M.R. Klauber; K. Schafer; M. Grundman; P. Woodbury; J. Growdon; C.W. Cotman; E. Pfeiffer; L.S. Schneider; L.J Thal. A controlled trial of selegiline, alpha-tocopherol, or both as treatment for Alzheimer's disease. The Alzheimer's Disease Cooperative Study [see comments]. *New England Journal of Medicine* 336, 17 (April 24, 1997): 1216–22.

Schreinemachers, Dina M. and Richard B. Everson. Aspirin use and lung, colon and breast cancer incidence in a prospective study. *Epidemiology*, 5 (1994): 138–46.

Seidell, Jacob C. The sagittal waist diameter and mortality in men: the Baltimore longitudinal study on aging. *International Journal of Obesity* 18 (1994): 61–67.

Simon, Alain; Jean-Louis Megnien; and Jaimie Levenson. Coronary risk estimation and treatment of hypercholesterolemia. *Circulation* 96, 7 (1997): 2449–52.

Spiegel, Karine. Impact of sleep debt on metabolic and endocrine function. *The Lancet* 354 (1999): 1435–38.

Theme Issue on Obesity. *Journal of the American Medical Association* 282 (1999): 1519–75.

Thune, Inger, et al. Physical activity and the risk of breast cancer. *New England Journal of Medicine* 336, 18 (1997): 1269–75.

Van Tol, A., et al. Changes in postprandial lipoproteins of low and high density caused by moderate alcohol consumption with dinner. *Atherosclerosis* 141, supp. 1 (1998): S101–S103.

Waples, M. D. Update on prostate cancer. *Wisconsin Medical Journal,* July/August 1999.

Wilson, P. W.; R. B. D'Agostino; D. Levy; A. M. Belanger; H. Silbershatz; and W. B. Kannel. Prediction of coronary heart disease using risk factor categories. *Circulation* 97, 18 (1998): 1837–47.

Mental Sphere

Ardelt, Monika. Wisdom and life satisfaction in old age. *Journal of Gerontology* 52, 1 (1997): 15–27.

Butler, S. M.; J. W. Ashford; and D. A. Snowdon. Age, education, and changes in the mini–mental state exam scores of older women: findings from the nun study. *Journal of the American Geriatrics Society* 44, 6 (1996): 675–81.

Dalack, Gregory. Perspectives on the relationship between cardiovascular disease and affective disorder. *Journal of Clinical Psychiatry* 51, 7, supp. (1990): 4–11.

Everson, Susan, et al. Anger expression and incident stroke. *Stroke* 30 (1999): 523–28.

Fava, G. A. Well-being therapy: a novel psychotherapeutic approach for residual symptoms of affective disorders. *Psychological Medicine* 28 (1998): 475–80.

Feldman, Jacob J., et al. National trends in educational differentials in mortality. *American Journal of Epidemiology* 129, 5 (1989): 919–33.

Fiscella, Kevin, and Peter Franks. Does psychological distress contribute to racial and socioeconomic disparity in mortality? *Social Science & Medicine* 45, 12 (1997): 1805–1909.

Glasser, Ronald, and Janice Kiecolt-Glasser. *Handbook of Human Stress and Immunity.* San Diego: Academic Press, 1994.

Glassman, Alexander H. Smoking, smoking cessation, and major depression. *Journal of the American Medical Association* 264, 12 (1990): 1546–49.

Hay, Louis L. *You Can Heal Your Life.* Hay House: 1999.

Kling, K. C.; M. M. Seltzer; and C. D. Ryff. Distinctive late-life challenges: implications for coping and well-being. *Psychology and Aging* 12, 2 (1997): 288–95.

Leigh, J. Paul, and James F. Fries. Education, gender, and the compression of morbidity. *International Journal of Aging and Human Development* 39, 3 (1994): 233–46.

Lowin, Bernard. Neuro- and psychologic mechanisms and the problem of sudden cardiac death. *American Journal of Cardiology* 39 (1977): 890–902.

Magni, Guido, et al. Chronic musculoskeletal pain and depressive symptoms in the national health and nutrition examination epidemiologic follow-up study. *Pain* 53 (1993): 163–68.

Marmot, M. G.; R. Fuhrer; S. L. Ettner; N. F. Marks; L. L. Bumpass; and C. D. Ryff. Contribution of psychosocial factors to socioeconomic differences in health. *Milbank Quarterly* 76 (3) (1998): 403–48.

McEwen, Bruce, and Eliot Stellar. Stress and the individual. *Archives of Internal Medicine* 153 (1993): 2093–101.

Nemeroff, M. D., et al. Depression and cardiac disease. *Depression and Anxiety* 8, supp. 1 (1998): 71–79.

Orth-Gomer, Krigina, et al. Relation between ventricular arrhythmias and psychological profile. *Acta Medica Scandinavica* 207 (1980): 31–36.

Penninx, B. W.; J. M. Guralnik; C. F. Mendes de Leon; M. Pahor; M. Visser; M. C. Corti; and R. B. Wallace. Cardiovascular events and mortality in newly and chronically depressed persons more than 70 years of age. *American Journal of Cardiology* 81, 8 (1998): 988–94.

Penninx, B. W.; J. M. Guralnik; L. Ferrucci; E. M. Simonsick; D. J. Deeg; and R. B. Wallace. Depressive symptoms and physical decline in community-dwelling older persons. *Journal of the American Medical Association* 279, 21 (1998): 1720–26.

Penninx, B. W.; S. Leveille; L. Ferrucci; J. T. van Eijk; and J. M. Guralnik. Exploring the effect of depression on physical disability: longitudinal evidence from the established populations for epidemiologic studies of the elderly. *American Journal of Public Health* 89, 9 (1999): 1346–52.

Peterson, Christopher, et al. Catastrophizing and untimely death. *Psychological Science* 9, 2 (1998): 127–30.

Rivara, F. P., et al. Alcohol and illicit drug abuse and the risk of violent death in the home. *Journal of the American Medical Association* 273, 7 (1997): 569–75.

Rumsfeld, John S., et al. Health-related quality of life as a predictor of mortality following coronary artery bypass graft surgery. *Journal of the American Medical Association* 281, 14 (1999).

Ryff, Carol D. Psychological well-being in adult life. *Current Directions in Psychological Science.* 4 (1995): 99–104.

Shekelle, Richard B., et al. Hostility, risk of coronary heart disease, and mortality. *Psychosomatic Medicine* 45, 2 (1983): 109–14.

Smith, Timothy. Hostility and health: current status of a psychosomatic hypothesis. *Health Psychology* 11, 3 (1992): 139–50.

Snowdon, D. A.; L. H. Greiner; J. A. Mortimer; K. P. Riley; P. A. Greiner; and W. R. Markesbery. Brain infarction and the clinical expression of Alzheimer's disease: the nun study. *Journal of the American Medical Association* 277, 10 (1997): 813–17.

Snowdon, D. A.; M. D. Gross; and S. M. Butler. Antioxidants and reduced functional capacity in the elderly: findings from the nun study. *Journals of Gerontology*, series A: *Biological Sciences and Medical Sciences* 51, 1 (1996): M10–M16.

Spiegel, David, et al. Effect of psychosocial treatment on survival of patients with metastatic breast cancer. *The Lancet* 344 (1989): 888–91.

Watson, M. Influence of psychological response on survival in breast cancer: a population-based cohort study. *The Lancet* 354 (1999): 1331–35.

Weeks, J. C.; E. F. Cook; S. J. O'Day; L. M. Peterson; N. Wenger; D. Reding; F. E. Harrell; P. Kussin; N. V. Dawson; A. F. Connors Jr.; J. Lynn; and R. S. Phillips. Relationship between cancer patients' predictions of prognosis and their treatment preferences. *Journal of the American Medical Association* 279, 21 (June 3, 1998): 1709–14.

Weiner, M. F.; C. M. Cullum; R. N. Rosenberg; and L. S. Honig. Aging and Alzheimer's disease: lessons from the nun study. *Gerontologist* 28, 1 (1998): 5–6.

Whooley, M. D., et al. Association between depressive symptoms and mortality in older women. *Archives of Internal Medicine* 158 (1998): 2129–35.

Kinship/Social Sphere

Berkman, Lisa F. Social network, host resistance, and mortality: a nine-year follow-up study of Alameda County residents. *American Journal of Epidemiology* 109, 2 (1979): 186–204.

Cohen, Sheldon. Psychosocial models of the role of social support in the etiology of physical disease. *Health Psychology* 7, 3 (1988): 269–97.

———. Social ties and susceptibility to the common cold. *Journal of the American Medical Association* 277, 24 (1997): 1940–44.

———. Stress, social support, and the buffering hypothesis. *Psychological Bulletin* 98, 2 (1985): 310–57.

Glass, Thomas A. Population based study of social and productive activities as predictors of survival among elderly Americans. *British Medical Journal* 319 (1999): 478–83.

House, James S. Social relationships and health. *Science* 241 (1988): 540–45.

House, James, et al. The association of social relationships and activities with mortality: prospective evidence from the Tecumseh Community Health Study. *American Journal of Epidemiology* 116, 1 (1982): 123–40.

Kaplan, Jay, et al. The effects of fat and cholesterol on social behavior in monkeys. *Psychosomatic Medicine* 53 (1991): 634–42.

LeVeist, Thomas A., et al. Extreme social isolation, use of community-based senior support services, and mortality among African-American elderly women. *American Journal of Community Psychology* 25, 4 (1997): 721–23.

Ljungquist, Birgit, and Gerdt Sundstrom. Health and social networks as predictors of survival in old age. *Scandinavian Journal of Social Medicine* 24, 2 (1996): 90–101.

Mechanic, David. Divorce, family conflict, and adolescents' well-being. *Journal of Health and Social Behavior* 30 (1989): 105–16.

Schoenbach, Victor J. Social ties and mortality in Evans County, Georgia. *American Journal of Epidemiology* 123, 4 (1986): 577–91.

Seeman, Teresa E. Impact of social environment characteristics on neuroendocrine regulation. *Psychosomatic Medicine* 58 (1996): 459–71.

Smith, Ken, and Cathleen Zick. Linked lives, dependent demise? Survival analysis of husbands and wives. *Demography* 31, 1 (1994): 81–90.

Tucker, Joan S., et al. Marital history at midlife as a predictor of longevity. *Health Psychology* 15, 2 (1996): 94–101.

Tucker, Joan S., et al. Parental divorce: effects of individual behavior and longevity. *Journal of Personality and Social Psychology* 73, 2 (1997): 381–91.

Uchino, Bert N. The relationship between social support and physiological process: a review with emphasis on underlying mechanisms and implications on health. *Psychological Bulletin* 119, 3 (1996): 488–531.

Vogth, Thomas M. Social networks as predictors of ischemic heart disease, cancer, stroke, and hypertension: incidence, survival and mortality. *Journal of Clinical Epidemiology* 45, 6 (1992): 659–66.

Yellen, Suzanne B., and David F. Cella. Someone to live for: social well-being, parenthood status, and decision-making in oncology. *Journal of Clinical Oncology* 13, 5 (1995): 1255–64.

Spiritual Sphere

Benson, Herbert, with Mark Stark. *Timeless Healing: The Power of Biology and Belief.* New York: Simon and Schuster, 1996.

Bly, Robert. *Iron John: A Book About Men.* New York: Random House, 1992.

Craigie, F. C., Jr., and R. F. Hobbs III. Spiritual perspectives and practices of family physicians with an expressed interest in spirituality. *Family Medicine* 31, 8 (1999): 578–85.

Dossey, L. Do religion and spirituality matter in health? A response to the recent article in *The Lancet* [see comments]. *Alternative Therapies in Health and Medicine* 5, 3 (1999): 16–18.

Ellison, Christopher G. Religious involvement and subjective well-being. *Journal of Health and Social Behavior* 32 (1991): 90.

Estés, Clarissa Pinkola. *Women Who Run with the Wolves.* New York: Ballantine, 1996.

Hamilton, D. G. Believing in a patient's beliefs: physician attunement to the spiritual dimension as a positive factor in patient healing and health. *American Journal of Hospice and Palliative Care* 15, 5 (1998): 276–79.

His Holiness the Dalai Lama. *Ethics for the New Millennium*. New York: Putnam Publishing, 1999.

————. *The Path to Tranquillity*. New York: Viking, 1998.

Hixson, K. A., et al. The relation between religiosity, selected health behaviors, and blood pressure among adult females. *Preventive Medicine* 27, 4 (1998): 545–52.

Kaczorowski, J. M. Spiritual well-being and anxiety in adults diagnosed with cancer. *Hospice Journal* 5, 3–4 (1989): 105–16.

Koenig, Harold G. *The Healing Power of Faith*. New York: Simon and Schuster, 1999.

Kübler-Ross, Elisabeth. *On Death and Dying*. New York: Macmillan, 1970.

Kushner, Harold S. *When Bad Things Happen to Good People*. New York: Schocken Books, 1981.

Maes, H. H.; M. C. Neale; N. G. Martin; A. C. Heath; and L. J. Eaves. Religious attendance and frequency of alcohol use: same genes or same environment: a bivariate extended twin kinship model. *Twin Research* 2, 2 (1999): 169–79.

McBride, J. L., et al. The relationship between a patient's spirituality and health experiences. *Family Medicine* 30, 2 (1998): 122–26.

Rasanen, J., et al. Religious affiliation and all-cause mortality: a prospective population study in middle-aged men in eastern Finland. *International Journal of Epidemiology* 25, 6 (1996): 1244–49.

Strawbridge, William J., et al. Frequent attendance at religious services and mortality over 28 years. *American Journal of Public Health* 87, 6 (1997): 957–61.

Waldfogel, S. Spirituality in medicine. *Primary Care: Clinics in Office Practice* 24, 4 (1997): 963–76.

Material Sphere

Aasland, O. G., et al. Health complaints and job stress in Norwegian physicians: the use of an overlapping questionnaire design. *Social Science and Medicine* 45, 11 (1997): 1615–29.

Brunner, E. J.; M. G. Marmot; K. Nanchahal; M. J. Shipley; S. A. Stansfeld; M. Juneja; and K. G. Alberti. Social inequality in coronary risk: central obesity and the metabolic syndrome. Evidence from the Whitehall II Study. *Diabetologia* 40, 11 (1997): 1341–49.

Calman, K. Lessons from Whitehall. *British Medical Journal* 317, 7174 (1998): 1718–20.

Carroll, D.; G. Davey Smith; D. Sheffield; M. J. Shipley; and M. G. Marmot. The relationship between socioeconomic status, hostility, and blood pressure reactions to mental stress in men: data from the Whitehall II Study. *Health Psychology* 16, 2 (1997): 131–36.

Davey Smith, George. Magnitude and causes of socioeconomic differentials in mortality: further evidence from the Whitehall Study. *Journal of Epidemiology and Community Health* 44 (1990): 265–70.

Harding, S.; A. Bethune; and M. Rosato. Second study supports results of Whitehall Study after retirement. *British Medical Journal* 314, 7087 (1997): 1130.

Hemingway, Harry, et al. The impact of socioeconomic status on health functioning as assessed by the SF-36 Questionnaire: the Whitehall II Study. *American Journal of Public Health* 87, 9 (1997): 1484–90.

Kaplan, George A., and Julian E. Keil. Socioeconomic factors and cardiovascular disease: a review of the literature. *Circulation* 88, 4, part I (1993): 1973–97.

Kawakami, N., and T. Haratani. Epidemiology of job stress and health in Japan. *Industrial Health* 37, 2 (1999): 174–86.

Kessler, Ronald, and Harold Neighbors. A new perspective on the relationships among race, social class, and psychological distress. *Journal of Health and Social Behavior* 27 (1986): 107–15.

Kogevinas, M. Socioeconomic differences in cancer survival. *Journal of Epidemiology and Community Health* 45, 3 (1991): 216–19.

Lantz, Paula. Health behaviors don't explain high death rates among poor—socioeconomic differences in mortality due to wider array of factors. *Journal of the American Medical Association* 279 (1998): 1745–46.

Luz, J., and M. S. Green. Sickness absenteeism from work—a critical review of the literature. *Public Health Reviews* 25, 2 (1997): 89–122.

Lynch, John W., et al. Do cardiovascular risk factors explain the relation between the socioeconomic status, risk of all-cause mortality, cardiovascular mortality, and acute myocardial infarction? *American Journal of Epidemiology* 144, 10 (1976): 934–42.

Marmot, M. G., and M. J. Shipley. Do socioeconomic differences in mortality persist after retirement? 25-Year follow up of civil servants from the first Whitehall Study. *British Medical Journal* 313, 7066 (1996): 1177–80.

Mein, G.; P. Higgs; J. Ferrie; and S. A. Stansfeld. Paradigms of retirement: the importance of health and aging in the Whitehall II Study. *Social Science and Medicine* 47, 4 (1998): 535–45.

National Census of Fatal Occupational Injuries, 1998. Bureau of Labor Statistics, August 1999, U.S. Department of Labor publication no. 99-208.

Pavalko, Eliza K., et al. Work lives and longevity: insights from a life course perspective. *Journal of Health and Social Behavior* 34 (1993): 363–80.

Power, Chris, et al. Inequalities in self-rated health in the 1958 birth cohort: lifetime social circumstances or social mobility. *British Medical Journal* 313 (1996): 449–53.

Rodin, Judith. Aging and health: effects of the sense of control. *Science* 233 (1986): 1271–76.

Stansfeld, S. A.; H. Bosma; H. Hemingway; and M. G. Marmot. Psychosocial work characteristics and social support as predictors of SF-36 health functioning: the Whitehall II Study. *Psychosomatic Medicine* 60, 3 (1998): 247–55.

Valat, J.-P., et al. Low back pain: risk factors for chronicity. *Revue du Rheumatisme* [English edition] 64, 3 (1997): 189–94.

Williams, Redford. Lower socioeconomic status and increased mortality. *Journal of the American Medical Association* 279, 21 (1998).

Index